Dementia Care

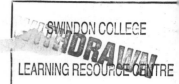
Trevor Adams PhD MSc RN Cert Ed CPN Cert
Lecturer in Mental Health, European Institute of Health and Medical
Sciences, University of Surrey, Guildford, UK

and

Jill Manthorpe MA
Reader in Community Care, School of Nursing, Social Work and
Applied Health Studies, University of Hull, UK

ARNOLD

A member of the Hodder Headline Group
London

First published in Great Britain in 2003 by Arnold,
a member of the Hodder Headline Group,
338 Euston Road, London NW1 3BH

http://www.arnoldpublishers.com

Distributed in the USA by
Oxford University Press Inc.,
198 Madison Avenue, New York, NY10016
Oxford is a registered trademark of Oxford University Press

Whilst the advice and information in this book are believed to be true and
accurate at the date of going to press, neither the authors nor the publisher
can accept any legal responsibility or liability for any errors or omissions
that may be made. In particular (but without limiting the generality of the
preceding disclaimer) every effort has been made to check drug dosages;
however, it is still possible that errors have been missed. Furthermore,
dosage schedules are constantly being revised and new side-effects
recognized. For these reasons the reader is strongly urged to consult the
drug companies' printed instructions before administering any of the drugs
recommended in this book.

British Library Cataloguing in Publication Data
A catalogue record for this book is available from the British Library

Library of Congress Cataloging-in-Publication Data
A catalog record for this book is available from the Library of Congress

ISBN 0 340 81020 3

1 2 3 4 5 6 7 8 9 10

Commissioning Editor: Georgina Bentliff
Development Editor: Heather Smith
Production Editor: Anke Ueberberg
Production Controller: Lindsay Smith
Cover Design: Amina Dudhia

Typeset in 9.5/13 pt Palatino by Phoenix Photosetting, Chatham, Kent
Printed and bound in Malta

What do you think about this book? Or any other Arnold title?
Please send your comments to feedback.arnold@hodder.co.uk

Contents

Contributors   v

Foreword   ix

Introduction   x

Section 1: Approaches to practice

1   Constructing dementia   3
Trevor Adams and Ruth Bartlett

2   Valuing people with dementia   22
Wendy Martin and Helen Bartlett

3   Policy and practice in dementia care   35
Jill Manthorpe and Trevor Adams

Section 2: Person-centred practice

4   Working with people in the early stages of dementia   51
Lindsay Royan

5   Managing language and communication difficulties in Alzheimer's dementia: the link to behaviour   69
Karen Bryan and Jane Maxim

6   Counselling people with dementia   86
Elizabeth Bartlett and Richard Cheston

7   Addressing the physical care needs of people with dementia   103
Roger Watson

8   Palliative care for people with dementia   114
Kay de Vries

9   Remembering and forgetting: group work with people who have dementia   136
Richard Cheston, Kerry Jones and Jane Gilliard

Contents

10 Positive communication with people who have dementia   148
    Jonathan Parker

11 Younger people with dementia: coming out of the shadows   164
    Maria Parsons

Section 3: Practice systems

12 Helping families cope with dementia   187
    Alison Marriott

13 Developing ethnically sensitive and appropriate dementia
    care practice   202
    Anthea Innes

14 Supporting and supervising in dementia care   213
    Mark Holman

15 Elder abuse and people with dementia   225
    Bridget Penhale

16 Maintaining quality in dementia care practice   240
    Dawn Brooker

Index   257

Contributors

Trevor Adams PhD MSc RN CertEd CPNCert has worked in dementia care nursing for over 25 years. During this time, Trevor has been involved in developing dementia care nursing through practice, education and research. He is currently Mental Health Pathway Leader for the MSc in Advanced Practice at the European Institute of Health and Medical Science, University of Surrey, UK.

Elizabeth Bartlett DipSocStud Relate Certificated Counsellor is Counsellor with the Salisbury and District Branch of the Alzheimer's Society, UK. Before establishing this branch of the society in 1985, she was a social worker and a Relate counsellor. The initial focus of Elizabeth's work was on practical services for people with dementia, but the need for counselling became increasingly apparent. As a result, she was in 1999 chosen to lead a pilot project on counselling for people with a diagnosis of dementia.

Helen Bartlett BA MSc PhD RGN RHV is Foundation Director and Professor of the Australasian Centre on Ageing, University of Queensland, Brisbane, Australia and was previously Professor of Health Studies at Oxford Brookes University, UK. Her research interests include quality measurement and policy issues in long-term care, especially in nursing and residential homes.

Ruth Bartlett RMN BA MA is Research Consultant at the Oxford Dementia Centre, Oxford Brookes University, Oxford, UK and a PhD student in the Sociology Department of Oxford Brookes University. She is researching the qualitative dimensions of social exclusion in relation to older people with dementia living in residential care. Ruth has also worked as a mental health nurse in a range of clinical areas.

Dawn Brooker BSc MSc PhD CPsychol(Clin) is currently employed by the Bradford Dementia Group at the University of Bradford, UK, where she is the Strategic Lead for Dementia Care Mapping. She was formerly Director of the Oxford Dementia Centre and has worked as a clinical psychologist. Dawn's research interests include the evaluation of service quality, organizational change, therapeutic interventions, person-centred care and emotional distress and coping in people with dementia.

Karen Bryan BSc PhD RegMRCSLT is a Speech and Language Therapist and Professor of Clinical Practice at the European Institute of Health and Medical Sciences, University of Surrey, Guildford, UK. Her research has addressed assessment and management of communication problems in people with dementia.

Richard Cheston MA PhD DipCPsychol is a Consultant Clinical Psychologist with Avon and Wiltshire Mental Health Partnership NHS Trust, Trowbridge, UK as well as a research fellow at Bath University. He has published extensively on the experiences of people with dementia and is the co-author with Mike Bender of *Understanding dementia: the man with the worried eyes*.

Kay de Vries RGN BSc(Hons) PGCEA MSc is Senior Lecturer at the Princess Alice Hospice, Esher, Surrey, and Research Fellow at the European Institute of Health and Medical Sciences, University of Surrey, Guildford, UK She is currently undertaking doctoral research into dementia and dying. Prior to working in the UK, Kay practised as a public health nurse in New Zealand.

Jane Gilliard BA CQSW FRIPH is Director of Dementia Voice, the dementia services development centre for south-west England, having worked with and for people with dementia for about 16 years as a social worker and a researcher. Jane chairs the National Network of Dementia Services Development Centres and is Visiting Professor in the Faculty of Health and Social Care at the University of the West of England.

Mark Holman MA RN works as a Community Mental Health Nurse in Derwentside, County Durham. He has been involved in supervisory relationships as both supervisee and supervisor for more than 12 years, 8 of which he has spent working in older people's services.

Anthea Innes BA MSc PhD is a Research Fellow at the Centre for Social Research on Dementia in Stirling. Her work has investigated the experiences of people with dementia, informal care-givers and care workers. Anthea's research and publications to date have focused on marginalized groups, such as minority ethnic groups, unqualified care staff and those living in rural areas.

Kerry Jones BSc(Hons) MA is a Research Officer at Dementia Voice, the dementia services development centre for southwest England. Kerry has worked for 17 years with various client groups including people with dementia. Trained in social and health care, and research and research management, Kerry has embarked upon a diversity of health and social care related research projects, prior to her work with Dementia Voice and the development of the Psychotherapeutic Groups for People with Dementia project. Kerry is presently part of a three-year Europe-funded project to assess the impact of technology on the quality of life of people with dementia in five European countries. She also teaches and develops workshops on dementia-specific issues in the UK and overseas.

Jill Manthorpe MA is Reader in Community Care at the University of Hull, where she specializes in research and teaching in gerontology. She has worked in the voluntary sector and is currently undertaking research into food and dementia, intermediate care and older nurses.

Alison Marriott BSc MSc CPsychol AFBPS is Consultant Clinical Psychologist, Manchester Mental Health and Social Care Trust, Manchester, UK and a UKCP-registered Family/Systems Therapist. She works clinically with older people and their families in Central Manchester and has published in a number of areas, including family therapy and psychological intervention for the carers of people with dementia.

Wendy Martin BSc MA RGN is Associate Lecturer at The Open University and a research student at the University of Warwick. She was previously a researcher for a project exploring the empowerment of older people with dementia in different care settings at the Oxford Dementia Centre. She has worked as a researcher on projects relating to ageing, bereavement, cancer care and family studies.

Jane Maxim MA PhD RegMRCSLT is Speech and Language Therapist, Head of Department and Senior Lecturer in Human Communication Science at University College London, UK. Her research has focused on language in normal and abnormal populations and communication training for care assistants.

Jonathan Parker BA(Hons) MA CQSW ILTM is Head of Social Work in the School of Nursing, Social Work and Applied Health Studies, University of Hull, UK. His research interests include dementia care and reminiscence, life story and biographical approaches. Before joining the university, Jonathan worked as a specialist social worker for people with dementia. He is also a cognitive behavioural psychotherapist.

Maria Parsons BA(Hons) CQSW PGCE MA, a social worker by profession, has over 20 years experience in practice, management and lecturing. She was instrumental in setting up the Oxford Dementia Centre, part of the Institute of Public Care at Oxford Brookes University. As Head of the centre, Maria is involved in consultancy, research and training in dementia care for health and social services and housing organizations, and in the care of older people with mental health needs.

Bridget Penhale BA MSc CQSW is Lecturer in Social Work and Applied Health Studies at the University of Hull, UK. She has specialized in work with older people since 1983. Bridget has published in the areas of decision-making and mentally incapacitated adults, social work and dementia, as well as extensively on elder abuse. Her principal research interests are elder abuse, domestic violence and mental health.

Lindsay Royan CPsychol BA(Jt Hons) DipDTh is Consultant Clinical Psychologist with North East London Mental Health NHS Trust, Essex, UK. She specializes in working with people in the early stages of dementia and co-wrote a document on the expanding role of memory clinics. She was a member of the mental health task group for the National Service Framework for Older People.

Roger Watson BSc PhD RGN CBiol FIBiol ILTM FRSA is Professor of Nursing in the Department of Nursing and Applied Health Sciences, University of Hull, UK, where he is responsible for leading research in nursing. Roger's clinical experience was gained working with older people with dementia, and he has a particular interest in the assessment of eating difficulty.

Foreword

It is a pleasure to write a piece for the start of this book, a book for those who are trying to support people in our position. We live at home, and about two years ago Robbie was diagnosed as having memory problems. In fact, he recognized that what was wrong could be related to his memory problem by reading a small article in a holiday magazine for older people. He rang our GP and pushed to be seen. Now Robbie is on anti-dementia drugs, and we are managing.

How would we like professionals to be? We would like them to be encouraging, and we would like them to give both of us information (which doesn't always happen). We appreciate it that if we need to see our community mental health nurse, we can telephone her and she will come to see us. And we do welcome people who are kind and helpful, not just those who work with memory problems, but all those who help with other difficulties.

When nurses and doctors carry out tests, it makes a difference if they do this in a certain way: it is best if they see the positives and don't keep emphasizing the mistakes or failures that are going on in one's head. We like it if people have a sense of humour, but that doesn't mean that we don't have bad days when we get cross with ourselves and each other. We like it if people are predictable and reliable: it helps, for example, to get letters about appointments. We would like, too, to be able to talk more to other people in our position.

There are some things that could be better, of course. We were very sad at the state of the hospital when one of us broke a bone. And we found we were booked for an assessment of an aspect of the condition when the drugs to treat it had already been started. And, as we have said before, putting us in touch with other people would be good.

We are able to share many good things from the past and still enjoy going out – bowling and on holiday. That doesn't mean we have forgotten the terrible things, the war in particular, but we are able to talk about the many good times of the past and to enjoy the present.

We know people are very rushed, but our final point is that we *do* value those who have time to listen to us and give us good advice, who are kind and pleasant.

We hope this book will equip people to support those in our position, both now and in the future. Our best wishes to you.

Robbie and Mollie Ness

Introduction

Over the past 20 years, there have been considerable changes in the provision of support to people with dementia, including a reorientation from institutional to community care, an increased reliance on families as the primary source of care, a discovery of the voice of the person with dementia and a shift from the monopro-fessional, medically orientated provision of care to multidisciplinary teamwork. The aim of this book is to provide professionals working with people who have dementia and their informal carers with an account of innovative practice, research and ideas on the contemporary provision of multidisciplinary dementia care.

Although, not so long ago, dementia care attracted little innovation, it has now become a dynamic and exciting area of professional development. Indeed, dementia care is probably one of the fastest developing areas of health and social care. These changes have not, however, been uniform throughout health and social care, and there are still many areas in which dementia care is firmly set within the 'old culture' of dementia care and all this conveys about institutional models of thinking, lack of imagination and a focus on paternalistic provision. We hope that this book will go some way to extending the 'new culture' of dementia care, contribute to the dissemination of good practice within dementia care and offer new ideas or support to those working or training in this area.

The book comprises three sections. The first is concerned with various over-arching approaches to practice within dementia care relating to such issues as the nature of dementia, ethical practice and health and social policy. In Chapter 1, Trevor Adams and Ruth Bartlett draw on recent developments within social constructionism and disability to provide a critical analysis of how dementia is understood within contemporary society. This chapter broadens current thinking about 'dementia' by calling for greater regard to how people with dementia may, in our view, be helped by seeing dementia as a disability.

Helen Bartlett and Wendy Martin, in the next chapter, look at the way in which people with dementia are constructed within a society that prevents their full participation. In the last chapter in this section, the editors, Jill Manthorpe and Trevor Adams provide a critical review of the policy developments that have underpinned dementia care practice in the UK. Each issue raised in this section is important and has considerable implications for the everyday work of health and social professionals working with people with dementia and their families.

The second section relates to 'person-centred approaches' to dementia care. In this section, the term 'person-centred approach' is adopted as it is used in the Department of Health's National Service Framework for Older People, and the contributors provide various accounts of therapeutic approaches that are now available within dementia care. The main aim of person-centred dementia care can appear to identify and address the needs of a range of people associated with the care of people with dementia. The individual with dementia must, however, be at the centre of this process, and this is one shift in emphasis that will be a yardstick for any evaluations of the National Service Framework and its impressive plans for improved service delivery systems in dementia care.

In this second section, Lyndsay Royan provides detailed insights into the early identification of people with dementia in the community and emphasizes that the effect of this shift is to facilitate swift intervention and support for people in the early stages of dementia and their families. Karen Bryan and Jane Maxim next address the neglected issue of communication and people with dementia, describing how practitioners can manage language and communication difficulties among people with Alzheimer's disease. Elizabeth Bartlett and Richard Cheston explore these processes of communication more fully in their chapter and examine various counselling strategies that health and social care professionals may use with people with dementia.

'Person-centred care' has, however, often been understood in psychological and social terms, but when people have dementia, their experience of dementia is embodied and affects how they experience their body. People with dementia may at various times feel tired, slow, wet or untidy. Indeed, having dementia is just as much a bodily as it is an emotional experience. This section therefore continues by examining the physical features associated with having a dementia. Roger Watson provides a review of the bodily needs of people with dementia. This importance of meeting the bodily needs of those with dementia is continued by Kay deVries, who develops a palliative care approach to people in the latter stages of dementia. Because of the tendency within a person-centred approach to marginalize people who are dying, the palliative care needs of people with dementia must not be neglected. People with dementia have bodies just as much as they have emotions, and people in the latter stages of dementia require the same standard of care as anyone else.

There is a tendency for the idea of person-centred care to fail to highlight various aspects of dementia care, one such area being working with groups of people with dementia. This omission is addressed in Chapter 9 by Richard Cheston, Kerry Jones and Jane Gilliard, who provide a description of a psychotherapeutic approach to groups of people with dementia.

The book's third section examines various systems associated with practice with people who have dementia and their families. In Chapter 12, Alison Marriott considers the various ways in which dementia care practitioners may help families to cope with dementia. Anthea Innes then addresses the issue of developing ethnically sensitive practice for people with dementia. The importance of the person with dementia is further developed by Jonathan Parker in Chapter 10 who develops the notion of positive communication. This chapter complements the earlier chapter by Karen Bryan and Jane Maxim and moves forward recent work by Tom Kitwood (1997) relating to positive person work. Finally, within this section, Maria Parsons highlights the needs of younger people with dementia and puts forward various responses that can be made to enhance their welfare.

In Chapter 14, Mark Holman examines how clinical supervision may be used to help practitioners to work with people with dementia and their families. This is an important chapter as working with people who have dementia is physically and emotionally demanding. Moreover, it frequently leads to practitioners becoming emotionally numbed to the pain that individuals with dementia experience. We would strongly argue that clinical supervision should be the part of the normal experience of dementia care practitioners and should make an important contribution to ensuring good practice.

The failure of service agencies to provide staff with effective clinical supervision may lead to staff abusing people with dementia. We believe that clinical supervision is one way in which abuse may be prevented. Bridget Pendale addresses the issue of abuse in dementia care more fully in Chapter 15, and finally Dawn Brooker examines an important means of ensuring quality in dementia care – dementia care mapping.

As much as anything, we believe that the response to people with dementia is multidisciplinary: whereas all professionals will have their own distinctive contribution, we believe that the future for dementia care lies in a multidisciplinary response in combination with medical diagnosis and to accompany treatment or to provide care when medication has no longer any benefit. We hope that this book will contribute to the continued development of this new culture of dementia care.

Trevor Adams and Jill Manthorpe

REFERENCE

Kitwood, T. 1997: *Dementia reconsidered: the person comes first*. Buckingham: Open University Press.

Approaches to practice

Constructing dementia

Trevor Adams and Ruth Bartlett

The first aim of this chapter is to examine recent approaches towards people with dementia, the second is to describe the way in which language constructs people with dementia, and the third is to provide a critical perspective on how people with dementia are understood and treated within society. Underlying the chapter is a social constructionist position by which the actions and language people use with respect to dementia are understood as constructing dementia (Burr 1995). The chapter addresses such questions as: How does society construct people who are chronically confused? How do these constructions influence the way in which people with dementia feel about themselves? To what extent do these disadvantage people with dementia? The approach adopted in this chapter criticises dominant oppressive and discriminatory forms of representing people with dementia and provides a positive means of reconstructing their identity in terms that are more advantageous to them.

DISCOURSE, SOCIAL PRACTICES AND THE CONSTRUCTION OF DEMENTIA

Language is a system of signs through which the social world is represented. Saussure (1974) argued that these signs comprise 'signifiers' and 'signified'. Take, for example, the two words 'bag' and 'big'. The signifiers are the marks that are made on the page, and the signified is the meaning made available by the signifier. Saussure argued that there is no natural or inevitable link between a signifier and a signified, and that signs do not possess any fixed or essential meaning. According to Saussure, the meaning that signifieds possess arises out of their difference from other signifieds. So 'bag' is a bag not because of its 'bagness' but because of its difference from other signifieds. This issue of 'marking a difference' is of particular interest since the way in which people with dementia are represented in talk, actions and the media affects how they are categorized and differentiated within society.

When people write, speak or do anything associated with people who have dementia, they draw upon a range of culturally and historically specific signifying practices that come together to form a discourse (Hall 1997). Foucault provides insights into how discourse is contained within social practices that give rise to the way in which social phenomena are understood. He defines discourses as 'practices which systematically form the objects they speak' (Foucault 1972, p. 49). Moreover, Foucault does not restrict discourse to refer to just verbal systems of representation, that is spoken discourse, but instead extends discourses to include people's behaviours and social practices. In this sense, discourse provides a way by which the knowledge about the social world comes to exist. Because there are many ways in which social phenomena may be described, there are many ways of talking and behaving with regard to people with dementia. The concern within this chapter is therefore how people with dementia are represented within the social world.

The relationship between social practices, discourse and the construction of social phenomena may be illustrated by an episode entitled *The Rat* that is taken from the television comedy series *Fawlty Towers*. The story line is that Manuel, the hotel porter, has acquired a rat that he keeps hidden away in his hotel room. Inevitably, the rat escapes just when a hotel inspector is due to visit the hotel. Throughout the episode, social practices occur relating to the rat, practices that contain certain discourses and are therefore called 'discursive practices'. Two sets of discursive practices are particularly evident. The first relates to love and affection, and provides the rat with the identity of something that Manuel adores. The second relates to hygiene and identifies the rat as a health hazard. The presence of one discourse rather than another makes certain features of a person (or, in this case, a rat) more visible than if another discourse were used. It is through the use of these discursive practices that people acquire knowledge about another. This is true of dementia: the availability and use of different discourses within social practices allow people to understand and experience dementia in particular ways and also give rise to their variable treatment in society.

Traditional ways of understanding identity that have arisen since the Enlightenment have assumed that a person's identity results from some essential feature associated with that person. An alternative argument has more recently developed in which identity is seen to be dependent not upon individuals themselves but rather upon their surrounding social setting (Antaki and Widdicome 1998). What is at issue here is the organization of conversational and discursive materials within people's talk and other social practices that gives rise to people occupying certain *subject positions* (*see* Wetherell 1998). The idea is that social practices within which discourses are contained allow people to occupy certain social positions within society.

It should also be noted that additional insights into the representation of people with dementia may also be gleaned from a further aspect of Saussure's work. The focus of attention here is that meaning is dependent upon marking the difference between signifiers. Thus, the meaning of the signifier 'dementia' arises through the difference between dementia and other social phenomena. The meanings associated with dementia are therefore understood in terms of their difference and relate to what it is not, leading to people with dementia being thought of as *not* rational and *not* normal. By marking out the difference between those who have dementia and those who do not, people with dementia are constructed as being different from the rest of society, as marginal and part of 'the Other'. This way of understanding people with dementia gives important insights into the injustice that people with dementia receive within society.

DEMENTIA AS A BIO-MEDICAL CONSTRUCTION

Towards the end of the nineteenth century, various discourses became available through the work of medical scientists that highlighted bio-medical features of dementia. It is important to note that these discourses did not exist prior to the work of medical science but rather arose from a particular way in which medical scientists saw people with dementia that did not exist prior to their work. One of these discourses highlighted the physiological nature of dementia and gave rise to experimental studies that led to such social practices as the identification of neurophysiological and neurochemical changes in the brains of chronically confused people, the classification of brain pathology and the publication of papers in acclaimed and prestigious scientific journals. Another discourse that became available at this time related to cognitivism. This discourse constructed chronic confusion in terms of the 'cognitive paradigm' in which dementia is primarily understood to affect people's cognitive functioning and give rise to memory failure (*see* Berrios and Freeman 1991).

Throughout the twentieth century, these two discourses were typically used to construct people with dementia. Kitwood argues that advances in technology in the 1960s and 70s, such as the development of computerized tomography, were used to support bio-medical discourses and gave rise to the closing down of psychosocial discourse about people with dementia (Kitwood 1987). In addition, various writers, notably Katzman and Bick (2000) and Fox (1989), describe the social and political processes that led to the increased public awareness of Alzheimer's disease in the 1980s and helped to transform it from an obscure, rarely applied medical diagnosis to a major cause of death.

Bio-medical discourses are contained in various social practices, such as the standard practice that professional bodies in medicine have of giving definitions of illnesses. The oft-quoted definition of dementia given by the Royal College of Physicians (1981), for example, defined dementia as:

the acquired global impairment of higher cortical functions including memory, the capacity to solve the problems of everyday living, the performance of learned perceptuo-motors skills, the correct use of social skills and the control of emotional reactions, all aspects of language and communication and the control of emotional reactions, in the absence of gross clouding of consciousness.

The constitution of people with dementia through the use of bio-medical discourses has been thought to lead to the depersonalization of people with dementia (Jonas-Simpson 2001). An example of this may be found in medical textbooks. Jacques and Jackson (2000, p. 99), for example, comment that 'At the final stages the patient may be assumed to have no real subjective awareness, no sense of self at all, and to be in this sense mentally "dead"'. Social scientists, Fontana and Smith (1989, p. 36) argue that:

> The Alzheimer's disease patients, in the early stages of the disease, continue to interact on the surface as if they were sentient beings. ... This self is increasingly devoid of content.

In publications for the wider public, the well-known evolutionary scientist Richard Dworkin (1993, p. 234) comments that:

> Demented people in the late stages have lost the capacity to recognize, appreciate or suffer indignity. ... It is expensive, tedious and difficult to keep seriously demented patients clean, to assure them space for privacy, to give them the personal attention they often crave.

This last quotation, perhaps more than any of the others, displays how the construction of people with dementia can affect their welfare. The constitution of people with dementia through bio-medical discourses alone constitutes people with dementia as having diminished and limited human value. Constructed in this way, bio-medical discourse identifies people with dementia as having no sense of self or any ability to make worthwhile decisions, thus allowing the possibility that they might be seen as having no worth and being an infringement on other people.

IMPLICATIONS FOR PRACTICE

When used in health and social care, bio-medical discourse positions people with dementia as having a severe mental illness – dementia, chronic brain syndrome or chronic brain failure. When dementia is understood as an illness, those with the condition themselves recede into the background, and the disease process itself is highlighted. This construction of dementia plays down the significance of, for example, psychosocial features of dementia which might have contributed to its development.

Moreover, bio-medical discourse highlights the relevance of physical treatments such as drug therapy and creates the impression that a cure may be just around the corner. In the absence of a cure, bio-medical discourses create therapeutic nihilism and 'warehousing', in which those with dementia cannot be offered a cure and are stored away in institutions in the hope that a cure may one day appear. The bio-medical discourse that often surrounds chronic confusion there-fore constructs the work of health and social care workers as a form of 'body main-tenance' in which the person with dementia is merely kept clean, fed and watered.

In addition, the failure of bio-medical discourse to construct people with dementia as sensate human beings may give cause for health and social care workers to develop practices that distance them from people with dementia. When this occurs, people with dementia are often treated as objects or objectified, and are more likely to be at risk of oppressive and discriminatory practices, including emotional and physical abuse.

The objectification of people with dementia was a consistent finding of numerous reports on mental hospitals in the 1960s and 70s, especially notable being *Sans Everything*, which focused specifically on older people. In *Sans Everything*, an acting chief male nurse reported that:

after six months in certain hospitals, there are ways in which psychiatric nurses are no longer like ordinary people. Their attitude to mental illness changes – as it does to old age, to cruelty, to people's needs, and to dying. It is as if they become numbed to these things (Robb 1967, p. 13).

In this way, people with dementia often found themselves placed in difficult and sometimes humiliating situations that led to their devaluation, disempowerment and marginalization by psychiatric nurses. One explanation why institutional practices such as these occurred may be the dominance of bio-medical discourses that identified people with dementia as being different from the rest of society and constructed them as marginal, as 'the Other'.

DEMENTIA AS A BEHAVIOURAL PROBLEM

Various discourses developed within the academic discipline of psychology have been applied to people with dementia. These have constructed people with dementia in terms of their behaviour rather than, as with bio-medical discourse, their diagnosis. They have given rise to dementia care practitioners regarding some of the behaviours of those with dementia, such as wandering and aggression, as a problem. This behaviour is typically seen to be the result of prior learning, which raises the possibility of changing problematic behaviour through techniques directed towards enabling people to relearn.

Such an approach may be seen in the work of Stokes (2000), who describes how 'problem behaviours' in people with dementia may be addressed by behavioural analysis. This technique is sometimes referred to as an ABC analysis, in which 'A' stands for antecedents (which activate the event or situation), 'B' stands for behaviour and 'C' stands for consequences (Stokes 2000).

Behavioural discourses are also present in another major intervention strategy – reality orientation – the main aim of which is to reduce disorientation. Reality orientation employs techniques that modify people's physical and interpersonal environment so that individuals who are disorientated develop a better degree of orientation (*see* Chapter 9 for a further discussion of this approach).

Implications for practice

Behavioural discourse highlights certain aspects of chronically confused people in preference to others. It provides a means of identifying the difficulties experienced by individuals and enables practitioners to develop strategies for their resolution. However, identifying the person with dementia as someone who is having problems gives rise to a number of serious difficulties. First, behavioural discourse highlights only the outward manifestation of dementia: what people do and what they say. It fails to highlight the inner personal world of people with dementia and leads to an assumption that people with dementia possibly do not have any inner world. Second, behavioural discourse does not allow people with dementia to be considered as possessing any interpretations, judgements or personal feelings about the outside world. Third, behavioural discourse positions people with dementia as a problem and does not allow people to see that their behaviour may be a reasonable response to others' unkind and unthoughtful behaviour.

DEMENTIA AS A SUBJECTIVE EXPERIENCE

Over the past 20 years, various discourses have highlighted the subjective experience of people with dementia. One such discourse relates to attachment and draws upon wider psychoanalytic discourses such as those developed by Bowlby (1969). This discourse brings into prominence the disturbed and demanding behaviour sometimes exhibited by people with dementia and identifies their behaviour to be the result of feelings of anxiety arising from an earlier attachment figure.

Another discourse that highlights the subjective experience of people with dementia relates to the significance of past events for the mental health. This discourse draws upon others that were developed in the twentieth century, initially by Freud (2002) and later by Erikson (1950). These discourses are present in the work of Butler (1963) relating to 'life review', in which the ability to take stock of one's life is constructed as an essential feature of good mental health in older people. They are also present in the work of Naomi Feil, who has developed validation therapy, which attends to people's past experiences rather than bringing people back to 'the here are now', as advocated by reality orientation (*see* Morton 2000, and Chapters 6 and 10).

Without doubt, the most important and significant discourse on dementia that has developed in the past 20 years relates to personhood. Kitwood set a discourse of personhood against what he called 'the standard paradigm', i.e. the bio-medical model of dementia, arguing that the bio-medical model leads to the depersonal-ization of people with dementia. To Kitwood (1997, p. 46), the depersonalization of those with dementia should not be blamed on any one individual but is instead part of our 'cultural inheritance' and of the stream of thinking that has developed since the Enlightenment.

Within this context, Kitwood saw dementia as a dialectical interplay between neurological impairment and malignant social psychology. Underlying his approach is the idea that the personhood of people with dementia remains intact throughout dementia, Kitwood arguing (1997, p. 51) that individuals with dementia are engaged in 'an involutionary spiral' that undermines their sense of personhood. As he comments: 'When self-esteem is lacking or damaged, a person is disastrously incapacitated in many ways, and easily falls into a cycle of discour-agement and failure' (Kitwood 1990).

This draws on discourses that had recently been made available by Sixmith et al. (1993) relating to 'rementia', i.e. the interruption of the involutionary spiral and the recovery of powers that were once lost. Moreover, other writers have drawn on discourses relating to rementia (Sabat 1994), and Kitwood (1997) puts forward 17 types of malignant psychology that can contribute to the involutionary spiral (Box 1.1).

In his later work, Kitwood applied his approach to organizations supporting people with dementia, his main concern once again being to maintain the person-hood of those with dementia. First, he developed a quality assurance tool, dementia care mapping, based on the idea of personhood (*see* Chapter 16). Second, he argued that there is increasing awareness of how much can be done for people with dementia. With this in mind, Kitwood proposed (1997) that a 'new culture of dementia' that is 'more strongly committed, more psychologically aware, more practical and more pragmatic than anything that has gone before is beginning to emerge'.

Kitwood's work has had an immense impact on dementia care, probably because of its ability to engage with popular feeling among people working in dementia care. After years of excessive institutionalization of individuals with dementia, many practitioners had become disillusioned with existing service provision and were looking for an alternative that would allow a compassionate and human approach with a focus on the person with dementia.

Box 1.1 Examples of manifestations of malignant social psychology in dementia care (from Kitwood 1997, 46–47)

Treachery – Using some form of deception in order to distract or manipulate a person, or force them into compliance.

Disempowerment – Not allowing a person to use the abilities that they do have; failing to help them to complete actions that they have initiated.

Infantilization – Treating a person very patronizingly (or 'matronizingly') as an insensitive parent might treat a very young child.

Intimidation – Inducing fear in a person, through the use of threats or physical power.

Labelling – Using a pattern of behaviour (e.g. smearer, stripper) or a category such as 'organic mental disorder', as the main basis for interacting with a person.

Stigmatization – Treating a person as if they were a diseased object, an alien or an outcast.

Outpacing – Providing information, presenting choices, etc, at a rate too fast for a person to understand; putting them under pressure to do things more rapidly than they can bear.

Invalidation – Failing to acknowledge the subjective reality of a person's experience, and especially what they are feeling.

Banishment – Sending the person away, or excluding them; physically or psychologically.

Objectification – Treating a person as if they were a lump of dead matter, to be pushed, lifted, filled, pumped or drained, without proper reference to the fact that they are sentient beings.

Ignoring – Carrying on (in conversation or action) in the presence of a person as if they were not there.

Imposition – Forcing a person to do something, over-riding desire or denying the possibility of choice on their part.

Withholding – Refusing to give asked for attention, or to meet an evident need; for example, for affectional contact.

Accusation – Blaming a person for actions or failures of action that arise from their lack of ability, or their misunderstanding of the situation.

Disruption – Roughly intruding on a person's action or inaction; crudely breaking their 'frame of reference'.

Mockery – Making fun of a person's 'strange' actions or remarks; teasing, humiliating, making jokes at their expense.

Disparagement – Telling a person that they are incompetent, useless, worthless, etc; giving them messages that are damaging to their self-esteem.

Although Kitwood's work has become an important means of changing previous ways of constructing people with dementia and their care, it has a number of drawbacks. First, it is largely anecdotal and rhetorical. Although Kitwood refers at various times to his own empirical work, he did not, with the exception of his study of Rose (Kitwood 1990), publish any research findings. This is a major failing of Kitwood's work. If he had established his research, he would have been able to support his findings with evidence and also provide helpful illustrations for his ideas.

Second, the methods that Kitwood used in his work were impaired. The data that Kitwood does reveal, from the larger body of work that Kitwood refers to but never formally published, concern a women with dementia called Rose. This information was collected during an open-ended interview with Rose's two daughters, an interview that covered large areas of their mother's life, including things that had happened long before they were born. It is therefore questionable whether their account could really be relied upon to give a reliable and accurate account of such events. In addition, there are a number of problems with dementia care mapping, notably the validity of its observational techniques and whether assumptions or inferences about people's level of personhood are possible (Adams 1996; Harding and Palfrey 1997).

The problems associated with Kitwood's work, particularly within the context of its acceptability as an ethical and compassionate response among progressively minded dementia care practitioners, pose as yet unanswered questions. These are concerned with the nature of, and the relationship between, theory, research and practice in dementia care, and include such questions as 'What methods should be used in research about people with dementia and their care?' and 'Should research underpin practice?'. These questions were only touched upon in Kitwood's work and have hardly been addressed outside this; moreover, it has to said that Kitwood's work sits uneasily within the present context of evidence-based practice.

IMPLICATIONS FOR PRACTICE

Discourses that highlight the inner experience of people with dementia raise the possibility that intervention by health and social care workers could be enhanced. This might be through the development of approaches that directly addressed the intrapsychic experience of people with dementia, such as with reminiscence therapy or validation therapy. Alternatively, Kitwood's construction of malignant social psychology provides a theoretical basis for developing practice that is sensitive to the feelings of people with dementia. Through his development of a 'new culture of dementia' and dementia care mapping, Kitwood takes his approach beyond the intra- and interpersonal approach and applies his work to organizations that deliver support to people with dementia.

DEMENTIA, VOICE AND CHOICE

Kitwood's work is mainly concerned with the links between neurological impairment and malignant social psychology and the way in which a person's sense of personhood is, through this interplay, determined. However, Kitwood's illumination of the subjective nature of dementia allows people to be constructed as having feelings that may be voiced or expressed by using appropriate methods and strategies.

In addition, a further discourse relates to the voice of people with dementia. There are two ways in which the voice has been used in recent work on dementia. The first approach focuses on the inner voice of people as they try to make sense of having dementia; the focus here is on the person's inner interpretation of dementia. The second focuses on the political exercise of voice, the way in which the voice maintains the power possessed by those with dementia and allows them to exercise personal choice.

Voice as a means of making sense

This discourse was initially developed in relationship to dementia by writers such as Robert Davis (1993) and Diane Friel McGowin (1993), who provide first-hand accounts of what it is like to have dementia. Following the interest stimulated by these writers, empirical work was published that illuminated the inner voice of people with dementia. This work uses data collected from a variety of sources: accounts of individuals with dementia (Keady and Gilliard 1999), support group discussions (Yale 1995), clinical experience (Balfour 1995; Mills 1998) and family experience (Crisp 1995). In addition, two books have been written about a close relative's experience of having dementia – by Linda Grant (1998) about her mother, and by John Bayley about his wife, the novelist Iris Murdoch (Bayley 1999).

Kitwood outlines seven 'access routes' through which insight into the subjective world of people with dementia may be obtained:

- Reading accounts by people with dementia
- Listening to people with dementia in a specially organized interview or group meeting
- Listening to people with dementia in ordinary conversation
- Observing the behaviour of people with dementia
- Talking to someone who has had an illness with dementia-like features
- Using poetic imagination
- Doing role play.

Cheston uses these access routes to describe a model of how people make sense of having dementia (Cheston 1996). In addition, Cheston examines how people with dementia use metaphors and stories to make sense of what is happening to them. In one example, Cheston describes a man with dementia who tells a story about being in a thick dense jungle in which he has 'difficulty of getting through the jungle, thick high grass and things like that'. Cheston argues that when the man is talking in this way, he is using a metaphor for his present experience through which he is making sense of what is happening to him.

Voice as a means of maintaining power

Various studies show that voice is a means by which personal control and power are exerted in the social world. They construct the person with dementia as someone who has wants and preferences and can participate in decision-making related to his or her own care. This way of constructing people with dementia draws on discourses that relate to voice and set the person with dementia within a socio-political context.

Goldsmith (1996) argues that the bio-discourse has constructed people with dementia as having little ability to make decisions about their own care. As a result of the dominance of the professions, health and social care workers expect that people with dementia are not able to make choices about the sort of care they want.

Implications for practice

Discourses relating to voice highlight the fact that the person with dementia is not silent and passive but has ideas and opinions and can express these. The implication is that health and social care practitioners should make it possible to hear the voice of individuals with dementia. At a practical level, this means preventing extraneous and distracting 'noise', which affects hearing what people with dementia are saying. In addition, it means developing ways of talking that help those with dementia to engage in conversation and implement their views.

DEMENTIA AS A DISABILITY

Discourses identifying people with dementia as having a disability may be found in various parts of Kitwood's work as he encourages people to think of dementia first as a disability (Kitwood 1997). The use of discourses that relate to disability makes it difficult for people to think of someone as a 'dementia sufferer' and gives rise to their being thought of as someone who not only has a diagnosable illness, but also encounters a diverse range of social restrictions and barriers. Discourses that identify people with dementia as having a disability lie, however, very much on the outskirts of dementia care. The aim of this latter part of the chapter is therefore to outline an approach to dementia that allows people with dementia to be constructed by themselves and others through disability discourses in ways that resist oppressive and discriminatory practices and lead to their empowerment.

Disability defined

Defining disability is not a straightforward issue. At the time of writing, the formal classification, supplied by the World Health Organization (WHO) and used since 1994, is under review as a result of sustained international pressure. Unlike previous classifications, the new WHO version of disability will incorporate 'contextual factors' such as the environment and personal circumstances, a move that will not only please critics who found previous definitions too negative and clinical, but also signal the extent to which disability is rapidly becoming understood as a social rather than a medical phenomenon. A full account of the changes can be found on the WHO website (http://www.who.int/icidh/index.htm).

In the UK, social problems such as unemployment and inaccessible public buildings have long been a part of disabled people's lives (Blaxter 1976), although since the Disability Discriminations Act (1995), it is now unlawful for large employers and service providers to discriminate against a person because of a disability. For legal purposes, disability is broadly defined as 'physical or mental impairment, which has a substantial and long-term adverse effect upon a person's ability to carry out normal day-to-day activities' (www.disability.gov.uk/dda/). People with dementia are therefore legally protected by the Disability Discriminations Act (1995) and could potentially use it as a protective tool if they wished, for example, to remain in a sheltered housing scheme. According to disability activists, however, a single piece of legislation is not in itself enough permanently to improve the lives of people with a disability as the social oppression they face is considered far too deep-seated for that (Charlton 1998).

Another popular way of defining disability is to see it as a form of social oppression, oppression in the sense that people experience isolation and exclusion not because they have a mental or physical impairment, but because society is designed in such a way as to privilege those without a disability (Priestly 2001). Steps and cobbled streets, for example, make getting around extremely difficult for a wheelchair user. Similarly, excessive noise and activity can make life intolerable for someone with dementia (Marshall 2001). The idea that society is essentially at the root of disabled people's problems is the basic premise of what is commonly known as the 'social model of disability' (Oliver 1995), and it is to this model that we now turn.

THE POLITICS OF DISABILITY

By introducing the notion of oppression into the debate on what disability means, disability activists also introduce the realm of politics. Like the feminism and gay rights movements, the personal becomes the political as people with a physical disability join forces to demand that society consider the disabling barriers and negative attitudes that people constantly face as a denial of their human rights.

During the 1980s, for example, people with a physical disability chained themselves to railings and buses to protest about how difficult it was to gain access to the world around them (Campbell and Oliver 1996). The fact that disabled people themselves are the driving force behind the movement reflects one of their most strongly held beliefs, that 'empowerment is not the gift of the powerful – empowerment is something that people do for themselves collectively – disabled people have decided to empower themselves' (Oliver 1995, p. 15).

This is an interesting global view of disabled people: have, and indeed can, *all* disabled people really decide to empower themselves? For people disabled by any degree of cognitive impairment, prescriptive accounts of how greater control should be achieved and who should instigate the process would certainly seem to disable them still further. The 'dementia' usefulness of this approach emerges, however, following consideration of the underlying philosophy.

One of the strongest strands running through disability studies is a belief in the 'collective experience of disability', i.e. the idea that as 'disabled people' face similar barriers, they are a more powerful force in the struggle against social oppression than any one individual with a disability (Oliver 1995). The dominant paradigm of 'individualism' in health and social care settings is therefore seen as 'a way of using power to oppress by separating each individual from the great body of humanity' (Ryles 1999, p. 605).

The relevance of this for people with dementia has been questioned: would not any devaluing of individuality turn back the clock of dementia care to the days of simply 'warehousing' older people with mental health problems? The point that disability writers make, however, is not that people with a disability should be *cared* for as an homogenous group but that while care practices are individualized, people with a dementia are unlikely to perceive their situation in any shared or collective sense. Moreover, their position in society will always be governed by *other people's* perceptions of what they need and ideas about how things could be improved.

Consider for a moment the benefits that older people have derived from uniting and being seen 'as one': a sizeable group of elderly residents recently protested in London about the closure of residential homes. Carers of people with dementia are also becoming a formidable group with the help of organizations such as the Alzheimer's Society, which exist to champion their rights. At present, however, those personally affected by dementia have a limited (if any) opportunity simply to come together and support each other (Gilliard 2000) and possibly develop a more powerful and positive group identity. A similar trend is developing in social research as individual interviews are being joined by focus groups, which have the potential 'to raise collective consciousness' (Kitzinger 1994, pp. 102–21) as popular methods of data collection. Individual assessments lead to individualized solutions, but whereas the new culture of dementia care undoubtedly raises the profile of personal worth, the approach can paradoxically reduce an individual's strength. In this sense, disability studies are useful as they highlights not only the advantages of a group identity, but also the reality of human *inter*dependence and reliance on one other (Bond 1999).

The myth of independence

Independence is a prominent feature of government strategy for older people with mental health problems (Audit Commission 2000). Voluntary organizations and older people themselves (Nystrom and Segesten 1994) obviously regard independence as an important aspect of a person's life that should be maintained regardless of age. Does independence have the same priority for people with dementia, though? Or are other possible outcomes, such as feeling safe or feeling a sense of belonging, more important (Davies et al. 2000)? From a disability perspective, this is a particularly important issue to understand as the notion of independence has the potential to stigmatize people who are not able to do everything for themselves.

Oliver (1995) argues that when professionals and people with a disability talk about independence, they are not necessarily talking about the same thing. Policy guidelines, for example, define independence in terms of an ability to self-care without assistance (Audit Commission 2000), whereas disabled people see it as 'the ability to be in control and make decisions about one's life' (Oliver 1995, p. 54). This difference of opinion is supported by Baltes (1996) who in a psychological study of older people found that older patients delegate control to others as a way of 'reserving energy', thus maintaining and optimizing the domains that they most value and that are in most danger of decline. Someone might, for example, prefer to use a wheelchair to go to an activities session, and thus avoid using up valuable energy walking, preferring to be socializing or doing something creative and interesting. Anecdotal evidence suggests that people with dementia are also making similar decisions about what areas of their life to 'let go of' and what activities it is important to concentrate on (Davis 1989). Disability studies invite us to think again about what independence means and to realize that if independence is defined strictly in terms of how much people are able to do rather than how much they are able to control, then people with any kind of impairment will inevitably be stigmatized.

Stigma and stereotypes

Earlier in this chapter, we argued that language and labels (such as 'acceptable behaviour' and 'dementia') reproduce people with dementia as somehow different or 'less normal' than everybody else. Disability writers are also concerned about the way in which society talks about and constructs an 'idea' of disability that is detrimental to those affected. For example, literary and film portrayals of 'hunchbacks' and 'cripples' as figures of fun and inherently villainous people are said to contribute to the social stigma associated with a disability (*see* Campbell and Oliver, 1996). The impact of popular representations of dementia on social attitudes has yet to be explored with quite the same vigour, although recent work reveals a welcoming interest in this area (McColgan et al. 2000).

Something that is known to affect those with dementia and their families is the label 'dementia'. The impact of this label is not dissimilar to the experiences of people diagnosed as having a learning difficulty in that whereas a diagnosis can open doors to specialist services and treatment provision, both classifications are over-arching diagnoses that can shape identities and exclude people from everyday opportunities (Gillman et al. 2000). People with dementia may, for example, not be able to articulate dissent or anger related to their situation, and if they do so, it is commonly viewed as symptomatic of the disease, so they are offered medication. Thus, direct public action may be seen as an appropriate response to social injustice for a person with a physical disability, but if a person has a mental health diagnosis, displays of anger or dissent are more likely to be viewed as symptomatic of his or her psychopathology (Sayce 2000).

The importance of place

One of the biggest decisions facing service developers in dementia care today is whether or not to provide separate housing and care facilities for residents with dementia. Such decisions are usually based on intuitive concerns and/or objective measures of the best long-term location for someone with a chronic and progressive illness. In other words, although much is known and felt about the features of 'quality care', little empirical work has been done on the long-term housing needs of those with dementia. In particular, we need to know more about whether people with dementia can, should or wish to live alongside those without any significant cognitive impairment.

Sociologically speaking, a consideration of where people live is important as 'place' is linked to matters of personal identity and a sense of belonging. Thrift (1997), for example, suggests that places 'form a reservoir of meanings, which people can draw upon to tell stories and thereby define themselves'. Unfortunately, little is yet known about how people with a diagnosis of dementia define themselves by the places in which they live because little has been asked. This may be because, in an increasingly mobile society, the importance of place can be forgotten in the process of making decisions about where older people should receive care (Reed et al. 1998).

From a disability perspective, the places in which people live and the way in which spaces are used in general terms are matters too important to overlook. Kitchin (1998) argues, for example, that by separating people with a disability from their peers and local communities (as was the case with 'special' schools in the 1970s and 80s), negative ideas are perpetuated about disabled people being 'out of place' in society and somehow different from other people. The relevance of this in terms of dementia care is that, in the short term, housing and care services should be based on barrier-free and inclusive principles rather than 'special' and excessively remedial initiatives, and that, in the long term, alternatives to institutional care should be explored. In addition, for people with dementia to be treated equally, with dignity and respect, education needs to tackle the negative attitudes held by other service users – who do not have a disability – as well as the training needs of care staff.

Bodily developments

Much of dementia care is 'body-work', a term favoured by medical sociologists to describe caring activities such as bathing (Twigg 2000). Faces are shaved, nails are cut, hair is brushed, and teeth are cleaned, to the extent that the presentation of well-ordered bodies comes to symbolize 'a job well done' (Lee-Treweek 1994). In this sense, the body functions as a site of social *meaning*, as well as pathology, in so far as people are defined by what their bodies can and cannot do (*see* Shilling 1993). The everyday life of a person with dementia is, for example, often described using expressions such as 'got up with minimal help', 'wandering' and 'repeatedly asking the same questions'. In other words, the emphasis is on how an individual's *body* seems to be affected by the cognitive impairment. The personal becomes the political as the language used to describe such individuals also often renders them docile, unproductive or disempowered (Hughes and Paterson 1997).

Since the early 1990s, disability writers have begun to challenge the 'social model of disability' on the basis that it excludes the individual's experience of impairment. Marks (1999), for example, argues that many people with a disability are oppressed more emotionally than socially or politically, calling for a 'mutually constitutive' explanation of disability. By this, Marks means that, in order to understand the true extent of oppression, a person's emotional and bodily state should be considered *in conjunction* with their political and social context.

Implications for practice

Defining dementia as a disability raises a number of important implications for service providers and health and social care practitioners. First, people with dementia are legally protected by the Disability Discriminations Act (1995); thus, treating those affected less favourably is not only bad practice, it is unlawful. In other words, people with dementia have a right to the same goods, services and facilities as other service users, so those affected should not be excluded from some activity or from going somewhere simply on the grounds of their dementia.

A second implication of thinking about dementia as a disability is that the

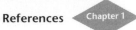

collective identity of those affected is both emphasized and regarded as a potential source of strength. It may seem counterintuitive within dementia care to see people as being part of a 'group' rather than individuals with unique needs. If, however, we also concentrate on what people with dementia have in common (such as a lack of alternatives to institutional care) and focus on the barriers that face *all* people with dementia (such as cognitive bias in wider society), those affected will perhaps have an increased opportunity to empower themselves.

A third and final implication for practice relates to how well people with dementia are supported through transitional phases of care. Little is known, for example, about the meanings that people with dementia attach to being assessed and monitored in a day hospital, or indeed about the extent to which residents with dementia regard the institution they are living in as 'home'. Disability writers remind us of the dangers of spatial segregation, of placing people with disabilities apart from the rest of society (Kitchin 1998) and particularly of the risk of people internalizing feelings of anger and resentment when this happens (Marks 2000). It is therefore imperative that people with dementia have an opportunity for extended meaningful conversation, particularly during times of transition. These conversations would of course not necessarily have to be with care staff, as opportunities could, for example, be created and sustained in partnership with other service users.

Finally, although these three suggestions have resource implications, the disablement of people with dementia relates to not only the quality of care, but also the politics of disablement and exclusion.

REFERENCES

Adams, T. 1996: Kitwood's approach to dementia and dementia care: a critical but appreciative review. *Journal of Advanced Nursing* **23:** 946–53.

Antaki, C. and Widdicome, S. eds. 2000: *Identities in talk.* London: Sage.

Audit Commission. 2000: *Forget me not: mental health services for older people.* London: Audit Commission.

Balfour, A. 1995: Account of a study aiming to explore the experience of dementia. *PSIGE Newsletter* **53:** July 15–19.

Baltes, M. 1996: *The many faces of dependency.* New York: Cambridge University Press.

Bayley, J. 1999: *Iris: a memoir to Iris Murdoch.* London: Duckworth.

Berrios, G.E. and Freeman, H.L. 1991: Dementia before the twentieth century. In: Berrios, G.E. and Freeman, H.L. eds. *Alzheimer and the dementias.* London: Royal Society of Medicine, 9–27.

Blaxter, M. 1976: *The meaning of disability.* London: Heinemann.

Bond, J. 1999: Quality of life for people with dementia: approaches to the challenge of measurement. *Ageing and Society* **19:** 561–79.

Bowlby, J. 1969: *Attachment and loss,* volumes 1–3. New York: Basic Books.

Burr, J. 1995: *An introduction to social constructionism.* London: Routledge.

Butler, R. 1963: The life review: an interpretation of reminiscence in the aged. *Psychiatry* **26:** 65–76.

Campbell, J. and Oliver, M. eds. 1996: *Disability politics: understanding our past, changing our future.* London: Routledge.

Charlton, J. 1998: *Nothing about us without us: disability, oppression and empowerment.* London: University of California Press.

Cheston, R. 1996: Stories and metaphors: talking about the past in a psychotherapy group for people with dementia. *Ageing and Society* **16:** 579–602.

Crisp, J. 1995: Making sense of the stories that people with Alzheimer's tell: a journey with my mother. *Nursing Inquiry* **2:** 133–40.

Davies, S., Ellis. L. and Laker, S. 2000: Promoting autonomy and independence for older people with nursing practice: an observational study. *Journal of Clinical Nursing* **9:** 127–36.

Davis, R. 1989: *My journey into Alzheimer's disease.* Amersham: Scripture Press.

Dworkin, R. 1993: *Life's dominion.* New York: Knopf.

Erikson, E. 1950: *Childhood and society.* New York: Norton.

Fontana, A. and Smith, R.W. 1989: Alzheimer's disease victims: the 'unbecoming' of self and the normalization of competence. *Sociological Perspectives* **32:** 35–46.

Foucault, M. 1972: *The archeology of knowledge.* London: Tavistock.

Fox, P. 1989: From senility to Alzheimer's disease: the rise of the Alzheimer's disease movement. *Millbank Quarterly* **67:** 58–102.

Freud, S. 2002: *Psychopathology of everyday life.* Harmondsworth: Penguin.

Gilliard, J. 2001: The perspectives of people with dementia, their families and their carers. In: Cantley, C. ed. *A handbook of dementia care.* Buckingham: Open University Press, 77–90.

Gillman, M., Heyman, B. and Swain, J. 2000: What's in a name? The implications of diagnosis for people with learning difficulties and their family carers. *Disability and Society* **15:** 389–409.

Goldsmith, M. 1996: *Hearing the voices of people with dementia.* London: Jessica Kingsley.

Grant, L. 1998: *Remind me who I am, again.* London: Granta.

Hall, S. 1997: The work of representation. In: Hall, S. ed. *Representation: cultural representations and signifying practices.* London: Sage/Open University, 13–64.

Harding, N. and Palfrey, C. 1997: *The social construction of dementia: confused professionals?* London: Jessica Kingsley.

Hughes, B. and Paterson, K. 1997: The social model of disability and the disappearing body: towards a sociology of impairment. *Disability and Society* **12:** 325–40.

Jacques, A. and Jackson, G. 2000: *Understanding dementia.* Edinburgh: Churchill Livingstone.

Jonas-Simpson, C.M. 2001: From silence to voice: knowledge values and beliefs guiding health-care practices with persons living with dementia. *Nursing Science Quarterly* **14**(4): 304–10.

Katzman, R. and Bick, K. 2000: The rediscovery of Alzheimer disease during the 1960s and 1970s. In: Whitehouse, P.J., Maurer, K. and Ballenger, M.A. eds. *Concepts of Alzheimer's disease: biological, clinical and cultural perspectives.* London: Johns Hopkins University Press, 104–115.

Keady, J. and Gilliard, J. 1999: The early experience of Alzheimer's disease: implications for partnership and practice. In: Adams, T. and Clarke, C. eds. *Dementia care: developing partnerships in practice.* London: Baillière Tindall, 305–24.

Kitchin, R. 1998: Out of place, 'knowing one's place': space, power and the exclusion of disabled people. *Disability and Society* **13:** 343–56.

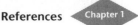

Kitwood, T. 1990: Understanding senile dementia: a psychobiographical approach. *Free Associations* **19:** 60–76.

Kitwood, T. 1997: *Dementia reconsidered*. Buckingham: Open University Press.

Kitzinger, J. 1994: The methodology of focus groups: the importance of interaction between research participants. *Sociology of Health and Illness* **16:** 102–21.

Lee-Treweek, G. 1994: Discourse, care and control: an ethnography of nursing and residential elder care work. Unpublished PhD thesis. Plymouth: University of Plymouth.

McColgan, G., Valentine, J. and Downs, M. 2000: Concluding narratives of a career with dementia: accounts of Iris Murdoch at her death. *Ageing and Society* **20:** 97–109.

McGowin, D. 1993: *Living in the labyrinth: a personal journal through the maze of Alzheimer's*. San Francisco: Elder Books.

Marks, D. 1999: Dimensions of oppression: theorising the embodied subject. *Disability and Society* **14:** 611–26.

Marks, D. 2000: *Disability*. London: Routledge.

Marshall, M. 2001: Care settings and the care environment. In: Cantley, C. ed. *A handbook of dementia care*. Buckingham: Open University Press, 173–85.

Mills, M. 1998: Memory, emotion, and dementia. In: Miesen, B.M.L. and Jones, G.M.M. eds. *Care-giving in dementia*. London: Routledge: 48–66.

Nystrom, A. and Segesten, K. 1994: On sources of powerlessness in nursing home life. *Journal of Advanced Nursing* **19:** 124–33.

Oliver, M. 1995: *Understanding disability: from theory to practice*. London: Palgrave.

Priestley, M. ed. 2001: *Disability and the life course: global perspectives*. Cambridge: Cambridge University Press.

Reed, J., Payton, V., Roswell, V. and Bond, S. 1998: The importance of place for older people moving into care homes. *Social Science and Medicine* **46:** 859–67.

Robb, B. 1967: *Sans everything*. London: Nelson.

Ryles, S. 1999: A concept analysis of empowerment: its relationship to mental health nursing. *Journal of Advanced Nursing* **29:** 600–7.

Sabat, S.R. 1994: Excess disability and malignant social psychology: a case study of Alzheimer's disease. *Journal of Community and Applied Social Psychology* **4:** 157–66.

Sayce, L. 2000: *From psychiatric patient to citizen: overcoming discrimination and exclusion*. London: Macmillan.

Saussure, F. 1974: *Course in general linguistics*. London: Fontana.

Shilling, C. 1993: *The body and social theory*. London: Sage.

Sixmith, A. Stillwell, J. and Copeland, J. 1993: Dementia: challenging the limits of dementia care. *International Journal of Geriatric Psychiatry* **8:** 993–1000.

Stokes, G. 2000: *Challenging behaviour in dementia: a person centred approach*. Bicester: Winslow Press.

Thrift, N. 1997: Re-imagining places, re-imagining identities. In: Mackay, H. ed. *Consumption and everyday life*. London: Sage, 159–212.

Twigg, J. 2000: *Bathing: the body and community care*. London: Routledge.

Yale, R. 1955: *Developing support groups for individuals with early-stage Alzheimer's disease: planning, implementation and evaluation*. Baltimore: Health Professions Press.

Wetherell, M. 1998: Positioning and interpretative repertoires: conversation analysis and post structuralism in dialogue. *Discourse and Identity* **9:** 387–412.

Valuing people with dementia

Wendy Martin and Helen Bartlett

The way in which people with dementia experience disempowerment is well documented (Goldsmith 1996; Kitwood 1997; Parker and Penhale 1998), and assumptions that they are not capable of making decisions or choices are commonplace. When people with dementia are not viewed as autonomous individuals, there is less opportunity for their own views and choices about care services and everyday life to be expressed. It is not only the illness that reduces control and influence for those affected – people with dementia experience a double disadvantage. First, dementia is frequently associated with old age. A person with dementia is therefore further challenged by the negative stereotypes, images and attitudes towards older people that prevail in an ageist society (Bartlett and Martin 2000). Second, a dominant view of disability as a personal tragedy can permeate many social policies and social interactions for the person with dementia (Oliver 1990). It is therefore not only the diagnosis of dementia that 'leads to lack of control and influence, but the attitude of others' (Parker and Penhale 1998, p. 203).

The discourses that surround dementia are complex, but a major shift in thinking has occurred over the past decade. Society is becoming more informed about dementia, and the importance of valuing people with dementia is being increasingly recognized within professional and family care domains. Dementia research is now addressing the psychosocial aspects of dementia, with the goal of increasing understanding of individuals' experience of the disease and their needs and preferences. The purpose of this chapter is to explore the implications of these developments for dementia care and the advancement of good practice. First, developments in the policy and social context of dementia care will be outlined to demonstrate how the perspectives of people with dementia have gained prominence. Second, selected studies that have involved people with dementia as active participants will be discussed. Third, barriers to involving people with dementia as active participants will be explored. Fourth, the challenges to researchers and practitioners when attempting to hear the voices of people with dementia will be examined by drawing on findings from a 2 year project (funded by the Community Fund) undertaken by the authors in partnership with the Oxford Dementia Centre and Anchor Trust. Finally, the implications for good practice will be considered.

THE POLICY CONTEXT

The increased attention paid to dementia can be located within the changing health and social care policy context, in particular that which relates to older people and community care (Cantley 2001a). Many of the recent policy reforms have direct relevance for those with dementia. Notions of consumerism, the empowerment of users, and individualized and responsive care have been promoted by a series of strategic and policy developments including *Caring for People* (Department of Health 1989), the NHS and Community Care Act 1990, the Royal Commission on Long Term Care (1999) and the *National Service Framework for Older People* (Department of Health 2001). Older people are no longer viewed as dependent on the welfare system but have become reframed as consumers and active participants of welfare. As Gilleard and Higgs (2000, p. 171) argue, 'Whenever possible, people's own choices are to shape the kinds of service they receive, not the paternalistic welfare state.' Within this context, the involvement of older people in choices and decision-making is therefore central. Less attention has, however, been paid specifically to promoting these concepts for people with dementia.

Ways of including individuals in the decision-making process have been identified (Killeen 2001). These can range from involvement in the development of services, in a representative and/or advocacy role, to having more control and influence as service recipients within their everyday lives. As many people with dementia are unaware of their diagnosis (Bartlett and Martin 2001a), the promotion of a collective voice for people with dementia has, however, its limitations. Furthermore, the diversity of voices of people with dementia needs to be recognized. Although an appropriate policy framework is essential, the challenge remains for practitioners and researchers to implement policy into practice and adopt inclusionary strategies.

DEVELOPMENTS IN DEMENTIA CARE

Dementia has been understood from a predominantly bio-medical perspective, but psychological and sociological models of dementia care are now also acknowledged (Bond 2001). The bio-medical view of dementia emphasized the disease and illness that was located within the individual. Those with dementia were objectified and denied the opportunity to be involved in decisions about their care (Clarke 1999). They were traditionally 'overlooked, ignored or assumed not to exist' (Parker and Penhale 1998, p. 203). Challenges to the medical discourses that previously surrounded a person with dementia (Harding and Palfrey 1997; Clarke 1999; Lyman 2000; Bond and Corner 2001) have opened up the possibility of involving people with dementia as active participants in their own care. In particular, Kitwood's psychosocial approach to dementia care has challenged previous assumptions that there is an erosion of the self and personality of individuals with dementia (Kitwood and Benson 1995; Kitwood 1997) and highlighted the importance of valuing their subjective experiences.

The social worlds of people with dementia were previously constructed and mediated via the views of care-givers and family members (Clarke 1999; Stalker et al. 1999). Now both practitioners and researchers increasingly aim to understand the perspectives of people with dementia. A tool for eliciting their perceptions, the dementia care mapping method, has been developed by Kitwood and Bredin (1994) as a means of assessing care standards. Its application has been favourably evaluated in practice (Williams and Rees 1997), although it has also been criticized both in terms of methodology and in relation to its reliability and validity (Adams 1996).

Whereas a greater emphasis on the individual sense of self, the rights of the person and valuing the perspectives of people with dementia has been noted (Downs 1997), the research nevertheless suggests that a more meaningful involvement of people with dementia in decisions and choices is possible (Adams 1999; Adams and Clarke 1999; Cantley 2001b; Wilkinson 2001a). To support this change, Cox et al. (1998) have developed a value framework to underpin dementia care that is based on the following five values:

1. Maximizing personal control
2. Respecting dignity
3. Enabling choice
4. Preserving continuity
5. Promoting equity.

The framework has been designed to demonstrate the centrality of those with dementia, their diverse and dynamic needs, and the differing perspectives within the care relationship.

Practitioners and service providers now increasingly aim to involve the person with dementia in the decision-making process. Researchers also seek to investigate the subjective perspectives of people with dementia and understand how they construct their social worlds. The various challenges faced when attempting to listen to the voices of people with dementia will be explored later, but first some of the insights from research that has involved people with dementia will be examined.

HEARING THE VOICES OF PEOPLE WITH DEMENTIA: INSIGHTS FROM RESEARCH

Until recently, social research into dementia focused almost exclusively on the needs of family and professional carers (Adams 1999). People with dementia are now, however, increasingly the focus of research that aims to understand not only how people with dementia construct and experience their own social worlds, but also how they mediate their way through the barriers and power relations within society (Wilkinson 2001b). Achieving this level of understanding inevitably requires direct engagement with the person with dementia, preferably using participatory methods, in which the person with dementia is actively involved in the research process.

Although there is a limited amount of empirical research in which people with dementia are involved, some important insights have been gained from recent studies (e.g., Gilles 1995; Goldsmith 1996; Gwyther 1997; Keady and Gilliard 1999; Bamford and Bruce 2000; Barnett 2000; Allan 2001; Wilkinson, 2001a). Key findings from a selected number of studies will now be summarized.

The importance of communication is highlighted by Goldsmith (1996), whose study involved interviews with service providers and people with dementia. Strategies to help health and social care professionals involve people with dementia in decisions concerning their care were identified. These included the development of diverse and effective communication skills, the recognition of verbal and non-verbal cues, group work, eliciting life stories and promoting an environment conducive to communication.

Keady and Gilliard (1999) undertook a study of people with an early diagnosis of dementia. The research showed how people with dementia used two interdependent strategies in order to cope with the inherent uncertainty of dementia, namely 'taking stock' and 'sharing the load'. The first strategy of 'taking stock' occurs when the person starts to become aware he or she has a problem. This can involve an intense and private process of adjusting to a new everyday reality, the development of a number of coping behaviours and the concealment of symptoms, for example through the use of lists and memory aids. In contrast, the strategy of 'sharing the load' is a process of unburdening in which those with dementia reveal their covert activities to a person close to them, who tends to be a family member rather than a health care professional. The work of Keady and Gilliard provides an important insight into how people with an early diagnosis of dementia construct their social worlds in the everyday context of uncertainty. Furthermore, the strategies developed by the participants suggested that they were aware of and responded to prevalent attitudes to dementia within society.

Barnett (2000) also sought to promote the participation of people with dementia in both research and decisions relating to their care. Of particular note to valuing the perspectives of people with dementia were the themes that emerged from the interviews of participants with dementia who either attended the day hospital or were residents in long-term care. Barnett was interested in the participants' own concerns, and she first explains the awareness of the participants – of themselves, of their memory loss, of their own situation and of important relationships. Other people were significant to their everyday lives, although the participants experienced this both positively and negatively. Many described further their own experiences of 'loss' and bereavement within their lives, in particular the loss of their home and of key relationships. Finally, the participants described their own subjective meanings associated with the experience of dependency. Although they recognized their dependence on others, the participants also spoke with concern and care about the people who cared for them, which, for Barnett, points to the interdependence of the care relationship. Moreover, Barnett suggests (2000, p. 129) that 'a new way of framing the care relationship, so that it is not about passive receipt but a two-way, mutual process' could be developed. Achieving this goal would certainly involve valuing the person with dementia as an active and important partner within the care relationship.

Ways in which staff can consult and promote the views and opinions of service users with dementia have been explored in a study conducted by Allan (2001). The research clearly shows the importance of diverse and individualized approaches to communication, through which important understandings and views can be elicited. Also highlighted was the value of promoting the staff's confidence and self-esteem, and of acknowledging the sophistication of their communication skills. As sustained and effective communication is emotionally demanding and consuming in terms of both time and energy, the support of staff was therefore a very significant issue for service providers. Although Allan promotes communication in the everyday worlds of service users with dementia, she also recognizes the tension that arises between individualized care and the everyday routines of organizations.

Identifying desired care outcomes from the perspective of the person with dementia has also been the focus of recent studies. Bamford and Bruce (2000), for example, consulted people with dementia and their carers about community care. A key outcome that they identified was maximizing a sense of autonomy. Their work highlights the limitations of relying solely on carers as proxy respondents. In another study, Gwyther (1997) identified a range of other outcomes relevant to people with dementia, including a sense of control, inclusion, reciprocity, meaningful activities, feeling safe and secure, maintaining self-esteem, and maximizing physical well-being through health care.

Although such studies are relatively few in number, they provide crucial insights into the experience of dementia and, importantly, illustrate the quality of the interactions that can be achieved between researcher and participant. Implicit in this is a focus on valuing people with dementia – their experiences and perspectives.

METHODOLOGICAL ISSUES

The term 'active participation' suggests a closer, honest and reciprocal relationship between researchers and participants. As a detached approach to the research relationship is increasingly being rejected, researchers now aim to involve participants in all aspects of the research process (de Laine 2000; *see also* Bartlett and Martin 2001a; Clarke and Keady 2001; Wilkinson 2001a, b). This promotion of active participation is an ethical stance in which researchers are explicit about their research goals, undertake a process of informed consent and respect the privacy of the respondents (de Laine 2000). It is further argued that participants may find the experience of participating in research to be empowering. Although research that involves people with dementia increasingly attempts to be participatory, it does not necessarily embrace the characteristics of emancipatory research (Wilkinson 2001b). Although both aim to be inclusive and democratic, and both question the power and expertise within the researcher–participant relationship, emancipatory research is part of a wider process in which the goal is the liberation of disabled people as active participants and citizens within society.

Involving people with dementia in the research process can be a considerable challenge for researchers. The issues are complex and there are no definitive guidelines, but a number of criteria can be formulated from the collective wisdom of researchers such as Bartlett and Martin (2001a, b), Bond and Corner (2001), Clarke and Keady (2001), Martin and Bartlett (2001) and Wilkinson (2001a, b):

1. Be creative and positive in the approach to data collection.
2. Allow people with dementia to articulate and express their own perspective and to ensure the data are trustworthy.
3. Develop rapport and mutual trust within the research relationship.
4. Allow plenty of time and ensure that an ongoing process of consent is maintained.
5. Be reflexive about the research process.
6. Pay attention to the research design, for example the use of multiple methods and/or maximizing engagement within the research relationship.
7. Be aware of verbal and non-verbal cues to ensure that the participant is not experiencing distress.
8. Value the person with dementia within the research relationship.

PRACTICE INSIGHTS FROM A STUDY OF EMPOWERMENT

A recent study completed by Bartlett and Martin will now be drawn upon to inform practice development. The purpose of this study was to explore how decisions are made for older people with dementia by focusing on these issues from the perspective of older people with dementia and their carers. The study was concerned with identifying the opportunities that exist for older people with dementia to be involved in how they live, the barriers to realizing these opportunities, and practices that can overcome these barriers. In particular, the aim was to examine how the rights and choices of people with dementia can be balanced with possible concerns that people have for their safety and well being. Comparisons were made between different care settings – residential homes, sheltered housing and the community. Eighteen case studies were completed, involving interviews with older people with dementia, participant observation, and focus groups with key staff and family members.

Involving participants in all aspects of the research process can be difficult to achieve, as this study found (Bartlett and Martin 2001a). In the process of negotiating access, multiple layers of protection surrounding the older person with dementia had to be penetrated. In addition to the usual requirement of ethics committee approval, a wide range of other gatekeepers, including senior and middle management, service providers, care staff and family members, were involved in giving permission to proceed with various stages of the study.

The process of obtaining informed consent required the active participation of the respondents. In this study, the question of competency obviously arose (Bartlett and Martin 2001a). Lack of competence to consent could not, however, be assumed just because the participants had a diagnosis of dementia. One participant had, for example, previously worked in a university and, when negotiating the process of informed consent, asked about funding, the key aims of the research and how the research would be written up. Although, because of her short-term memory loss, she needed on a return visit to be reminded about the purpose of the research, it was evident that she was active in the process of informed consent. A well-designed information sheet also assisted with this process. The process of informed consent is, therefore, ongoing rather than a single event.

Another issue in obtaining informed consent is whether or not individuals are aware of their diagnosis (Bartlett and Martin 2001a). When introducing the project, we used the term 'memory problems' rather than dementia for fear of causing undue distress and harm to the potential participant. True participation is therefore less likely when a participant may not be aware of the real focus of the study. At the same time, there is an ethical obligation for researchers not to cause harm. It was therefore necessary to balance the opposing notions of 'empowerment' – involving the older person with dementia in the decision-making process – and 'risk' – by being aware of potential harm and distress.

CHALLENGES TO PARTICIPATION IN PRACTICE

The partnership model of dementia care promotes the active participation of the person with dementia within the care relationship. This represents an ethical stance in which the voice of the person with dementia is valued. It is therefore important to develop practices that are inclusionary, attention being given to hearing the diverse and dynamic voices of people with dementia. Examples of inclusionary practice, and challenges to achieving this ideal, will be illustrated by extracts from interviews with older people with dementia, and focus groups with health and social care staff, that have been taken from the empowerment project.

The first illustration explores a participant's perspective on her case review when a decision was made for her to move from her own home to a nursing home. Christine was a 74-year-old retired shop owner who had recently been diagnosed with dementia. She had been a widow for many years and had lived in the same village for most of her life, where she had always been actively involved in community activities. She had one married daughter who lived nearby. The interview took place in a hospital setting 1 week after her case review.

Christine had found the case review meeting especially difficult and upsetting. Despite being articulate and able to express her views effectively, she felt that her voice had not been heard. First, she described the reason why a decision had been made for her to move into a nursing home: 'They said I was not fit to be left all night, I couldn't be left, I suppose that is it.' At the same time, she questioned the reasons given for moving accommodation: 'I was diagnosed as short term memory – short term memory and that was one of those things, but I didn't think it was enough – just short term memory but apparently it was ... I was able to manage up to then.'

Although Christine was included in the case review meeting, she felt that she had not been prepared. Her own view had not been represented, she had been disempowered by the number of staff present, and she had not felt involved in the decision-making process. Although her family members were present, she had not realized the difficulty they were finding in taking care of her. The following extract describes her experience of the case review meeting:

> People I had never seen before. I suppose it was quite fairly done but I didn't think it was. I know the doctor was on my side because he said he wanted to thank me for being so brave about it all. But I wasn't brave, but I just didn't say anything because I didn't know what was going to happen.

Christine clearly felt unable to voice her opinion at the meeting and felt that she had not been able actively to participate in a key decision about her future.

The second illustration involves a 69-year-old widow called Sue who lived in a residential home and details the extent to which she felt involved in decisions related to participating in organized activities. Sue first described how she enjoys participating in organized activities:

> *Interviewer*: I saw you doing some gardening a couple of weeks ago.
> *Sue*: Oh, I like doing that.
> *Interviewer*: You like doing that?
> *Sue*: Well yes, I have always done it.

Sue's enjoyment of gardening and her involvement in other activities organized by the residential home did not mean, however, that she wished to participate in all the activities:

> *Interviewer*: Do you like art as well?
> *Sue*: No, I don't really. But they are making me come and do it now.
> *Interviewer*: They make you do it?
> *Sue*: Well, they come and ask me and I can't say no.

Despite being consulted on making a decision regarding her everyday life, Sue felt unable to voice her opinion and found it difficult to say 'no' within the social context of the residential home.

In the study, health and social care staff, family members and older people were interviewed in focus groups and were asked how people with dementia participated in decision-making, as well as being asked to describe possible barriers to their involvement. The staff raised a number of issues, highlighting circumstances that made it difficult to involve people with dementia. A key theme identified was the tension between ideal and reality when involving older people with dementia in decisions about their care and everyday life. The interviews included the use of prompt cards covering key decision-making areas (Brown and Benson 1997) such as 'Eating food you like', 'Choosing how you spend the day' and 'Having someone to represent your interests when important decisions are made about your life'. Of particular interest was the discussion about the interview prompt card 'Having people talk over your head as though you are not there'. Some responses by staff to this prompt were as follows:

> Not intentionally, we don't do it on purpose but . . . you are discussing something, so you tend to get on and talk, and then forget that the resident is listening.
> I think one of the things that make it difficult is because of how mentally impaired our residents are. So that just in an ordinary personal everyday way . . . when you are setting out your work, it can be quite lonely if you are

working with somebody that you can't actually speak to about anything social, ... but you always try to focus it through this other person, but they are not always able to join in.

Well, because they take longer to give out what they want to say sometimes you feel there isn't time to spare, and so sometimes you can have a conversation that doesn't include them. So it does happen. It shouldn't but it does.

Although the staff were aware of good practice and of the importance of involving older people with dementia in decision-making, there were significant barriers to achieving these goals. The barriers included staff shortages, daily communication patterns between staff, the routines of institutional life, lack of time and the emotional stress of communicating with and involving older people with dementia. The working environment and staff practices can in such ways affect the extent to which older people are actively involved in decision-making. It is therefore important to recognize the barriers to good practice. In this way, the gap between research and practice, between ideal and reality, can be reduced and the quality of life of older people with dementia promoted.

CONCLUSION

The way in which people with dementia are considered and the care they receive have undergone significant change. The work of Kitwood and others has had a major influence on promoting person-centred care, and social research has empha- sized the importance of valuing the person with dementia as a participant in the research process. New insights into the capacity of people with dementia to engage in decision-making have been revealed, and some progress in practice development has been documented. Nevertheless, further education and support, in particular the translation of theory into practice, are still needed for practi- tioners and the carers of people with dementia. Good practice can be built only if there is an understanding of the individual's rights, of how to balance empower- ment and individual risk, of the importance of gaining appropriate consent and of assessing competence in everyday situations.

A number of good practice principles that promote valuing people with dementia can be formulated from both the research literature and recent practice developments:

- Understand the stages of dementia and the nature of the social worlds of people with dementia.
- Acknowledge that people with dementia have their own perceptions of self, memory loss and ageing.
- Promote the rights of the individual person with dementia.
- Recognize individual diversity, and don't assume that everyone is the same.

- Seek to locate individuals within the context of their life history and become familiar with their life interests and skills through biographies.
- Focus on the strengths that people with dementia still have rather than on their losses and dependency.
- Foster communication through group work, life stories and a conducive environment.

- See all forms of behaviour, including verbal and non-verbal cues, as communication.
- Encourage people with dementia to articulate and express their own perspectives.
- Allow sufficient time for effective interactions.
- Balance the pursuit of empowerment and the avoidance of risk-taking with the needs and desires of the person with dementia.

Several key points for managers can also be identified:

- Develop strategies that promote the involvement of people with dementia in decision-making and choices about their services, their care and their everyday lives.
- Consider how staff can be supported to promote communication with people with dementia.
- Develop a value framework for care and service provision that promotes the involvement of people with dementia.
- Be aware of barriers to involving people with dementia in decision-making and choices.

- Provide ongoing education and training for staff on how to value people with dementia.
- Balance the tensions between individualized care and the organization of institutional life, as well as between 'risk' and 'empowerment'.
- Be familiar with the research evidence to inform practice.
- Value the person with dementia within the partnership of care.

REFERENCES

Adams, T. 1996: Kitwood's approach to dementia and dementia care: a critical but appreciative review. *Journal of Advanced Nursing* **23:** 948–52.

Adams, T. 1999: *Recent developments in dementia care. Nursing Times Clinical Monographs no. 33.* London: Nursing Times Books.

Adams, T. and Clarke, C. eds. 1999: *Dementia care: developing partnerships in practice.* London: Baillière Tindall.

Allan, K. 2001: *Communication and consultation: exploring ways for staff to involve people with dementia in developing services.* Bristol: Policy Press.

Bamford, C. and Bruce, E. 2000: Defining the outcomes of community care: the perspectives of older people with dementia and their carers. *Ageing and Society* **20:** 543–70.

Barnett, E. 2000: *Including the person with dementia in designing and delivering care.* London: Jessica Kingsley.

Bartlett, H. and Martin, W. 2000: A balancing act. *Guardian Society*, 6 September, p. 127.

Bartlett, H. and Martin, W. 2001a: Ethical issues in dementia research. In: Wilkinson, H. ed. *The perspectives of people with dementia: research methods and motivations.* London: Jessica Kingsley, 47–62.

Bartlett, H. and Martin, W. 2001b: Decision-making and older people with dementia: findings from a UK study in sheltered housing and residential care settings. *Australasian Journal on Ageing* **20** (suppl. 1): 38.

Bond, J. 2001: Sociological perspectives. In: Cantley, C. ed. *A handbook of dementia care.* Buckingham: Open University Press, 44–61.

Bond, J. and Corner, L. 2001: Researching dementia: are there unique methodological challenges for health services research? *Ageing and Society* **21:** 95–116.

Brown, S. and Benson, S. 1997: *Quality lifestyles for older people with dementia: training workshops for staff based on the principle of normalisation.* Brighton: Pavilion.

Cantley, C. 2001a: Understanding the policy context. In: Cantley, C. ed. *A handbook of dementia care.* Buckingham: Open University Press, 220–239.

Cantley, C. ed. 2001b: *A handbook of dementia care.* Buckingham: Open University Press.

Clarke, C. 1999: Dementia care partnerships: knowledge, ownership and exchange. In: Adams, T. and Clarke, C. eds. *Dementia care. Developing partnerships in practice.* London: Baillière Tindall, 5–36.

Clarke, C. and Keady, J. 2001: Getting down to brass tacks: a discussion of data collection. In: Wilkinson, H. ed. *The perspectives of people with dementia: research methods and motivations.* London: Jessica Kingsley, 25–46.

Cox, S., Anderson, I., Dick, S. and Elgar, J. 1998: *The person, the community and dementia. Developing a value framework.* Stirling: Dementia Services Development Centre.

de Laine, M. 2000: *Fieldwork, participation and practice. Ethics and dilemmas in qualitative research.* London: Sage.

Department of Health. 1989: *Caring for people. Community care in the next decade and beyond.* London: HMSO. Cm 849.

Department of Health. 1990: *National Health Service and Community Care Act 1990.* London: HMSO.

Department of Health. 2001: *The national service framework for older people.* London: Stationery Office.

Downs, M. 1997: The emergence of the person in dementia research. *Ageing and Society* **17:** 597–607.

Gilleard, C. and Higgs, P. 2000: *Cultures of ageing. Self, citizen and the body.* Harlow: Pearson Education.

Gilles, B. 1995: *The subjective experience of dementia: a qualitative analysis of interviews with dementia sufferers and their carers and the implications for service provision.* Stirling: Dementia Services Development Centre.

Goldsmith, M. 1996: *Hearing the voice of people with dementia: opportunities and obstacles.* London: Jessica Kingsley.

Gwyther, L. 1997: The perspective of the person with Alzheimer disease: which outcomes matter in early to middle stages of dementia? *Alzheimer Disease and Related Disorders* **11** (suppl. 6): 18–24.

Harding, N. and Palfrey, C. 1997: *The social construction of dementia: confused professionals?* London: Jessica Kingsley.

Keady, J. and Gilliard, J. 1999: The early experience of Alzheimer's disease: implications for partnership and practice. In: Adams, T. and Clarke, C. eds. *Dementia care. Developing partnerships in practice*. London: Baillière Tindall, 227–56.

Killeen, J. 2001: Involving people with dementia and their carers in developing services. In: Cantley, C. ed. *A handbook of dementia care*. Buckingham: Open University Press, 278–94.

Kitwood, T. 1997: *Dementia reconsidered. The person comes first*. Buckingham: Open University Press.

Kitwood, T. and Benson, S. eds. 1995: *The new culture of dementia care*. London: Hawker Publications.

Kitwood, T. and Bredin, K. 1994: *Evaluating dementia care: the DCM method*. Bradford: Bradford Dementia Research Group.

Lyman, K. 2000: Bringing the social back: A critique of the biomedicalization of dementia. In: Gubrium, J.F. and Holstein, J.A. eds. *Aging and Everyday Life*. Oxford: Blackwell, 340–56.

Martin, W. and Bartlett, H. 2001: Empowerment: theory and practice in dementia research. In: Gubrium, J. and Holstein, J. eds. *Quality in later life: rights, rhetoric and reality. Conference Proceedings. British Society of Gerontology. August–September 2001*. Stirling, University of Stirling, 158–9.

Oliver, M. 1990: *The politics of disablement*. London: Macmillan.

Parker, J. and Penhale, B. 1998: *Forgotten people: positive approaches to dementia care*. Aldershot: Ashgate Publishing.

Royal Commission on Long Term Care 1999: *With respect to old age: long term care – rights and responsibilities*. London: Stationery Office.

Stalker, K., Gilliard, J. and Downs, M. 1999: Eliciting user perspectives on what works. *International Journal of Geriatric Psychiatry* **14**: 120–34.

Wilkinson, H. ed. 2001a: *The perspectives of people with dementia: research methods and motivations*. London: Jessica Kingsley.

Wilkinson, H. 2001b: Including people with dementia in research: methods and motivations. In Wilkinson, H. ed. *The perspectives of people with dementia: research methods and motivations*. London: Jessica Kingsley, 9–24.

Williams, J. and Rees, J. 1997: The use of 'dementia care mapping' as a method of evaluating care received by patients with dementia – an initiative to improve quality of life. *Journal of Advanced Nursing* **25**: 316–23.

Policy and practice in dementia care

Jill Manthorpe and Trevor Adams

A chapter on policy needs to be selective so this chapter will focus on three themes. It presents a chronology of policy at national level, placing reports and legislation in a time line (Box 3.1), but policy debates have been grouped around three key themes:

1. The place of people with dementia
2. Dementia and decision-making
3. Dementia at the frontier.

These themes have been chosen because they allow a study of dementia in contexts broader than simply those of health and social care delivery. Other chapters in this book also touch on policy since the way in which services are thought about and systems are organized relates to the implementation of policy at local or agency level. Policy in welfare is also strongly influenced by organizational control over what is translated into local service delivery. In dementia care, professional groups have played an important part in developing service responses, to which was added the organized voice of families during the 1980s. Similarly, at the turn of the century, there is some evidence that people with dementia are themselves beginning to influence the policy process.

At the time of writing, two important areas are emerging, which will be briefly considered. These are a growing appreciation of the need to take into account national and regional variations in the UK (*see* Payne and Shardlow 2002 for a discussion of social work in the British Isles) and an exploration of policy at European level (*see* Warner et al. 2002). Both of these need to be set in the context of global initiatives such as the new International Plan of Action on Ageing

Box 3.1 A chronology of policy

1946	Foundation of the National Health Service
1947	*Old People*: Report of a Committee of Enquiry established by the Nuffield Foundation (Chair: Seebohm Rowntree)
1948	National Assistance Act
1959	Mental Health Act
1962	The Hospital Plan
1967	Publication of *Sans Everything* (Robb, 1967)
1975	White Paper *Better Services for the Mentally Ill*
1979	Foundation of the Alzheimer's Disease Society (now the Alzheimer's Society), which currently covers England, Wales and Northern Ireland
1979	Green (Consultative) Paper *A Happier Old Age*
1983	The *Rising Tide* report (Health Advisory Service) and the Mental Health Act 1983
1984	Alzheimer's Disease International founded (in the USA)
1985	Mental Health Act (Scotland)
1988	Sharpen Report (Scottish health priorities for the 1980s and 90s); first dementia services development centre established, in Stirling
1989	White Papers *Caring for People: Community Care in the Next Decade and Beyond* and *Working for Patients*
1990	National Health Service and Community Care Act 1990
1993	Final implementation of the National Health Service Community Care Act
1994	Alzheimer's Scotland – Action on Dementia launched; merger of Scottish Action on Dementia/Alzheimer's Society in Scotland
1995	Carers (Representation and Services) Act
1997	*Who Decides? Making Decisions on Behalf of Mentally Incapacitated Adults* (Lord Chancellor's Department 1997)
1999	Report of the Royal Commission on Long Term Care of the Elderly (Chair: Sir Stewart Sutherland); *Caring for the Carers: National Strategy for Carers* (HM Government)
2000	National Service Framework for Mental Health (Department of Health)
2001	Adults with Incapacity (Scotland) Act; NHS Plan; Adults with Incapacity Act (Scotland); National Service Framework for Older People (Department of Health)
2002	Care Standards Act; Health and Community Care (Scotland) Act

following the second World Assembly on Ageing, held in Madrid in 2002. Thinking about policy and dementia calls for links to be made between family and local experiences, and the broader global scene. Dementia policy-making occurs at various levels, and multidisciplinary responses to dementia need to engage with more than the usual welfare 'suspects'. As this chapter shows, dementia care practitioners need to understand and communicate with lawyers, ethicists, scientists

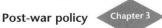

and voluntary and pressure groups, as well as to forge alliances with others working in disability services and provision for older people. The chapter starts with a consideration of 'place' and dementia, arguing that notions of where dementia is situated have formed a long debate within welfare and beyond.

POST-WAR POLICY

This first section explores policy developments in the UK, starting with the period after the Second World War. This is not to say that many of the responses to people with dementia, as with other groups of disabled people, did not have their origin in earlier periods. The watershed of the Second World War provides, however, an opportunity to focus on the welfare state since much of its formative legislation and service structures have proved remarkably resilient.

Dalley (1998) has usefully elaborated on the 1947 Committee of Enquiry, chaired by Seebohm Rowntree and established by the Rowntree Foundation, on the needs of older people. In this, 'senile dements' were seen as being appropriately placed in 'special institutions', large asylums, whereas those who were classed as 'slightly senile' could be transferred from home to a public assistance institution or work-house if they started 'annoying other people' (Dalley 1998, pp. 2–3). As with many older people in poor health or poor circumstances, the embryonic welfare state struggled to find places for those with chronic health conditions, and public assistance institutions were regarded as providing 'little more than food and shelter in a near-Dickensian environment' (Foot 1973, p.108).

The 1950s, as analysed by Means and Smith (1998), were a period during which debates about older people who were mentally 'infirm' centred around the (in)appropriateness of mental hospitals as a location for their care or treatment. Means and Smith note that 'infirmity' was a broad concept employed to cover dementia, other mental health problems and physical disabilities, and even being 'awkward'. Discussion ranged around whether older people in such circumstances should be the responsibility of local authorities rather than the National Health Service (NHS), in particularly that of long-stay psychiatric hospitals. As might be expected, this was not because older people might benefit from local authority care, although it was accepted that the stigma of certification under the Lunacy Acts was ill received by many families. Instead, hospital services were to be freed from any responsibility to care for 'chronic sick' older patients to concentrate on 'cure', treatment and higher-status work. Older patients who were mentally infirm could, it was argued, be adequately cared for in hostels and residential homes.

As Means and Smith (1998) demonstrate, however, 'care of the senile' was never satisfactorily classified as either a health or a welfare authority responsibility. Health authorities were to be responsible for those 'senile confused' who were 'unfit to live a normal community life in a welfare home' (p. 184). Distinctions between the 'senile' and 'senile confused' were inevitably imprecise. During the 1960s, a small number of specialist residential homes for the elderly confused were opened, and it is possible to see these as a pragmatic attempt to bridge the service gap created by the twin edifices of NHS and local authority post-war provision. An absence of nursing homes (left out in the creation of the welfare state) in particular may account for this effort to provide an institutional response for those 'misplaced' in residential or hospital provision. Whether residential provision for people with dementia should be segregated or specialist is an example of a matter that continues to receive mixed policy messages (Norman 1987; Marshall and Archibald 1998).

It was not, however, only those with dementia who were seen as being wrongly placed. Much criticism in the 1960s related to the 'dumping' of older people into mental hospitals. As one editorial in a nursing magazine (*Nursing Times*, quoted in Robb 1967, p.10) reported:

> A very great number of elderly people sit waiting for death in mental hospitals where they have no place to be. .... We cannot dodge the accusation that we, as an advanced and civilized country are treating a very great number of our old people in a manner that is far worse than barbarous.

Such opinion was built upon evidence supplied mainly by doctors, whose debates made much of the fact that older people with mental infirmity, as well as those without, were misplaced in hospital wards (Robb 1967).

What is important from this focus upon hospitals and their patients is the concentration on care in an institutional setting and the fact that there is little recognition of the support provided by the families of older members. Largely hidden from professional debates and often classified as bedridden or infirm, most people with possible dementia were supported by their families. For some, with financial resources, alternatives to their families or the care of the local authority were provided by small private residential and nursing homes, but again we know little of this apart from some interesting later observations from novelists such as Bailey (1967) and Taylor (1971).

Historians such as Thane (1998) have illuminated the role of social surveys from the post-war period in presenting views of older people in the context of family life. As she reports, Townsend (1957) observed, through an examination of the records of a geriatric hospital and of London County Council Homes, that older people who were accommodated in such services were very unrepresentative and appeared to be characterized by living alone and being childless, particularly lacking a daughter. Although such surveys do not identify those with dementia as a distinct group, references to mental infirmity and those needing nursing care from relatives suggest that a hidden population of people with dementia existed and only rarely came to the attention of services. Sheldon's study (1948), for example, of older people in Wolverhampton, noted some families in which high levels of care were provided by daughters, often combining work and caring in 'almost a slave' routine (Thane 1998, p.184).

The placing of dementia within policy contexts therefore touches upon many areas of community care and services for older people in particular. The discovery of caring within informal family networks that emerged during the 1980s continues a theme observed by Sheldon and others that the care and support of older people were generally the responsibility of families rather than professionals. Family policy is as much central to dementia care as are service and professional boundaries and responsibilities.

The discovery of carers drew on many accounts – mainly by women – about the work involved in providing care to a sick or disabled relative. Most such accounts were grouped together to provide a testament of women's experiences as daughters and wives. Some were incorporated within feminist literature, and it takes a detailed reading to see that some of the early experiences described probably relate to the care of people with dementia. Carpenter (1985), for example, discussing her life, mentions her home help work for a retired doctor who was later found 'wandering' and who had to be taken into a geriatric hospital. At the same time, she was looking after her father-in-law, who needed nursing and supervision: 'He was senile and very difficult, and had turned into a horrible man' (1985, p. 44).

Accounts such as these both fuelled demands for social and health care services to be more responsive to the needs of families and stimulated self-help groups for families caring for people with a variety of conditions. In relation to dementia, the Alzheimer's Disease Society (now the Alzheimer's Society), founded in 1980, was explicitly designed to operate as a pressure group or campaigning body, as well as an association of relatives providing each other with support and information.

Family policy is an area that allows a discussion of dementia in a context wider than just health and social care services. Much of the early work on informal care, for example, drew on debates over the lack of social recognition of informal care as work and the impact of caring on women's current and future incomes (Equal Opportunities Commission 1982). These critiques included campaigns against discriminatory social security provision that initially failed to acknowledge the caring work of 'housewives' and the continued lack of financial recognition of older carers, many of whom were involved in the care of spouses with dementia (Milne et al. 2001).

The place of people with dementia within policy thus brings together a number of strands of formal and informal support. What is thought of as care in the community, as summarized by the White Paper *Caring for People: Community Care for the Next Decade and Beyond* (Department of Health 1989), has its roots in family care as a norm of behaviour. These rest upon feelings related to the obligations and transfers between spouses and between parents and their children. Only in a minority of instances do older people with dementia enter full-time care, and then, as the recent debates surrounding payment for long-term care have illustrated, many of them pay for this support (Sutherland 1999). In the 1990s, the movement of older people with dementia, many classed as 'psychogeriatrics', from NHS hospital care to private sector nursing homes and residential homes continued a process of finding the right 'place' for people with dementia.

Finally, it is worth observing that this focus on 'place' usefully draws attention to the interface between social and health care, and housing policy and provision. Housing has generally been viewed as an afterthought in debates about community care, related housing policy concentrating on adaptations to the environment for people with physical disabilities. Recent attention to housing issues suggests the value of understanding how a convenient, comfortable and warm home, in good repair, can contribute to the support of those with dementia. McClatchey et al. (2001), for example, have tried to bridge the gap between those working in schemes providing repair and improvement services to older people and those working in dementia services. Their research found that the implications of dementia for housing often went unrecognized by housing workers, but, similarly, dementia services often failed to realize that housing improvements could be funded, arranged and supervised by housing support staff. The growth in owner-occupied housing among older people and policy objectives that people should age in place for as long as possible, rather than entering long-stay care or leaving their supportive networks, makes this link between housing and social and health personnel highly pertinent.

DEMENTIA AND DECISION-MAKING

This section discusses dementia and decision-making, placing some of the policy debates in a more individualized context. It makes more of the link between dementia and mental health policy, and the way in which dementia is sometimes seen as part of systems that relate to mental incapacity. Indeed, some of the calls for a change in the law relating to decisions made by those with mental incapacity explicitly cite the growing number of people with dementia as a reason for a change in laws that were established some time ago. Elderly people with dementia suffer a progressive loss of mental capacity, so that an increasing number of decisions about their personal care, health care and finances inevitably fall to be made by others (Law Commission 1995, p. 21).

Dementia does not, however, involve only legal decisions over civil liberties and property ownership, although these raise a number of ethical issues. The law relating to decision-making relates to daily behaviour and the rights and risks of people who are adults but whose adult status is seen to be compromised. Decision-making therefore often has much to do with risk.

Individuals with dementia are one of a number of groups for whom mental health policy has evolved to provide some form of protection, as well as some form of control. Protection is usually seen as a response to people's growing inability to provide care for themselves, perhaps through self-neglect. In the early days of the welfare state, public health measures that existed in some areas before the Second World War were brought under the umbrella of the National Assistance Act 1948 (section 48). These permitted the compulsory removal of people from their own homes if they were aged, infirm or unable to care for themselves and living in, for example, insanitary conditions. Such powers were rarely used, but they provided a form of control over people who might be causing concern to neighbours, family or services but who did not appear to be suffering from mental illness. Although this legislation might not have entailed the stigma of lunacy, it had very limited appeal mechanisms and increasingly became seen as a symbol of the ways in which legal powers could take away rather than protect the rights of people with dementia or similar conditions (Age Concern England 1985).

Decision-making involves a consideration of the workings of mental health legislation, and in England and Wales many of the calls for a reform of mental health law have had little to do with the legal problems encountered by people with dementia and those supporting them. Recent reform agendas have instead focused on community treatment for people with psychotic illness against a background of concern over homicides committed by those who have been under the care and treatment of the mental services (Stanley and Manthorpe 2001). Older people with dementia have largely been excluded from this debate, although it will be important to consider whether new legislation might help to provide a better framework for decisions that may currently be taken informally and without any input from a person with dementia and his or her advocate. For those with dementia, although there are plans to change the law on mental incapacity in England and Wales, reform recently occurred in Scotland with the passing of the Adults with Incapacity Act 2000. It will be important for this to be evaluated so those lessons can be learned and applied elsewhere.

Much of the debate surrounding mental capacity reform draws for its examples on decisions relating to money or property. In England and Wales, the current systems of enduring power of attorney and the Public Trust Office provide some structure for decision-making. The former permits people to plan for the future by nominating a person or people to act on their behalf should they become mentally incapacitated, but this covers only the area of finance and resources. The second system has its roots in protecting the resources of individuals with mental incapacity, and there have been many debates over the extent to which such a system fully meets the best interests of the person with dementia in terms of care and living arrangements.

One way of thinking about such systems is to explore the ways in which they encourage people to be involved in their own care and decisions about the future.

This is not to say that elements of protection may not be necessary (*see* Chapter 15). Charters of rights for people with dementia are one way of outlining what might be good practice in this area; the King's Fund Centre (1986) developed an early version of these that has stood the test of time (Box 3.2).

These principles draw on philosophies of normalization that have been influential in community care services and attitudes to disability (Malin et al. 1999). These might today be joined by the language of social inclusion, but the values they espouse may well be ones with which people in services would agree and, more importantly, may accord with the desires of those with dementia themselves (Litherland and Robson 2001). The charter of principles for the care of people with dementia and their carers developed by Alzheimer's Disease International, the umbrella organization for national Alzheimer's associations, provides a similar set of demands (Box 3.3) but, interestingly, combines the rights of people with dementia with those of their carers.

The Alzheimer's Disease International principles present a picture of family care in which the interests of those with dementia and their carers are indivisible and coincide. In the UK context, this perspective has been criticized, notably from the viewpoint of the disabled people's movement. It has argued that people with disability need support more than they do care and that a disabling environment adds to the difficulties of individuals with mental health or physical health problems. The influence of the disability movement has so far been limited in the area of dementia politics and service philosophies. As Barnes (1996) has observed, user groups of people with mental health problems of whatever form face particular

Box 3.2 The five principles of care (King's Fund 1986)

1.	People with dementia have the same human value as anyone else irrespective of their degree of disability or dependence
2.	People with dementia have the same varied human needs as anyone else
3.	People with dementia have the same rights as other citizens
4.	Every person with dementia is an individual
5.	People with dementia have the right to forms of support which don't exploit family and friends

Box 3.3 Summary of Alzheimer's Disease International (1999) *Charter of Principles*

1.	Dementia has a profound impact on those affected and their families
2.	A person with dementia has dignity, worth and deserves respect
3.	People with dementia need a safe environment and protection from abuse
4.	People with dementia need information and services
5.	People with dementia should be involved in decisions
6.	Family carers should have their needs recognized
7.	Resources should be available to meet the needs of people with dementia and their carers
8.	Those supporting people with dementia need information, education and training

problems in presenting their own cause because they are seen to lack insight. Added to this, the difficulties of many old people in terms of making their voice heard may help to explain why organizations of people with dementia have been hard to start and sustain.

At the level of individual decision-making, we are also beginning to see how a diagnosis of a dementia can reduce people's autonomy as those around them become overcautious and overprotective. Goldsmith has, for example, used the phrase the 'doctor's dilemma'(1999, p. 82), but it might also be a dilemma for other practitioners and family members when sharing the diagnosis of a dementia with the individual concerned. Although organizations such as the Alzheimer's Society (Cayton 1995) argue that diagnosis-sharing is a right, there are many who see this approach as difficult if it places the individual in a position of despair, or if the family disagree that sharing the diagnosis is in the person's best interests. Whereas such decisions about informing people of their diagnosis may appear to be a matter for medical practitioners, it is clear from other contributions to this book that many professionals have to work with the realization of a dementia among the people they support on a regular basis.

Early diagnosis can also reveal some of the gaps in the legal and policy context for those with dementia as legal and financial planning are still complex and incomplete systems of support. Although it might be possible to make some choices on future care, this does not guarantee that good-quality care is available or affordable. Social services support is, for example, rationed and discriminates against older people in both overt and covert forms (Help the Aged 2002). A care package that might support a person with dementia may be seen as too expensive for an older person with dementia, whereas it might be funded for a younger person. Similarly, older people with dementia, like other disabled adults using social care services, will be charged for these.

Making decisions as a result of receiving an early diagnosis of dementia thus reveals many of the limits on choice and empowerment. In the conclusion to this chapter, we focus on future challenges for policy-makers and those practitioners who implement, interpret and translate policy into human services.

DEMENTIA AT THE FRONTIER

The publication of the NHS Framework for Older People (Department of Health 2001) set a new 10 year plan for service development in the NHS and social care services. Standard 7 outlines aspirations for mental health services (interestingly, older people's mental health was not included in the framework on mental health). This standard suggests that social services commissioning care should require providers to ensure that their staff can recognize mental health problems and make timely and appropriate referrals. Specialist mental health teams are proposed, and these should link with colleagues in primary care. Training for work with older people from different cultures should be provided. Such policies, now grouped under the title of a service standard, should also link with other elements of the framework, notably its tacit admission that care for older people generally has often been discriminatory and of low quality.

The general insistence on person-centred care is one way in which developments in dementia care have apparently begun to influence broader services for all older people, and it is this aspect of policy and practice that we will use to conclude this chapter. 'Person-centred care' (standard 2 of the National Service Framework) may seem a familiar term to those working in dementia support. It has provided a value base for practitioners working in dementia care and unites almost every professional group in every professional setting. To see it translated into a mission statement for all older people's services can, to a degree, be welcomed. The problem lies, however, in the plasticity of the term – almost anyone can be the person, the older person or the carer. The term is also highly individualized and leaves out many of the wider policy problems associated with dementia, for example the unequal distribution of resources between people with dementia and other groups, and the reasons why dementia appears to be related to socio-economic status. Equally, the position of the balance between the needs of people with dementia and those of their families may have to be considered in the context of resource shortages rather than as a attempt to improve the behaviour of undervalued staff working in difficult conditions.

Person-centred care needs to be set in a resource context. As Marshall and Archibald (1998) have argued, one of the characteristics of long-stay care for people with dementia has been the cost-shunting of responsibility between different parts of the welfare state and different levels of government. Dementia is one area in which the cost has been borne largely by people with dementia themselves or their families. Such issues do not sit comfortably with notions of person-centred care unless we are to see this as confirming an individualized response to the problem of supporting people with dementia. Many of the early discussions of dementia tried to provoke action and research by stressing the 'demographic time-bomb' (Robertson 1991) or the 'rising tide' of older people with mental health problems and all that this would entail in terms of resource pressures (Health Advisory Service 1983). In a context of increasingly individualized responsibility for care, 'person-centred care' may suggest that people with dementia operate as individuals and should be responsible for their own support, their family acting as proxy consumers in the care market or in the choice of medication and therapy.

New developments in terms of gene therapy and medication advance have as yet had little impact on the world of support for people with dementia. Hard choices will, however, have to be made at the level of teams and primary care trusts making decisions on the balance of expenditure between medication and care. In a context of evidence-based practice, it may be difficult to argue against medication that provides some hope, and people with dementia and their carers may well see this as an appropriate use of resources. So far, although we have begun to consult with people about care services and aspects of community care delivery, we have less information on where people with dementia would set their priorities. The pharmaceutical industry will no doubt be keen to argue that medication deserves priority in terms of development. Few of us working in support services for people with dementia encounter the influence of this industry, although a general look at the advertisements of the trade press will illustrate its power.

That is not to say that those in social and health care support services are either inevitably against mediation or that dementia support needs to take more than its fair share of resources. Although those working within dementia support inevitably focus on the condition, many are well aware that the overall number involved is small, although people may be severely disabled by the syndrome, and many will be affected for several years. One of the difficulties in arguing the cause of dementia is the tendency that, to make its claims legitimate, it is necessary to refer to a large number and to the economic burden of the condition.

This chapter has argued that policy in relation to dementia is as complex as the condition itself. There are many layers of policy relevant to the support of those with dementia and many interests operating at the level of support. One of the challenges for those working in a multidisciplinary context, whether in the dementia teams proposed by the National Service Framework, or in primary care, social care or other service environments, will be to look beyond narrow health and social care confines. Although organizational turbulence does not always make this an easy task, one of the policy challenges for the twenty-first century in dementia support will be listening to the views and experiences of those with dementia related to what structures and systems they desire, and setting these in the context of citizenship for all older people, other people with mental health problems and disabled people generally. All these groups have much to contribute to our understanding of which policy responses work and which do not. It will also be important for those in dementia circles to offer ideas to policy debates instead of simply reacting to others' agendas.

REFERENCES

Age Concern England. 1985: *The law and vulnerable elderly people*. Mitcham: Age Concern England.

Alzheimer's Disease International. 1999: *Charter of principles*. London: ADI.

Bailey, P. 1967 *At the Jerusalem*. London: Jonathan Cape.

Barnes, C. 1996: Institutional discrimination against disabled people and the campaign for anti-discrimination legislation. In: Taylor, D. ed. *Critical social policy, a reader*. London: Sage, 95–112.

Carpenter, V. 1985: Looking after three generations. In Hemmings, S. ed. *A wealth of experience: the lives of older women*. London: Pandora, 41–52.

Cayton, H. 1995: Diagnostic testing: who wants to know? *Journal of Dementia Care* **3**: 12–13.

Dalley, G. 1998: Changing attitudes, practice and numbers: 50 years of improving the lives of an increasingly ageing population. In: Centre for Policy on Ageing *Dementia in focus: research, care and policy into the 21st century*. London: CPA, 1–6.

Department of Health. 1989: *Caring for people: community care in the next decade and beyond.* London: HMSO. Cm 849.

Department of Health. 2001: *National service framework for older people.* London: Stationery Office.

Equal Opportunities Commission. 1982: *Caring for the elderly and handicapped: community care policy and women's lives.* Manchester: EOC.

Foot, M. 1973: *Aneurin Bevan: a biography*, volume 2, *1945–1960*. London: Davis-Poynter.

Goldsmith, M. 1999: Ethical dilemmas in dementia care. In: Adams, T. and Clarke, C. eds. *Dementia care: developing partnerships in practice*. London: Baillière Tindall, 79–94.

Health Advisory Service. 1983: *The rising tide*. Sutton: HAS.

Help the Aged. 2002: Age discrimination. In: *Public policy: a review of the evidence*. London: Help the Aged, 40.

King's Fund Centre. 1986: *Living well into old age*. Project Paper no. 23. London: King's Fund Centre.

Law Commission. 1995: *Mental incapacity. Report of the Law Commission*, no. 231. London: HMSO.

Litherland, R. and Robson, P. 2001: Involving people with dementia in service development and organisational change. Paper presented to the 7th Researching the Voluntary Sector Conference, 5 September, NCVO, London.

McClatchey, T., Means, R. and Morbey, H. 2001: *Housing adaptations and improvements for people with dementia*. Bristol: University of the West of England.

Malin, N., Manthorpe, J., Race, D. and Wilmot, S. 1999: *Community care for nurses and the caring professions*. Buckingham: Open University Press.

Marshall, M. and Archibald, C. 1998: Long-stay care for people with dementia: recent innovations. *Reviews in Clinical Gerontology* **8**: 331–43.

Means, R. and Smith, R. 1998: *From poor law to community care*, 2nd edn. Bristol: Policy Press.

Milne, A., Hatzidimitriadou, E., Chryssanthopoulou, C. and Owen, T. 2001: *Caring in later life: reviewing the role of older carers*. London: Help the Aged.

Norman, A. 1987: *Severe dementia: the provision of longstay care*. London: Centre for Policy on Ageing.

Payne, M. and Shardlow, S. eds. 2002: *Social work in the British Isles*. London: Jessica Kingsley.

Robb, B. 1967: *Sans everything: a case to answer*. London: Thomas Nelson.

Robertson, A. 1991: The politics of Alzheimer's disease: a case study in apocalyptic demography. In: Minkler, M. and Estes, C.L. eds. *Critical perspectives on aging: the political and moral economy of growing old*. Amityville: Baywood Publishing, 135–50.

Sheldon, J.H. 1948: *The social medicine of old age*. Oxford: Radcliffe Medical Press.

Stanley, N. and Manthorpe, J. 2001: Reading mental health inquiries: messages for social work. *Journal of Social Work* **1**: 77–99.

Sutherland, S. 1999: *The Royal Commission on the care of the elderly*. London: Stationery Office.

Taylor, E. 1971: *Mrs Palfrey at the Claremont*. London: Virago.

Thane, P. 1998: The family lives of old people. In: Johnson, P. and Thane, P. eds. *Old age from antiquity to post-modernity*. London: Routledge, 180–210.

Townsend, P. 1957: *The family life of old people*. Penguin: Harmondsworth.

Warner, M., Furnish, S., Longley, M. and Lawlor, B. eds. 2002: *Alzheimer's disease: policy and practice across Europe*. Oxford: Radcliffe Medical Press.

Person-centred practice

Working with people in the early stages of dementia

Lindsay Royan

In recent years, increasing attention has focused on meeting the psychological needs of people who have only recently received a diagnosis of dementia. This has been made possible partly by a rise in the number of people actively seeking help for their memory and other cognitive problems. Most dementia services report that they are now generally referred people at an earlier stage in the condition than was the situation a decade ago. This is due, at least in part, to the increase in public knowledge and understanding of dementia through media coverage of recent research findings. The introduction of the so-called 'anti-dementia' drugs has meant, perhaps for the first time, that many people see some point in obtaining a diagnosis if there are medications that might help to modify the effects of dementia.

There is no doubt that developments in dementia care have suffered neglect because the people most affected are old and, generally, a non-vociferous section of society. Ageism has still not been satisfactorily challenged in health care, as illustrated by the fact that anti-ageist policies have their own standard (Standard 1) in the *National Service Framework for Older People* (Department of Health 2001). The publicity surrounding high profile individuals diagnosed as having Alzheimer's disease – Rita Hayworth, Ronald Reagan and Iris Murdoch, for example – has helped to bring dementia to public notice and challenge some popular misconceptions. The tragic news footage of young people with new variant Creutzfeld–Jacob disease (CJD) has alerted the world to the fact that dementia is no respecter of age. Research has also brought a greater public awareness that dementia affects people regardless of gender or cultural group (*see* Chapter 13).

Current dementia services are also witnessing a 'cohort shift': the oldest members of the community grew up in a world that broadly accepted the (false) notion of memory loss as an inevitable consequence of ageing. The term 'senile', which simply means 'pertaining to old age', had become synonymous with a 'failing, aged brain'. For much of their lives, this view went largely unchallenged by the medical profession (Lyman 1998), and their own elders had not reached a great age in sufficiently large number to provide evidence to the contrary. Furthermore, this pre-National Health Service generation was brought up with very different attitudes towards and expectations of health care (e.g., a fear of the expense, exhortations not to 'bother' the doctor and a mixture of gratitude and shame for services received).

Not so their children, who have experienced a very different set of circumstances. 'Young' pensioners have lived most of their adulthood with a National Health Service and the expectation of free and accessible health care across the lifespan. They can expect to enjoy many years of healthy retirement, have had greater access to education and information than their forebears, and have been more inclined to question authority and the status quo. This trend has been accompanied by an increasing value being placed on the individual as a consumer able to expect and make personal choices that affect lifestyle and well-being. As a result, succeeding generations of people reaching retirement will be ever more likely to expect and demand good public services regardless of their age or condition (Barnett 2000).

Memory clinics

Another development that can claim some role in promoting the early detection and treatment of dementia is the establishment of memory clinics, initially set up primarily as research centres to investigate the early stages of dementia and carry out drug trials, the first UK clinic being set up at St Pancras Hospital in London in 1983. These clinics helped to challenge notions that dementia is always a severe, global condition for which institutional care is the only realistic option. Researchers such as Una Holden (1988) concluded that many cognitive, behavioural and psychological skills are preserved in the early stages of dementia.

Unfortunately, in those early days, few clinics were funded or equipped to work remedially with their clients, as they were only assessment centres. To make matters worse, few statutory or voluntary sector facilities were set up to work with people in the early stages of dementia as they focused their efforts mainly on supporting people in the later stages and on providing respite care for family carers. This left the memory clinic staff in the unenviable position of giving individuals a diagnosis of dementia and then, effectively, adding that they would not be eligible to receive services until their condition had deteriorated, perhaps 2 or 3 years into the future. It is only comparatively recently that the concept of dementia 'treatment' has been added to that of dementia 'care'.

Although the introduction of the so-called 'anti-dementia' drugs has had an impact on the public and professional perspective of dementia, particularly since the publication of the National Institute for Clinical Excellence (NICE) guidelines in 2001, a cure for the condition is evidently still some years away. It is critical that services and researchers still work towards developing non-pharmacological interventions that meet a number of psychosocial needs. A well-developed service for those in the early stages of dementia should be able to offer:

- Psychological support and therapy for individuals, families and groups
- A range of activities that provide cognitive stimulation and rehabilitation
- Targeted and appropriate advice and information
- Opportunities to engage the individual in decision-making and choice.

All such activities must be grounded in a philosophy that promotes what Kitwood (1997) called 'personhood'. To be in a positive state of personhood, one must have opportunities to attain the highest level of well-being possible and to be treated as a full citizen in a community that also recognizes and adapts to the various disabilities that inevitably accompany a progressive condition such as dementia. The challenge for the community is to have the flexibility to adapt to changing needs and to minimize the creation of secondary social and psychological disabilities that may arise from a failure to meet the challenge of positive care. We can only hope to appreciate what is required by attempting to understand what it might be like to experience dementia and by acknowledging what our own needs might be in a similar situation (Kitwood 1997; Cassidy 1988). This person-centred approach is the cornerstone of approaches being developed for those in the early stages of dementia, and this chapter provides an introduction and critical overview to some of the key areas.

POST-DIAGNOSTIC INTERVENTIONS

Once a diagnosis of probable dementia has been made, health and social care practitioners need to be aware of possible psychological reactions when planning interventions. As with any life-challenging condition, there will almost inevitably be a period of mourning for the person and his or her family, who have to come to terms with news that will irrevocably change their lives. Families and individuals may experience some or all of the stages of grief that various writers have described – denial, anger, bargaining, depression and acceptance (Kübler-Ross 1969). Some will receive the diagnosis with surprise or shock; for others, it will confirm a long-held fear or suspicion. Some even express an initial relief on discovering a physical explanation for their difficulties. Later, many will seek an explanation for the dementia, perhaps blaming themselves or expressing anger towards the Fates.

Individuals and families may have a unified approach to tackling the challenges that face them. It may, however, also be the case that the person and the family may have different ideas and expectations related to the diagnosis. This can sometimes lead to widely divergent needs for services. Some people with dementia will, for example, want to maintain an unchanged and 'normal' lifestyle for as long as possible, whereas their family may immediately respond by making plans for the long-term future and will put care packages in place sooner rather than later. In other families, the opposite may be true. Some people seek extensive information about the condition and its probable course; others prefer to have the least amount of knowledge necessary. There may be differences of opinion within families too, some of which can have long-term and devastating consequences as each member finds his or her own way of coping. Professionals must attempt to steer a path through these complex and varied needs and be aware that needs may also change many times over the period of involvement with the person and his or her family.

One of the most frequent complaints from families is the tendency of professionals to divert their communication and focus from the person concerned to a carer immediately on receiving the diagnosis. This usually results in individuals with dementia feeling sidelined and isolated as they are not included in discussions about their own future. It is rarely the case that such an approach is justified. Most people in the early stages of dementia are capable of engaging in insightful discussion and decision-making. It may, however, be necessary for professionals to adapt their usual style of communication and provide more time for explanations and responses. We should be prepared to examine the effectiveness of our communication skills, and should remove as much jargon as possible without creating a misleading impression (*see* Chapter 10). We should also regularly check the person's comprehension. Time spent profitably in the early days after diagnosis will help to reduce distress and crisis situations in the future.

Many people receiving a diagnosis ask for support in three main areas:

- Advice and information
- Medication
- Self-help tips.

Advice and information

Experience of working in an early-intervention service suggests that people with dementia rarely want much involvement of services from the outset. There is a frequently expressed desire to 'get on as normally as possible for as long as we can'. Many ask for information about services for possible future use. It is generally helpful to support any verbal information with clear, concise written information. Services are most often asked to supply information about the condition, financial help (such as attendance allowance), the handling of finances (such as enduring power of attorney) and local facilities, including support groups, voluntary bodies (Alzheimer's Society, Age Concern and so on) and specialist contact numbers.

Medication

People are increasingly receiving their diagnosis at a clinic specifically designed to prescribe medication to suitable candidates. They will therefore already have an expectation of some medical intervention and should be given the opportunity to discuss, with their doctor and family, the probable outcome of taking drugs for their dementia. Currently, the only prescription drugs specifically designed for dementia are only for Alzheimer's disease. In 2001, NICE gave its approval for the prescribing of acetylcholinesterase inhibitor medication by consultant psychiatrists, neurologists and geriatricians to those of their patients who meet certain criteria. The drugs are recommended for people with mild-to-moderate Alzheimer's disease and those with a carer to ensure that they are taken regularly. Some physical conditions or treatments, such as heart disease, may deter the consultant from prescribing this medication. Regular reviews of progress are required, and each service should work out its local arrangements for supporting individuals taking the drugs.

Pre-prescription counselling is also advised as there is no guarantee of who will benefit and to what extent. Experience has shown that some of the greatest improvements occur in motivation, mood and interest in the environment, general concentration and the ability to carry out everyday tasks. Others may experience a smaller improvement, and some may seem no different but may feel that the medication is slowing their decline. It is also important to stress that current medications are not able to effect a 'cure'. It is extremely likely that, at some unspecified time in the future, the medication will cease to be effective as the Alzheimer's disease will progress to a point beyond the scope of the drug.

Decisions about commencing or withdrawing medication need to be made, as far as possible, in collaboration with the person with dementia and the family, and all team members should be aware of those decisions. Discussions related to medication can be delicate and difficult, and can arouse powerful feelings, as exemplified by recent communications from carers in the Alzheimer's Society newsletters. Some are strongly opposed to any medication that prolongs the condition without curing it as they believe this merely prolongs the agony for all concerned. Others refer to the drugs as 'buying time', providing the opportunity to enjoy more months and years of quality living than would otherwise be possible. Families are often divided in their views and will seek advice from staff, so it is important for professionals to keep themselves informed about relevant issues, particularly the cognitive and non-cognitive benefits derived from, and cautions associated with, the drugs. The NICE guidelines (2001) highlight the need for both aspects of functioning to be taken into consideration at review and also stress the value of assessing the individual's overall quality of life or sense of well-being.

There is some evidence from clinical practice that acetylcholinesterase inhibitors help to improve mood and motivation, and restore a degree of skill to activities of daily living. These effects may be greater than cognitive improvements seen, as measured on mental test scores, and may be valued more highly by those with dementia and their families. Others experience such an increase in their quality of life that they or their families wish to continue the medication long after there is any clear clinical evidence of its continuing efficacy with regard to, for example, memory function.

Not surprisingly, there is considerable research interest in pharmacological treatments for Alzheimer's disease and other forms of dementia, paralleled by an increasing body of knowledge on the causes of dementia. The next generation of drugs to become available are likely to be those which arrest the disease process and prevent it developing further. These will be followed by drugs capable of stopping the process and returning the person to health, and these may even be available prophylactically to people with a high risk of developing dementia. Such treatments lie, however, some way off; in the meantime, staff need to find a balance between being positive about current treatments and not raising false hopes.

Self-help

Increasingly, professionals are being asked for advice on self-help. More people are aware of 'off-the-shelf' treatments that have been identified as providing support for dementia and other memory problems, such as herbal treatments, complementary therapies, exercise and general lifestyle changes.

Herbal treatments and nutritional supplements

There is currently much research interest in naturally derived products that can be shown to slow the decline in dementia, particularly Alzheimer's disease. The herbal treatments *Gingko biloba* and *Panax ginseng* are the two most commonly cited, but manufacturers also supply a number of products that contain a combination of ingredients thought to be helpful in slowing dementia. *Gingko biloba*, particularly in combination with *Panax ginseng*, has been shown in some studies (e.g. Le Bars et al. 1997) to be as effective as acetylcholinesterase inhibitors.

There is also good evidence to suggest that an adequate intake of anti-oxidants, especially vitamin E (preferably in food but also in preparation form), not only has a preventative function, but also is also useful in the early stages of Alzheimer's disease (American Psychiatric Association 1997). Anti-oxidants are also commonly found as vitamins A and C and in trace elements such as selenium. Other naturally occurring substances have also been implicated in maintaining healthy function after dementia has been diagnosed. These include the B vitamins, iron and certain homeopathic treatments. Other complementary therapies such as reflexology and acupuncture are beneficial for some people. As it is beyond the scope of this chapter to give details on the potential of each treatment, practitioners are recommended to update themselves on the latest research findings in this area in order to be able to provide accurate information.

COGNITIVE REHABILITATION

Another area gaining interest among both service users and psychologists is the role of memory re-training or cognitive rehabilitation in early dementia. Recent research has shown that many techniques used to help people recover from the effects of head injury can be adapted for people with early or mild dementia. These techniques include:

- Vanishing cues
- Expanding rehearsal
- Associative learning
- Errorless learning.

Vanishing cues

This approach relies on the fact that visual cues aid recognition memory, an aspect of memory that is generally better preserved than recall alone. A person is given an appropriate piece of information in full, perhaps a name that they would like to remember. This name is written on a card and the person is taught to look at it each time he or she wishes to remember the name. Once this has been successfully established, another card is used that omits the final letter. The person practises remembering the name in the same way until another letter can be removed. This process continues until a blank card can trigger recall. Should the person encounter difficulties at a particular stage, the last letter is replaced until success is attained. In this way, the individuals achieves far more successful recollections than failures. This can have a tremendous effect on well-being and perhaps reverse the psychological effects of continually experiencing memory problems.

Expanding rehearsal

This technique can be very helpful for people who repeatedly ask the same questions as a result of rapid forgetting. The psychologist will first establish the frequency of the question and then ask the carer to give the answer, followed by the question, at intervals slightly less than this. If, for example, a person with dementia asks every 5 minutes on a car journey, 'Where are we going?', the carer will say every 4 minutes, 'We are going to our daughter's. Where are we going?' Although this initially involves more work for carers, many report that they feel they are at least taking some control of the conversation rather than waiting tensely for the question yet again. Those with dementia will feel reassured by these regular reminders, especially if they sense that their carer is less irritated. Having reached this stage, the carer then lengthens the time of giving and asking for the information at a pace that is demonstrably successful. Some people have been able to increase the interval from 2 to 30 minutes, with a considerable allevi-ation of carer stress (Clare and Woods 2001).

Associative learning

Psychologists have long understood that humans learn best by associating things, grouping pieces of information and finding patterns in their experience. This fact can be exploited in dementia care. Many people report attempts to support memory by writing notes to themselves. Although this approach can be very helpful and should indeed be encouraged, a significant proportion report forget-ting the location of the paper on which the note has been written. Keeping all notes in one place is an obvious solution, but there needs to be some technique that aids the recall of that location. One approach that has been used successfully is learning to associate memory with the colour of, for example, a diary in which the infor-mation is stored. This reduces the burden on memory to one association. If the diary is red, the person thus learns that 'memory is red'. Once the diary has been placed in an obvious place where it can be spotted, individuals will learn to retrieve both the book and the memories stored within it.

Similarly, should a person wish to re-learn how to use a video recorder, coloured stickers appropriate to function can be placed around the buttons. To maximize association learning, a green sticker can indicate 'play' ('go') and a red sticker 'stop'. It is important to attempt to re-train only within the person's ability; it might therefore be necessary not to try to teach all the video functions but only those which are most important to the person and will provide a feeling of success and autonomy.

Errorless learning

The term 'errorless learning' refers to the underlying philosophy of all these approaches. Learning without making mistakes not only breeds an atmosphere of success and encourages a sense of self-worth, but also ensures that errors are not learned instead. Many people in the early stages of dementia tend to repeat an error and have difficulty correcting themselves. One explanation for this is that as the world becomes an increasingly confusing and rather bizarre place, a person will naturally tend towards any information or knowledge that feels most familiar and safe. In essence, if the person is asked the current year and responds with '1974', this is more likely to be retained than the correct response given by the questioner. The year 1974 may have a special significance for the person; more commonly, however, it is that hearing an incorrect response in one's own voice creates a greater feeling of familiarity that the correct response given in a less familiar voice. The more frequently individuals hear their own response, the more it will become established and be harder to shift. Errorless learning attempts to deal with this by discouraging people from giving any response until they are reasonably confident that it is the correct one. In this way, there is no competition in terms which version of information is stored.

Other techniques are also being developed; for further information; the reader is referred to the work of Linda Clare (see the references at the end of the chapter).

PSYCHOTHERAPEUTIC INTERVENTIONS

Although there seems to be more dialogue between those working in specialist dementia services and those with dementia than was previously the case, many people who have just received a diagnosis will not explicitly request help with their emotional response to the news. Staff frequently collude with this apparent silence, often justifying their behaviour on the grounds that dementia denies someone the capacity for adequate self-awareness. Just because a person does not outwardly display signs of distress does not mean that he or she is not experiencing a whole variety of emotional responses. Many people with dementia report that they do not like to share their feelings because they feel guilty that their carer already has enough to cope with. They choose to protect the carer, often a family member, from their distress (Gisser 1994). Others say that they are afraid they will not be able to contain their feelings once they have expressed them. They may also believe that no-one will wish to listen to what they have to say.

These, and other, experiences have been usefully described in Pratt and Wilkinson's (2001) report to the Mental Health Foundation on the implications of sharing the diagnosis of dementia. The experience of dementia certainly does not make comfortable listening because it forces us to consider what it might be like progressively to lose all those attributes which we attach to human identity. The capacity for self-determination, awareness, independence, recall, self-expression, reflectiveness, problem-solving, planning, organization, language and social functioning are all undermined in dementia. Exploring these areas in depth with an affected human being demands huge reserves of humanity and courage on the part of the listener (Kitwood 1997). Sharing the distress and sense of loss that inevitably arises in such circumstances tests our capacity to share pain to the limit. As we attempt to find an empathic response to such emotion, we cannot divorce ourselves from the thought that we might be hearing about our own future. As Kitwood has so eloquently described in *Dementia Reconsidered* (1997), we all too often protect ourselves by erecting a wall that separates 'us' from 'them', creating an illusion that only the people with dementia are 'damaged' or 'deficient' whereas we remain whole and invulnerable.

A number of psychologists have explored the importance of the 'talking therapies' for people in the early stages of dementia. Cheston and Bender (1999) have written extensively on the need to attend to the non-cognitive aspects of dementia. There is a danger that so much attention is paid to memory problems in dementia that the emotional elements are ignored. Many writers in addition to Cheston and Bender have, however, stressed the need to develop psychological therapies for use in dementia. The work of each will be described separately, but it is worth noting that a common theme runs through their approaches. Feil's validation therapy (1993) picks up a theme from Holden and Woods' (1982) work on reality orientation from their stressing the need to respond to the emotional aspects of a person's 'confused' talk (*see* Chapter 9). Kitwood (1997) developed a person-centred approach based on his work of trying to understand the world from the emotional perspective of the person with dementia and psychologists such as Moniz-Cook (Moniz-Cook et al. 1998) and Sutton (1994) have explored how psychosocial and psychotherapeutic interventions that acknowledge the centrality of emotional reality can be introduced into mainstream dementia services. Each writer describes a wealth of opportunities for psychotherapeutic intervention. Some of their findings can be summarized as follows:

- It is the task of the therapist to 'decode' the meaning of the emotional expression of the person with dementia and find ways of reflecting and exploring the issues raised.
- It may be that conventional psychotherapy is not always appropriate; the person with dementia may have problems with verbal communication and may need more time to process ideas and experiences.
- Therapeutic sessions may need to be more flexible in length to compensate for fluctuating abilities of concentration.
- The therapist may need to meet with the person more frequently as memories of previous sessions fade more rapidly.
- The language of therapy may need to be modified to maximize understanding and allow for a tendency for thinking to become more concrete and less abstract.
- The setting of therapy may be significant; it is likely that the therapist will have to travel to the people's homes rather than meet in the clinic. Changing the setting also changes the dynamics of the meeting. Other people may, for example, share the person's home and have an influence on how sessions take place. Arriving at an individual's front door may make it harder for the

person to decline therapy than if he or she had to choose to travel to the therapist.

- People may need multiple reassurances of the confidentiality of their disclosures, especially if all other aspects of their care are openly discussed with family and professionals.
- The person may want to protect him- or herself, and the therapist, from the experience of dementia; such resistance may be an important coping strategy and should be treated sensitively.

Whereas the psychotherapeutic approach is discussed in Chapters 6 and 9, it is particularly pertinent here as this work is most likely to be useful when begun in the early stages of the condition. Not only does the person have more cognitive and emotional resources to make use of psychotherapy at this point, but there is also, hopefully, less work to do on repairing the effects of poor therapeutic care. Some of the work developed by people in this field is outlined below.

Validation therapy

Feil (1993) devised this approach in response to what is now recognized as a serious misinterpretation of an earlier model known as reality orientation. This earlier approach was designed to encourage interest in the present through giving people pertinent information about the day, date, time, place and matters of current interest. This was, however, unfortunately extended to include correcting people's misinformation and misperceptions, and confronting them with the 'truth'. This was explicitly advised against by early practitioners in reality orientation (see Holden and Woods 1982) but nevertheless became standard practice in a large number of care settings.

Many people, including Feil, became appalled at the apparent insensitivity of this approach as it blatantly failed to take into account anything of the emotional world of the person with dementia. Even though reminding an older woman of the death of her husband or the absence of her children, for example, clearly did nothing to relieve her distress, and frequently heightened her anxiety and grief, institutions seemed reluctant to change their strategy. Validation therapy adopted the neglected advice of reality orientation and advocated listening to the emotional meaning of a person's words rather than the words themselves.

Words are merely a tool of communication – meaning lies in their expression and use. We can only understand the woman who is looking for her dead husband if we take into account what we know of her, her previous relationship, how she is expressing the desire to see him (tone of voice, physical actions and so on) and the context in which she is expressing herself. This information might reveal a sense that she is bored, worried, grieving or feeling useless, or has recently been upset by someone else; a whole host of possible interpretations exist. The validation therapist tries to decide which is most likely on the basis of knowledge, intuition and a response from the person. Training for this work equips the therapist with skills to find meaning in behaviour and respond in a way that demonstrates a recognition of the emotional truth of the person's experience and helps to resolve conflicts and concerns from the past. The 'truth' of individuals' words are, in this technique, not disputed. Validation therapy uses a range of approaches depending on the individual concerned and the stage of his or her dementia. Although techniques may vary, other approaches share the underlying philosophy of entering and accepting the emotional world of the person with dementia.

Resolution therapy

Stokes and Goudie (2002) suggest that, in attempting to understand the meaning to be found in behaviour, it is important to consider what present circumstances may be contributing to a person's distress. They recognize that those with dementia register and respond to their emotional environment even when this may not always be immediate or obvious. Confused messages may be an attempt to make sense of the world, to seek help, comfort or explanation. The onus to provide a suitable response lies within the person's living environment. Care staff need to examine their practice and ask what they can do to reduce confusion and distress, and enhance understanding. This requires a preparedness to accept that practices or approaches may exist that, unwittingly or otherwise, contribute to confusion and misunderstanding.

Person-centred approach

Kitwood (1997) coined the phrase 'personhood' to describe all the varied attributes that define the human condition. He also used the term 'malignant social psychology' to illustrate the variety of ways in which personhood might be denied. Kitwood listed 17 ways in which people with dementia might be treated differently and not accorded the treatment one could expect as a full citizen in society. Like the work described above, much of his study was based on the experiences of people in the later stages of dementia. He pointed out, however, that the process of denying personhood to another can begin as soon as a diagnosis is confirmed.

Kitwood describes the problem of 'outpacing', in which a professional does not allow enough time for the person to process the news of the diagnosis, or fails to try to explain it in a way that can be understood by a person with dementia. Healthy adult communication usually involves an equal exchange between two parties. Dementia denies people the ability to maintain their part so others must make the extra journey to make contact. Kitwood stresses that the person, rather than the diagnosis, should come first. If personhood is maintained in the early stages of the condition, there is less risk of developing secondary (non-neurological) aspects of dementia that progressively exclude the person from the world of which they are still a part.

Psychotherapy and life review

The idea that people with dementia can benefit from psychotherapy may seem strange, especially to those influenced by Freud's notion that few beyond middle age retain the mental elasticity to participate in therapy. Some people, even in the early stages of dementia, lose some capacity for reflection but can nevertheless achieve a degree of closure and peace of mind from telling their story to a non-judgmental listener. The process of life review provides one structure by which this can occur (Haight and Burnside 1993; Garland and Garland 2001).

Life review is based on the view that development continues across the lifespan, that human beings have a need to make sense of their lives and, sometimes, to share that meaning with others, and that past experience shapes and influences our present and future selves. It encourages story-telling that explicitly challenges unhelpful assumptions and helps people to draw more positive conclusions about themselves. It helps to uncover key points in a person's life that may be causing difficulties in the present. It allows for some reconstruction of a life that might appear fractured. For Erikson (1960), a review of one's life in old age brings with it the challenge of finding a sense of integrity of self as opposed to a sense of despair. Talking about the source of their distress in a supportive environment may help some people who are troubled by the past. Exploring issues that are most important may also help not only to resolve the past, but also to prepare for the future. In many respects, life review creates a bridge between psychotherapy and reminiscence. Although not unique to dementia work, life review, psychotherapy and reminiscence all have a role to play in piecing a life together.

Reminiscence

Reminiscence and life review are not often considered in the early stages of dementia. Such activities are popular in day and residential services for people with moderate-to-severe dementia, where they are often nostalgia-based activities designed to create a sense of comfort and enjoyment through familiarity. Reminiscence may, however, have a useful function in the early stages by helping to involve the person with dementia in planning future treatment and care. It is well understood that, at times of change in our lives, we find strength from looking back to remind ourselves how we have coped before in similar circumstances and, more generally, to reinforce our memories of our skills and attributes (Woods and McKiernan 1995). This is particularly true for those with dementia. Some individuals may find the past a more attractive place as the present becomes increasingly difficult to comprehend and the future may be filled with increasing uncertainty. In the early stages of dementia, people may also feel the desire to record their lives and experiences in some way while they are able to take editorial control. Not everyone, however, wants a permanent record of their story; for some, sharing tales with another is enough.

The following list offers some possible functions of reminiscence at this time:

- To identify personal strengths and coping strategies
- To maintain conversational skills
- To explore change and loss
- To express personal feelings and process past conflicts
- To produce a life history
- To rediscover fun.

It is clear from this list that many aspects of reminiscence closely match the aims of psychotherapy. Both reminiscence work and psychotherapy involve an exploration of personal stories, fantasies and desires. Both aim to build on the individual's strengths, sometimes by resolving issues from the past or by changing the perception of past events. The main differences in dementia work will relate to the training of the therapist and the depth at which the work takes place.

To identify personal strengths

Most people choose to tell positive stories about themselves. A personal story may serve as shorthand for how the teller would like to be regarded by the listener. Tellers provide a story that portrays them as intelligent, attractive, witty, cunning, brave or whatever quality they value highly. The story-teller is highly conscious of the listener and will adapt the story to achieve the desired effect. The listener can promote or inhibit the story by his or her prompts and reactions. It may not, however, always be enough to encourage someone simply to recall past experiences; it is also necessary to find elements of the reminiscence that can be used to cope with present adversity. If, for example, a person's stories reveal that he or she has used humour to cope with difficult situations, it may be possible to continue using that strategy, with support from others.

To maintain conversational skills

Many people in the early stages of dementia report difficulty following conversations, because they are too fast, because the subject matter changes too frequently or because too many people are involved. Talking about him- or herself gives the speaker control over the pace and content, and is most effective on a one-to-one basis or in small groups. It is understood that conversational skills, even in people without cognitive impairment, will deteriorate quickly without regular practice. If people can be encouraged to talk on a familiar topic through reminiscence, this can slow the deterioration and help to keep people engaged in the present. A study covering various groups across Europe – the Remembering Yesterday, Caring Today project for people with dementia – found that general communication levels improve after reminiscence sessions. More details on how this project was set up and how it can be replicated elsewhere can be found in Schweitzer (2000).

To explore change and loss

Dementia brings multiple losses, losses of skills, memory, independence and confidence in the future, to name but a few. Therapeutic reminiscence can help people to grieve for what was and what now may never be. The process of sharing stories can help to express feelings about the life lived, celebrate achievements and bring a degree of closure to past events and experiences. The first step may be simply to ask people how they feel (Wilkinson 2002).

To produce a life history

Many people wish to record their lives, thoughts and preferences to speak for them when they cannot. Life histories can take a variety of forms – diaries, biographies, pictorial records, tapes or 'memory boxes' – and can be created with family members and professionals over a period of time. The material included will be at the owners' discretion and could include guidelines on how they are to be treated should they enter formal care. To this end, life histories often accompany the person through their care journey.

To rediscover fun

The experience of dementia is for many people one of increasing failure in tasks once accepted as second nature. By utilizing the best-preserved aspects of memory, reminiscence can offer respite from this experience and reinstate the person in an expert role. The relief of using old skills again brings much laughter and relaxation to well-constructed reminiscence sessions. If such sessions can be demonstrated to have a value beyond personal diversion, such as by being used to contribute to a local school's living history project, the enjoyment is even greater.

Reminiscence can also play a role in personalizing care by exploring the values, beliefs and habits that shape a person's life. The reasons behind behaviour are multifaceted, and many people will not be aware of their influence. By discovering an individual's values in the early stages of dementia, it can become possible to understand apparently 'irrational' or 'challenging' behaviour later on. A gentleman who would never been seen in public without being washed, shaved and dressed in a suit and tie might, for example, be expected to react if a well-meaning member of staff were to persuade him to take breakfast unshaven and wearing a dressing gown. He might resist entering the dining room, reject any food offered him, avoid eye contact with others and use physical effort to express his discomfort. Without a knowledge of his personal standards, his subsequent behaviour might well become defined as 'challenging'.

Superstitious beliefs may also play a prominent role in behaviour. Superstition exists to explain phenomena that appear to have no rational explanation. Superstitious behaviour often involves a simple ritual to ward off bad luck; this helps to reduce anxiety by creating a sense of control in difficult or uncertain circumstances. Its use increases with the perceived level of crisis or uncertainty. It is no coincidence that the professions most fraught with danger and uncertainty are also the most superstitious (e.g., mining, fishing, sports and the theatre), and older people have generally been more exposed to superstitious beliefs than their descendents. The nature of dementia brings crisis and uncertainty, and may trigger superstitious behaviour in an attempt to regain a sense of control. An older person from a high-risk profession who has dementia may have an increased propensity for superstitious behaviour.

Moniz-Cook et al. (2000) have found that a wide variety of superstitious beliefs can account for so-called challenging behaviour. One man who was prone to pushing others downstairs was discovered to have had a lifelong superstition about passing people on the stairs. Because he was no longer able to rationalize his feelings or wait for others to use the stairs, he developed this worrying behaviour as a means of controlling his own anxiety. Once this was understood, staff were able to help him use the stairs safely at appropriate times. Reminiscence can be used to elicit these beliefs and frequently makes an enjoyable topic for discussion.

This chapter has provided a brief introduction to a range of exciting new developments in the treatment and care of people in the early stages of dementia. There is a growing interest in research in this area, and the future should see this work shaping clinical practice. It is clear that services need to be informed by a bio-psychosocial model in order to develop holistic treatment and care programmes that meet the complex and diverse needs of their clients. Biological, or physical, needs are being addressed with drug treatments, both conventional and alternative, complementary therapies, diet and exercise. In the future, drugs may be able to stop, reverse and even prevent the condition, and nutritional supplements may be routinely prescribed to slow the effects, or reduce the risk of onset, of dementia. Lifestyle will come under closer scrutiny as research reveals more insights into environmental factors. Psychological treatments are becoming increasingly more sophisticated; cognitive rehabilitation techniques will become more targeted and individualized to utilize a person's particular strengths. Therapeutic interventions should become more widely available and acknowledge both the desire and capacity of many people to talk about their experience of dementia (Pratt and Wilkinson 2001).

Those with dementia should be placed at the centre of their own care, whereas those family members and friends who provide care should also have their needs

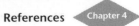

assessed and, where possible, met. An assessment of needs should acknowledge the importance of social networks, and services must find creative means of supporting people with dementia and their carers in maintaining valued areas of their lives for as long as possible. It is unlikely that one type of service can meet all these needs; the Audit Commission (2000) recommends multiagency services, preferably located on one site, as a useful development. Local dementia services development centres are a useful resource for information on good, evidence-based practices. There is scope for imaginative service development and many excellent examples of innovation around the country.

REFERENCES

American Psychiatric Association. 1997: Practice guidelines for the treatment of patients with Alzheimer's disease and other dementias of later life. *American Journal of Psychiatry* **154:** 1–39.

Audit Commission. 2000: *Forget me not: mental health services for older people.* London: Audit Commission.

Barnett, E. 2000: *Including the person with dementia in designing and delivering care.* London: Jessica Kingsley.

Cassidy, S. 1998: *Sharing the darkness.* London: Darton, Longman & Todd.

Cheston, R. and Bender, M. 1999: *Understanding dementia: the man with the worried eyes.* London: Jessica Kingsley.

Clare, L. and Woods, R.T. 2001: *Cognitive rehabilitation in dementia.* Hove: Psychology Press.

Department of Health. 2001: *The national service framework for older people.* London: Stationery Office.

Erikson, E. 1960: *Childhood and society.* Harmondsworth: Penguin Books.

Feil, N. 1993: *The validation breakthrough: simple techniques for communicating with people with Alzheimer's-type dementia.* Baltimore, Maryland: Health Professions Press.

Garland, J. and Garland, C. 2001: *Life review in health and social care.* Hove: Brunner-Routledge.

Gisser, N. 1994: Keeping a focus on the quality of life. *Alzheimer Association Cleveland Chapter* July: 10–14.

Haight, B.K. and Burnside, I. 1993: Reminiscence and life review: explaining the differences. *Archives of Psychiatric Nursing* **7:** 91–8.

Holden, U.P. 1988: *Neuropsychology and ageing: definitions, explanations and practical approaches.* London: Croom Helm.

Holden, U.P. and Woods, R.T. 1982: *Reality orientation: psychological approaches to the confused elderly.* Edinburgh: Churchill Livingstone.

Kitwood, T. 1997: *Dementia reconsidered: the person comes first.* Buckingham: Open University Press.

Kübler-Ross, E. 1969: *On death and dying,* London: Tavistock.

Le Bars, P.L., Katz, M.M., Berman, N. et al. 1997: A placebo controlled double blind randomised trial of an extract of Gingko Biloba for dementia. *Journal of the American Medical Association* **278:** 1327–32.

Lyman, K.A 1998: Living with AD: the creation of meaning among persons with dementia. *Journal of Clinical Ethics* **9:** 49–57.

Moniz-Cook, E., Agar, S., Gibson, G. et al. 1998: A preliminary study of the effects of early intervention with people with dementia and their families in a memory clinic. *Aging and Mental Health* **2:** 199–211.

Moniz-Cook, E., Woods, R. and Gardiner, E. 2000: Staff factors associated with perception of behaviour as 'challenging' in residential and nursing homes. *Aging and Mental Health* **1**(4): 48–55(8).

National Institute for Clinical Excellence 2001: *Technology appraisal guidance number 19. Guidance on the use of Donepezil, Rivastigmine and Galantamine for the treatment of Alzheimer's disease.* London: Nice.

Pratt, R. and Wilkinson, H. 2001: *No diagnosis has to be your whole life: the effect of being told the diagnosis of dementia from the perspective of the person with dementia. Final Report to the Mental Health Foundation.* London: Mental Health Foundation.

Schweitzer, P. ed. 1984: *Can we afford the doctor?* London: Age Exchange Publications.

Schweitzer, P. ed. 2000: *Reminiscence with people with dementia.* London: Age Exchange Publications.

Stokes, G. and Goudie, F. eds. 2002: *The essential dementia care handbook.* London: Winslow Press.

Sutton, L. 1994: What it is like to lose one's mind. Paper presented at the 10th International Conference of Alzheimer's Disease International, University of Edinburgh.

Wilkinson, H. ed. 2002: *The perspectives of people with dementia.* London: Jessica Kingsley.

Woods, R.T. and McKiernan, F. 1995: Evaluating the impact of reminiscence on older people with dementia. In: Haight, B.K and Webster, J.D. eds. *The art and science of reminiscing: theory, research, methods and applications.* Washington DC: Taylor & Francis, 233–42.

Managing language and communication difficulties in Alzheimer's dementia: the link to behaviour

Karen Bryan and Jane Maxim

Mrs Bailey is a 94-year-old woman living in a residential home who has reduced mobility. She has Alzheimer's disease and is usually friendly and talkative. Staff say Mrs Bailey conveys limited information and appears confused but is a model resident until the drug trolley appears. They try to ensure that she is out of the way before the trolley arrives as if she sees it, she tries to push the trolley and remove drugs from it, shouting and grabbing at staff who try to stop her. Mrs Bailey sometimes kicks and pinches but then gets very upset and cries. In desperation, staff have asked a visiting speech and language therapist, Jane Green, to see her. Jane's standard assessment shows the following:

- Mrs Bailey's speech is fully intelligible.
- A significant part of what she says is unexpected or inappropriate.
- She has a significantly reduced ability to name objects.
- When given tests of verbal expression, Mrs Bailey has low scores, indicating difficulty in listing female names, describing objects and re-telling a story or event.
- She shows inconsistent orientation to time, place and person.

Jane tape-records her conversation with Mrs Bailey. Jane encourages her to talk, her comments being validated (i.e. taken at face value as correct and not challenged). Mrs Bailey frequently switches topics; Jane does not challenge this but, as information emerges, provides gentle encouragement to say more. A discourse analysis of the content shows a number of references to 'nursing'. Mrs Bailey talks several times about college while pointing to herself. When asked 'Were you a nurse?', she says yes but attempts a long explanation and becomes very frustrated. Jane asks staff what is known about Mrs Bailey's past working life. No-one appears to know even though she has been a resident for 8 years. Could she have been a nurse? Staff feel it is unlikely – surely they would have known? Checks are, however, made and it is found that she was. Furthermore, a chance call from Mrs Bailey's daughter, who lives abroad, reveals that her mother nursed during the Second World War and later gained a nursing qualification.

Mrs Bailey's behaviour with the drugs trolley now makes more sense; clearly, the trolley is a concrete and salient object that triggers memories. Mrs Bailey wants to be part of the drug round and, as a trained nurse, may resent being 'sent away'. Jane suggests that Mrs Bailey be given a task as part of the round, one during which she will not be a risk. She is therefore assigned the job of following the trolley with a bag to collect discarded wrappings and so on. This is sufficient to engage Mrs Bailey. After this, she takes part every round and is her 'normal' self during the activity. As an added bonus, her mobility increases a little.

This scenario shows that communication with and by people with a dementia should be both accepted and valued. Steps need to be taken to understand what people are trying to say even though this may be difficult, and a careful analysis of what they say in context can be revealing. This chapter explores:

- How the ageing process may affect language and communication
- How problems associated with a dementia may further undermine the capacity to communicate effectively
- How an awareness of communication difficulties and a willingness to explore communication can be used to understand behaviours labelled as 'problematic' in people with dementia.

Communication is the process by which people convey information to one another. It can be verbal or non-verbal but is frequently a combination of the two. There are four components to communication:

1. A sound and rhythm system (phonology and intonation)
2. A grammatical system (syntax)
3. The meaning of words, phrases and larger units of language (semantics)
4. A system for the use of language such as rules for turn-taking and appropriateness, which are to some extent culturally determined and which represent the interface between communication and behaviour (pragmatics).

For communication to be fully successful, people need to have a shared code (or language), adequate motor skills for talking and listening, some memory for knowledge and a common code of behaviour, including body language (Stevens and Ripich 1999).

Aspects of the normal ageing process can, however, change language and communication skills. These need to be considered in relation to people with a dementia but not to be 'pathologized'. As we age, for example, it is normal occasionally to experience 'tip of the tongue' states in which people struggle to recall a word that they know, for example, 'Oh you know, that woman, what's her name, long hair and always carries a green bag, Cynthia no Mary, that's it Mary Smith.' This type of behaviour is not, however, only part of the normal ageing process but may be caused by any context in which language performance (here the ability to produce a name quickly in conversation) is made more difficult by external or internal factors (e.g., noise, stress or fatigue).

Research shows that some spoken language tasks (e.g., naming objects) and language-mediated tasks (such as defining words and explaining concepts) do not change greatly as we age, although a slower response may be seen. Understanding complex grammatical structures, ambiguous sentences and inferences does show some decline (Kemper and O'Hanlon 2000), but what is meant here by 'decline'? Older people tend to be slower to respond or may, on occasions, fail to understand a complex sentence. Sensory and environmental factors may also have a secondary effect on a person's ability to communicate.

HEARING

The hearing system undergoes a number of age-related changes that reduce the efficiency of hearing. As an adaptation to hearing loss, the older person may learn to supplement heard information with information from lip-reading and, in doing so, switch from normal eye contact to lip watching. Listening and understanding are affected by the hearing loss, and the person's own speech may be affected by loss of feedback, as a result becoming louder. An awareness of mis-hearing can also lead to anxiety about what others might be saying. It is important, where possible, to assess hearing in older people and be aware of possible reductions in hearing. Useful strategies include:

- A reduction of background noise
- Gaining the person's attention before speaking
- Facing the person to allow lip-reading
- Ensuring that light is on your face when speaking
- Speaking at a normal volume and speed (not a fast or very slow speed, and not raising your voice as this will distort the speech signal).

Hearing loss can exacerbate the difficulty of people with a dementia to access information through language and can encourage feelings of suspiciousness or paranoia if the person is aware of not being able to hear. In the early stages of a dementia, people may report problems with understanding as 'difficulty in hearing'.

VISION

The visual system undergoes changes associated with age that, for example, slow down the ability to focus and reduce the ability to distinguish colours. In addition, pathologies such as glaucoma and cataracts, which further reduce visual acuity, are common in older people. As well as disrupting both verbal and non-verbal communication (conveyed by gesture and facial expression), visual difficulties reduce contact with the outside world by making television and written language (books or magazines) less accessible. Useful strategies include:

- Using touch to alert the person to communication
- Providing extra verbal information to compensate for the loss of non-verbal information (e.g., stating that a family member looks tired rather than expecting the older person with visual difficulties to notice)
- Using larger print or pictures, clear text, a contrast between background colour and print and alternatives such as tape-recorded books and newspapers.

Many older people have visual and hearing difficulties in parallel with a dementia, increasing the effect on communication.

ENVIRONMENT

The environment has a strong influence on communication. Opportunities to interact with others create mental and physical stimulation, which in turn help naturally to foster communication. In other words, if there is nobody to talk to or nothing to talk about, communication will be reduced. Many older people may be socially isolated partly as a result of mobility problems, this being exacerbated by a reduction in their social network. Entry into residential care can remove people entirely from their social network, and a 'communication-impaired environment' exists in many homes (Lubinski 1991). Constant loud television will stifle any attempt to communicate and will make hearing more difficult. The classic 'chairs round the wall' layout in many residential settings reduces the opportunity to talk to others. Holden (1995) described a good communication environment as providing:

- Private and recognizable space in which people can talk at ease
- Active, interesting public spaces where there are things to see, touch and do

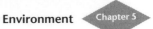

- An encouragement to self-care and an involvement in the activities of daily living
- An involvement in making choices, for example in terms of meals and activities
- Interesting things to do
- Information to update individuals, such as clocks and calendars.

If communication is a problem, sensory and environmental concerns need to be addressed as a first step:

1. Is the person able to hear?
2. If the individual has a hearing aid, is it working and being used?
3. Can the person see? Are spectacles clean, accessible and in use? Does the person need a reminder to put them on?
4. Is the individual wearing any dentures needed (as a lack of teeth compromises intelligibility)?
5. Does the individual need environmental change or encouragement to communicate?

Communication can be disrupted in older people by specific language disorders thath are not necessarily part of the dementia process. *Aphasia* (sometimes called dysphasia) refers to a loss of language, most frequently caused by a stroke (Parr et al. 1999). The ability to communicate verbally and the ability to understand may both be compromised. One aspect of language can be affected without the other: people may, for example, be able to speak with a reduced understanding of what others say, or they may have enormous difficulty expressing themselves verbally while fully understanding what others say. As part of aphasia, the ability to use language in print and to write may be compromised. Aphasia may be present in people with a vascular (multi-infarct) dementia.

Dysarthria is a difficulty in the production of speech, which results in a reduction in intelligibility. Dysarthria is a common problem in some neurological disorders such as Parkinson's disease and motor neurone disease. Dysarthria can also be produced as a drug side-effect, particularly in response to major tranquillizers and anti-psychotic medication.

The fact that communication, language and speech may all change during the normal ageing process and may, in addition, be disrupted by common health problems such as stroke or Parkinson's disease make this a complex area. We should therefore not assume that all the language changes seen in an older individual who has a dementia are necessarily 'caused by' that dementia. To take this line of argument further, we should not assume that all of the difficulties apparent in a person with dementia are caused by the dementia and therefore irreversible. Cleaning spectacles or a blocked hearing aid may have as dramatic an effect for someone with a dementia as they would for a person of any age.

Similarly, we need to view individuals in the context of their language skills, which will include their life experiences, their interests, their preferred communicative style (chatty, quiet, likes to be the centre of attention, never likes to be in groups and so on) and their personality, with its inherent likes and dislikes. This may seem 'trite', but its importance quickly becomes apparent when older people react in ways that are expected or unexpected. A large friendly dog from the local pat-a-dog scheme may, for example, cause a former dog-lover to be very responsive and unusually cheerful, wheras a former police-dog handler may start shouting instructions; conversely, somebody who has always hated dogs following an attack as a small child may become very upset.

What about the effects of a dementia? The impact on language and communication varies with individual patterns of difficulty and preserved skills. Factors that contribute to the variation across individuals are:

- The type of dementia
- The severity of the dementia
- Any underlying sensory reductions (hearing and vision)
- The presence of any other speech and language difficulties
- A person's pre-exiting language abilities, level of education and language style.

ALZHEIMER-TYPE DEMENTIA

Alzheimer's disease is one of the most common types of dementia, impairment in more than two areas of cognition, for example memory, language, abstract thinking and judgement, usually being present. The diagnosis is essentially one of exclusion so many older people are assumed to have Alzheimer's disease. For this reason, the term 'probable Alzheimer's disease' (pAD) will be used in this chapter.

Symptom variation and disease progression

It is now widely recognized that variation exists within the disease entity of pAD, but there is considerable debate over why this variation occurs and over its relationship to the neuropathology affecting brain structures. Schwartz (1990, p.143) describes this heterogeneity as:

each patient presents a landscape of eroding cognitive and functional capacities, but the landscape contains peaks and valleys. One patient may be seen with particularly severe visuospatial confusion (where objects seen visually are distorted or not recognised) and little language disturbance; another patient may show the reverse. Patients may have frontal lobe symptoms to a greater or lesser extent. They may have marked extra-pyramidal motor signs (parkinsonism). More typically most patients show simultaneous dissolution across several domains.

Martin et al. (1986), in an analysis of the performance profiles of 43 people with pAD, found that the majority had a profile in which retrieval and the use of semantic knowledge and visuo-constructional skills both showed deficits, but one subgroup had severely impaired naming skills with relatively preserved visuo-constructive skills, whereas another showed the opposite pattern. This finding has been extensively replicated, and we must now recognize that not everyone with pAD presents a uniform pattern of impairment. Furthermore, we must acknowledge the specific patterns of deficits for individuals with pAD.

Language processing and disease progression

Maxim and Bryan (1996) have presented a checklist of functions (language, cognition and personality) that shows deficits and spared skills at different stages of the disease and which is primarily applicable to late-onset Alzheimer's disease (Box 5.1). If taken at face value, however, this information provides a misleading impression of disease progression as being homogenous. Some aspects of language are usually compromised at all stages of pAD, but there is an enormous variation in deficits as well as retained functions among individuals in the pAD population, as well as differences in the rate of disease progression. Bayles et al. (1992) provide extensive information on language functions linked to stages of the disease measured on the Global Deterioration Rating Scale (Reisburg et al. 1982) in comparison to normal age- and education-matched controls; *see* also Kempler (1995) and Nebes (1992) for excellent overviews of language and cognition in pAD.

One of the key features of pAD is a semantic deficit in parallel with a relative preservation of other levels of language such as grammar and the sound system. The impact of this semantic deficit can be heard in the conversations of people with pAD. They usually produce language fluently, but there is often a paucity of specific nouns, a greater use of pronouns and generic nouns (e.g. 'thing', 'someone' or 'that') are used, and reference (specific words that link the meaning in different parts of an utterance) is underspecified so that it can be difficult for the listener to understand, for example, who or what is the focus of that conversation:

Well some people call it a, a straight pin, but I've never used that expression. I call it a stick pin, but this is an unusually stout one. They're usually finer, and it's grey, greyish metal. Is that alright?

This is a description by a man with mild Alzheimer's disease of an object placed in his hand – a nail. Once the reader knows that the item in question is a nail, the

Box 5.1 Checklist of functions in late-onset Alzheimer-type dementia

---

Early-stage Alzheimer's disease

Language	Low-frequency word-finding impaired
	Circumlocution in conversation
	Word fluency impaired
	Composite picture description incomplete
	Repetition on Boston Diagnostic Aphasia Examination low-frequency sentences poor
	Utterance completion poor in conversation
	Auditory and written complex sentence comprehension impaired
	Single word recognition maintained
Cognition	Episodic memory impaired
	Specific autobiographical memory impaired
	Time orientation impaired
	Naming of famous faces impaired
	Attention impaired
	Time orientation impaired
Personality	Change of affect
	Avoidance/denial strategies
	Increased anxiety
	Depression

Mid-stage Alzheimer's disease

Language	Naming deficits on high-frequency items
	Semantic paraphasias
	Reference deficit in pronoun use
	Errors in complex sentence production
	Occasional phonemic paraphasias
	Semantic cuing response decreased
	Sentence reading aloud poor
	Single regular word reading aloud retained
	Decreased use of gesture
	Repetition on Boston Diagnostic Aphasia Examination high-frequency sentences poor
	Single word recognition impairment
	Simple sentence comprehension impairments
Cognition	Working memory impaired
	Knowledge of current events decreased
	Ideational perseveration
	Time and place orientation impaired
	Calculation deficits
	Visuospatial and perceptual deficits
Other	Wandering and exit-seeking behaviour
	Increasing apathy
	Sleep disturbance
	Assistance needed in activities of daily living

Box 5.1 – *continued*

Late-stage Alzheimer's disease

Language	Language initiation decreased/ceases
	Noun use non-specific/non-existent
	Phonemic paraphasias on repetition
	Stereotypical utterances
	Verbal perseverations
	Echolalia possible
	No use of gesture
Cognition	Time, place and person disorientation
	Face recognition poor
Other	Dependent for activities of daily living
	Eye contact poor
	Social behaviour inappropriate
	Mobility poor
	Motor movements purposeless
	Incontinence
	Feeding and swallowing disorder

man's attempts at meaning are clear, but without the context, this is not so easy. The semantic or meaning system is described below to show the complexity and to illustrate some of the many reasons why a variation in communication ability occurs in dementia – a name recalled one day but not the next, a simple term forgotten but a complex label recalled.

The semantic system in pAD

Is the semantic system a structure in the brain that can be seen rather than a system that we conceptualize? What is known from brain imaging studies is that tasks that activate the semantic system show a differentiated picture: depending on the task, different parts of the brain appear to function. In other words, current imaging studies suggest that aspects of meaning and knowing are widely distributed across brain structures.

How does the semantic system change in pAD? Two central ideas have been put forward in an attempt to explain some of the deficits in meaning and knowing that are prevalent in pAD:

1. Does the semantic system become less accessible as the disease progresses, or is the disease destroying the semantic system?
2. Is it the language system that changes, or is it the ability to process information in the visual domain that becomes the problem?

What makes naming difficult in Alzheimer's disease?

Difficulty in finding words that are appropriate and specific to their context is one of the most noticeable features of pAD and may be reported early on in the disease by family members, although deficits in specific tasks such as picture-naming are not always an early feature of the disease process (Huff et al. 1986; Bayles et al. 1992). Deficits in word fluency (the ability to generate as many words from a given category, such as 'animals', in a given time) are often a presenting feature (Dick et al. 1989). The ability to name pictures or objects may also have little relation to disease severity. Bayles and Trosset (1992) found that, in a large group of 102 people with pAD, disease severity did not correlate with naming ability, the authors concluding that difficulty in naming in pAD was not closely related to general cognitive function. The exploration of naming and the knowledge of concepts (what we know about a name or an object, e.g. that a table is a piece of furniture, is most often found made of wood in a kitchen and has four legs) has usually occurred through a selection of the following range of tests:

- Object naming
- Word fluency/word generation
- Word-to-picture matching
- Category tasks
- Picture-naming
- Word definitions
- Picture-to-picture matching
- Probe questions on semantic features.

Complexity in language can make something either more difficult or easier to process. If complexity adds more information to the search for a specific word, it may make the word easier to name. If, however, the degree of complexity requires information from competing sources to be evaluated and processed before a specific word can be retrieved, this may add to the processing load in a way that makes the task more difficult.

The mechanisms causing a breakdown at the level of semantics are only partially understood, but there is evidence that, even in the early stages of the disease, access to the semantic system makes naming difficult (Bayles et al. 1992; Hodges et al. 1992). As the disease progresses, specific items appear to be lost altogether from what remains of the system (Funnel and Hodges, 1990; Hodges et al. 1992; Lambon-Ralph et al. 1997). Despite this evidence of deterioration, the semantic system at a single-word level (the ability to understand or name a single item) may remain partially intact up to a relatively late stage in the disease process. Bayles et al. (1992) evaluated consistency as a factor in naming. Testing repeatedly across the same tasks, they found that some people with pAD were consistently unable to name items whereas others were inconsistent in the ability to name them (Kempler et al. 1990).

Another factor in picture- and object-naming is that people with pAD may misperceive visual specifications of the target, the perceptual specification of the target having been shown to alter the success of naming (Grist and Maxim, 1992). The order of ease of naming is the same as that for older people without Alzheimer's disease: a real object, a coloured line drawing, a black and white line drawing, with equivocal results for coloured drawings versus photographs. People with pAD find that the visual degradation of such stimuli causes a significant difficulty in naming and that the visual complexity of drawings may lead to naming failure, those drawings which are identifiable from a characteristic outline being easier to name than those with a more complex outline (Grist and Maxim 1992).

There may also be an interaction between visual processing and the semantic system. If the semantic representation is difficult to access or is lost, visual stimuli will be interpreted using information that is accessible (Chertkow and Bub 1992). People with pAD produce naming errors that have a relationship with the target, for example:

- A category name ('animal' for horse)
- A semantically related name ('chair' for table)
- A semantic/visual mix ('worm' for snake).

The semantic feature system may deteriorate in pAD, more specific features being lost first. Studies in this area (e.g. Nebes 1992) have typically used tasks that require the person to answer questions such as:

- Is this a piece of furniture? (Category)
- Do you clean your teeth with this? (Functional attributes)
- Is this sharp? (Feature attribute).

Studies using large groups of people with pAD patients have concluded that the understanding of single words is better than naming (*see* e.g., Bayles et al. 1992). When, however, the same items are used in both naming and comprehension tasks, small group studies have found item consistency across both tasks and similar patterns of impairment. Some research has suggested that people with pAD find it easier to understand and to produce words that are more frequently used.

How can the semantic system be accessed?

If people with pAD find it difficult to access words, is there any way that access may be facilitated? Does context have an effect on phrase- or sentence-processing?

People with pAD show naming behaviours that may reflect changes to the semantic system. Several studies describe the use of phrases such as 'cutting blade', 'hand bell', 'ink pen' and 'drinking cup', which are added on to the object name; alternatively, object names may be replaced by a phrases that describe the function of the object. Bayles and Tomoeda (1983), for example, found that over a quarter of incorrect naming responses demonstrated correct contexts or functions. Such behaviour suggests that people with pAD have some ability to monitor and change their language behaviour in context.

One characteristic of language use in pAD is the repeated use of specific words, phrases or even short sentences, either in monologues or in conversational language. Such language use is sometimes perseverative, but words and phrases may be used as markers when other lexical items are not available. Such intrusions or even confabulations may be produced if correct information appears to be inaccessible (Dalla Barba and Wong, 1992; Dalla Barba et al. 1992).

In conversation, people with pAD may be said to adapt to their deficits by using retained skills (Perkins et al. 1998). How they do so will depend on their pre-morbid language skills and conversational style, their current level of language and their conversational partner. The research that informs this view has taken place using different theoretical frameworks within linguistics: discourse analysis, pragmatics and conversation analysis (Ulatowska et al. 1981; Perkins et al. 1998; Ripich and Terrell 1988). The ability to take turns is important in a conversation and requires the conversational partners to listen carefully for the end of a turn or find a way of alerting their partner to their wish to take over a turn. In early pAD, turn-taking rules are maintained in conversation, although they may later on be violated (Hutchinson and Jensen, 1980; Hamilton, 1994).

People with pAD may, early on in the disease process, change the topic of conversation when they cannot respond appropriately because they have not understood (Hutchinson and Jenson 1980; Ska and Guenard 1993). This causes their conversation to move rapidly from one topic to another. In the middle to later stages, however, they may be unable to start a new topic of conversation, or, if they do, they may not be able to orientate their partners, that is they do not alert them to this new topic (Causino Lamar et al. 1995; Garcia and Joanette, 1995).

Another aspect of language, which is important in conversation, is the ability to repair when we speak. We sometimes need to rephrase what we have said to clarify meaning, or we may hear ourselves make a mistake in pronunciation, the structure of a sentence or word choice. The ability to monitor our own language and to correct (repair) mistakes is a normal part of language function. But what happens when pAD is present? Repair to conversation does take place in pAD but may become increasingly scarce as the disease progresses (Hamilton 1994).

Pragmatics can be defined as the use of language in context. The ability of some people with pAD to use certain restricted styles of language may be retained until late on in the disease process, with an appropriate use of language in everyday contexts such as greeting, mealtimes and birthday celebrations (Chapman and Ulatowska 1991; Hamilton 1994). When we speak, we also need to alert listeners to reference points in conversation so that they are clear about the topic, the person and the time frame. This referential aspect of language use also shows deficits in pAD. There is, in addition, evidence that people with pAD react differently with different conversational partners, suggesting that they have residual abilities that should be used (Lubinski 1991; Hamilton 1994; Ramanthan-Abbott 1994). Finally, research shows that access to language can be improved in the early stages by use of different strategies, and drug interventions may also offer hope of mediating access and delaying the permanent loss of semantic information (Maxim et al. 2000).

The role of speech and language therapy in the management of people with dementia has been documented in relation to the UK and the USA (Griffiths and Baldwin 1989; Tanner and Bryan 1996; Stevens 1999; Stevens and Ripich 1999). Maxim and Timothy (2001) summarize the role of the speech and language therapist in relation to dementia as:

- Assessing language and communication for differential diagnosis
- Providing detailed information on language abilities and difficulties for patients, carers and multidisciplinary teams, ensuring that carers and other professionals are aware of the limits imposed on language and communication by any particular individual's dementia
- Providing specific advice to help to sustain or increase optimal language and communication abilities, utilizing cues and minimizing the disruption to communication caused by impairments by using alternative forms of communication such as drawing
- Reducing communication stress and the burden imposed on care-givers
- Providing specific language and communication therapy programmes for both individuals and groups
- Monitoring and reviewing abilities and difficulties over time and updating information as the dementia progresses
- Contributing to multidisciplinary problem-solving and liaison (as communication may, e.g., have a relevant role in behavioural difficulties)
- Educating and training staff, carers and those with dementia in communication-related skills and providing a resource for multidisciplinary student training in these areas
- Advising residential homes and other care settings on the optimum environment for communication and on how to achieve effective communication with individuals who may have complex communication needs associated with their dementia
- Promoting good practice to achieve effective communication with people who have communication difficulties associated with dementia.

Communication and behaviour

Communication is a vital part of our overall behaviour. It also has a mediating function. We are taught that shouting or even quietly using an expletive is better than hitting someone. Anger-management techniques often involve teaching appropriate ways to express anger verbally. The verbalization of frustration may not be possible for those with dementia, or their communication difficulties may cause them to express information in ways that require considerable under-standing on the part of the listener. For example, 'You stole my bag?' said in a pleasant, questioning way may be a way of asking 'Have you seen my bag?' The same utterance said in the context of a confused and anxious facial expression may indicate 'Please help, I can't find my bag.' The same utterance shouted at a carer along with an attempt to push or slap may, if the trail of events is followed, reflect frustration that previous attempts to get help have been ignored or misunder-stood.

Key messages for those supporting people with dementia include:

- Be sensitive to the different ways in which people speak.
- Be aware of how you yourself are speaking.
- Don't jump to hasty assumptions about people just because of how they sound.
- Listen actively (keeping eye contact, nodding, smiling and using filler phrases such as 'um' and 'uhuh').
- Listen reflectively. (Listen to how the person sounds and respond to or mirror the emotion that is being expressed using facial expression or words, particu-larly if you cannot extract the message from the words that you are hearing.)
- Respond and describe what you understand ('You seem upset', 'I wonder if you're upset').
- Show an appreciation of the individual and all the life experience that he or she has.

Using these techniques may allow the person with pAD to respond with more appropriate language, although this does not always work. These techniques, which have come to be known as 'validating' techniques, have a long history in counselling and psychoanalytic theory but have been subject to relatively little research.

Carers may report problems with swearing. Swear words may be used when other vocabulary cannot be accessed, and swearing may occur in a person who previously abhorred it, making the behaviour more difficult for carers to accept. In the context of residential care, swearing may give a superficial impression of aggression, but it is important to analyse the behaviour. Mr Andrews, for example, is an isolated man living in a residential home. He has dementia of Alzheimer type, his memory is poor, and he tends not to join in activities. At times, he is overtly disorientated and confused about where he is and what is happening. Staff complain that when they approach him, he swears loudly at them. An analysis of who approaches him and why quickly shows that he is approached only when people need him to do something. Staff who just say hello to him are rewarded with Mr Andrews swearing quietly. If they try chatting about something concrete for a minute or so, he initially swears but quickly stops and looks interested.

The staff set out to develop a management plan involving longer periods of talking with him and explanation of what is going to happen before any request is made. Within 3 months, Mr Andrews is much more amenable; he does swear, but staff do not interpret this in a negative way. A chance visit by a distant relative offers an opportunity to find out more about him, and a life story book left by his chair gives staff who do not know him well a means of initiating conversation if this proves difficult.

Finally, it is worth remembering that most of us have a preference for communicating in small groups or with individuals, respond to a social atmosphere, enjoy some nostalgia, use the occasional expletive when frustrated and do not always make the emotional content of our communication crystal clear. Everyone who cares for or works with people who have a dementia has a range of experience of human interaction that they can apply to the particular needs of those with dementia. Killick and Allan (2001) quote a woman with dementia discussing communication: 'You and I, John, we speak the same language only you speak it straight and I speak it upside down.' The challenge for everyone who supports people with dementia is to engage fully with the 'upside-downness' of the language to achieve a level of meaningful communication.

REFERENCES

Bayles, K, A. and Tomoeda, C.K. 1983: Confrontation naming impairment in dementia. *Brain and Language* **19**: 98–114.

Bayles, K.A. and Trosset, M.W. 1992: Confrontation naming in Alzheimer's patients: relation to disease severity. *Psychology and Aging* **7**: 197–203.

Bayles, K.A., Tomoeda, C.K. and Trosset, M.W. 1992: Relation of linguistic communication abilities of Alzheimer's patients to stage of disease. *Brain and Language* **42**: 454–72.

Bryan, K. and Maxim, J. eds. 1996: *Communication disability and the psychiatry of old age.* London: Whurr.

Causino Lamar, M.A., Obler, L.K., Knoefel, J.E. and Albert, M.L. 1995: Communication patterns in end-stage Alzheimer's disease: pragmatic analyses. In: Bloom, R.L., Obler, L.K., De Santi, S. and Enrhich, J.S. eds. *Discourse analysis and applications: studies in adult clinical populations.* Hillsdale: Lawrence Erlbaum Associates, 217–36.

Chapman, S.B. and Ulatowska, H.K. 1991: Nature of language impairment in dementia: is it aphasia? *Texas Journal of Audiology and Speech Pathology* **17**: 3–9.

Chertkow, H. and Bub, D. 1992: Constraining theories of semantic memory processing: evidence from dementia. *Cognitive Neuropsychology* **9**: 327–65.

Dalla Barba, G. and Wong, C. 1992: Encoding specificity and confabulation in Alzheimer's disease and amnesia. *Journal of Clinical and Experimental Neuropsychology* **3**: 378–92.

Dalla Barba, G., Wong, C., Parlato, V. and Boller, F. 1992: Encoding specificity, anosagnosia and confabulation in Alzheimer's disease and depression. *Neurobiology of Aging* **13**: 4–5.

Dick, M.B., Kean, M-L. and Sands, D. 1989: Memory for internally generated words in Alzheimer-type dementia: breakdown in encoding and semantic memory. *Brain and Cognition* **9**: 88–108.

Funnell, E and Hodges, J. 1992: Progressive loss of access to spoken word forms in a case of Alzheimer's disease. *Proceedings of the Royal Society of London B* **243**: 173–9.

Garcia, L.J. and Joanette, Y. 1995: Conversational topic-shifting analysis in dementia. In: Bloom, R.L. Obler, L.K., De Santi, S. and Enrhich, J.S. eds. *Discourse analysis and applications: studies in adult clinical population*. Hillsdale: Lawrence Erlbaum Associates, 185–200.

Griffiths, H. and Baldwin, B. 1989: Speech therapy for psychogeriatric services: luxury or necessity? *Psychiatric Bulletin* **13**: 57–9.

Grist, E. and Maxim, J. 1992: Confrontation naming in the elderly: the Build-up Picture Test as an aid to differentiating normals from subjects with dementia. *European Journal of Disorders of Communication* **27**: 197–207.

Hamilton, H.E. 1994: *Conversations with an Alzheimer's patient*. Cambridge: Cambridge University Press.

Hodges, J.R., Salmon, D.P. and Butters, N. 1992: Semantic memory impairment in Alzheimers disease: failure of access or degraded knowledge? *Neuropsychologia* **30**: 301–14.

Holden U. 1995: *Ageing, neuropsychology and the 'new' dementias*. London: Chapman & Hall.

Huff, F.J., Corkin, S. and Growden, J.H. 1986: Semantic impairment and anomia in Alzheimer's disease. *Brain and Language* **28**: 235–49.

Hutchinson, J.M. and Jensen, M. 1980: A pragmatic evaluation of discourse communication in normal and senile elderly in a nursing home. In: Obler, L.K. and Albert, M.L. eds. *Language and communication in the elderly*. Lexington, Massachusetts: D. Heath.

Kemper, S. and O'Hanlon, L. 2000: Semantic processing problems of older adults. In: Best, W., Bryan, K. and Maxim, J. eds. *Semantic processing: theory and practice*. London: Whurr, 125–49.

Kempler, D. 1995: Language changes in dementia of the Alzheimer type. In: Lubinski, R. ed. *Dementia and communication*. California: Singular, 98–114.

Kempler, D., Anderson, E., Hunt, M. and Henderson, V. 1990: Linguistic and attentional contributions to anomia in Alzheimer's Disease. *Journal of Clinical and Experimental Neuropsychology* **12**: 398–406.

Killick, J. and Allan, K. 2001: *Communication and the care of people with dementia*. Buckingham: Open University Press.

Lambon-Ralph, M.A., Patterson, K. and Hodges, J.R. 1997: The relationship between naming and semantic knowledge for different categories in dementia of Alzheimer's type. *Neuropsychologia* **35**: 194–9.

Lubinski, R. 1991: Learned helplessness: application to communication of the elderly. In: Lubinski, R. ed. *Dementia and communication*. Philadelphia: B.C. Decker, 142–51.

Lubinski, R. 1995: State of the art perspectives on communication in nursing homes. *Topics in Language Disorder* **15**: 1–19.

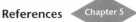

Martin, A., Brouwers, P., Lalonde, F., et al. 1986: Towards a behavioural typology of Alzheimer's patients. *Journal of Clinical and Experimental Neuropsychology* **8:** 594–610.

Maxim, J. and Bryan K. 1996: Language, cognition and communication in the older mentally infirm. In: Bryan, K. and Maxim, J. eds. *Communication disability and the psychiatry of old age.* London: Whurr, 37–79.

Maxim, J. and Timothy, C. 2001: Services for older people in mental health settings. In: France, J. and Kramer, S. eds. *Communication and mental illness.* London: Jessica Kingsley, 192–207.

Maxim, J., Bryan, K. and Zabihi, K. 2000: Semantic processing in Alzheimer's disease. In: Best, W., Bryan, K. and Maxim, J. eds. *Semantic processing: theory and practice.* London: Whurr, 150–179.

Nebes, R.D. 1992: Cognitive dysfunction in Alzheimer's disease. In: Craik, F. and Salthouse, T.A. eds. *The handbook of ageing and cognition.* Hillsdale, New Jersey: Lawrence Erlbaum Associates, 373–446.

Parr, S, Pound, C., Byng, S. and Long, B. 1999: *The aphasia handbook.* Leistershire: Ecodistribution.

Perkins, L., Whitworth, A. and Lesser, R. 1998: Conversing in dementia: a conversation analytic approach. *Journal of Neurolinguistics* **11:** 33–53.

Ramathan-Abbott, V. 1994: Interactional differences in Alzheimer's discourse: an examination of AD speech across two audiences. *Language in Society* **23:** 31–58.

Reisberg, B., Ferris, S.M., de Leon, M. and Crook, T. 1982: The global deterioration scale for assessment of primary degenerative dementia. *American Journal of Psychiatry* **139:** 1136–9.

Ripich, D.N. and Terrell, B.Y. 1988: Patterns of discourse cohesion in Alzheimer's disease. *Journal of Speech and Hearing Disorders* **53:** 8–15.

Schwartz, M.F. 1990: *Modular deficits in Alzheimer type dementia.* Cambridge, Massachusetts: MIT-Bradford.

Ska, B. and Guenard, D. 1993: Narrative schema in dementia of the Alzheimer's type. In: Brownell, H.H. and Joanette, Y. eds. *Narrative discourse in neurologically impaired and normal aging adults.* San Diego, CA: Singular, 299–316.

Stevens, S. and Ripich, D. 1999: The role of the speech and language therapist. In: Wilcock, G.K., Bucks, R.S. and Rockwood, K. eds. *Diagnosis and management of dementia.* Oxford: Oxford University Press, 137–57.

Stevens, S.D. 1999: The role of the speech and language therapist in dementia care. *Speech Therapy in Practice* **4:** 9–10.

Tanner, B. and Bryan, K. 1996: Service delivery in the UK. In: Bryan, K. and Maxim J. eds. *Communication disability and the psychiatry of old age.* London: Whurr, 144–59.

Ulatowska, H., North, A.J. and Macaluso-Haynes, S. 1981: Production of narrative and procedural discourse in aphasia. *Brain and Language* **13:** 345–71.

Chapter 6

Counselling people with dementia

Elizabeth Bartlett and Richard Cheston

The main aim of this chapter is to show how people who have received a diagnosis of dementia can be helped by a modified counselling technique, referred to as dementia counselling. The chapter also shows how people who are undertaking such counselling will need to interact with other professionals caring for the person with dementia, especially with the principal family carer if there is one. A number of techniques that can be used by dementia counsellors are described. Issues and the effects of counselling are illustrated by quotations from people with dementia who have received this type of support.

BACKGROUND

This chapter is based on observations made mainly as part of a national project called Learning to Live with Dementia, but experience gained from working with people with dementia for a number of years has also been used. The Learning to Live with Dementia project was initiated by the Alzheimer's Society and sponsored by Zurich Financial Services Community Trust. The overall aim of the project was to gather views from people with dementia themselves and to empower them to make decisions about their own future. This aim is consistent with Standard Two of the *National Service Framework for Older People* (Department of Health 2001), which is to give person-centred care and specifically to enable older people to make their own choices and be more involved in their own care.

The particular part of the project that provides the principal sources of evidence for this chapter began in Wiltshire and Hampshire in April 2000. It was designed to look at ways of working with people who were aware of their own diagnosis. Individuals were referred to the project by consultant psychiatrists, general practitioners, members of community mental health teams and the Salisbury and Lymington branches of the Alzheimer's Society. Most were referred to the project shortly after diagnosis. The work involved talking to people and discovering more about their feelings and ways of coping with the losses brought about by their dementia. The aim was to find effective ways of supporting people as they lived through this experience.

Fifty people ranging in age from 56 to 85 years were seen under the terms of the project. Approximately one fifth of the group were under the age of 65 years, and another fifth were over 80. There were roughly equal numbers of men and women in the younger age groups, but women were predominant among the older participants. Approximately one third of the people who took part in the project lived alone, the majority of the rest living with family carers – usually their husband or wife. Most people were seen for about 1.5 hours every 2 weeks, most of the interviews being conducted in people's own homes. In some cases, however, the interview was found to be more appropriate in a more relaxed environment, such as walking in the countryside or going for a drive in the car. As their dementia progressed – or as other illnesses intervened – some people dropped out of the project. Others continued to participate for over 24 months.

No significant differences were observed in the need for dementia counselling across the range of people seen. Nor was a significantly different approach found to be necessary for different groups of people, although it was of course essential to treat each person as an individual.

GENERAL PRINCIPLES OF COUNSELLING PEOPLE WITH DEMENTIA

The need for creativity and flexibility

A counselling approach can be very effective with people with dementia who are aware of their own diagnosis but who have to deal with huge emotional changes as well as the loss of skills and a fear of the future (Cheston and Bender 1999). Those who engage in this work therefore need to be very flexible and creative, while still adhering to the basic principles of counselling. Thus, Gardner (1993, p. 38) comments:

Creativity will be required to deal with some of the complicated problems that arise. Workers should not be bound by the traditional constraints of counselling, but, at the same time, they should observe the well accepted basic frameworks and principles which underpin the helping process.

In the same paper, Gardner points out that counselling people with dementia requires workers to 'integrate a large range of skills and roles to produce a generic service which is able to respond to the many, varied and rapidly changing psychosocial needs' (p. 38). He also emphasizes the need for people who work in this flexible way to make sure that their work is based on 'solid assessments' and that they have 'access to quality supervision'. These recommendations are whole-heartedly supported by experience gained through the Learning to Live with Dementia project, which states that:

> It is therefore strongly recommended that people who wish to offer coun-selling and support to people with dementia should have received good training in conventional counselling principles and techniques. They should also have clinical supervision.

Dilemmas in counselling

There are some significant dilemmas for anyone counselling people with dementia.

Tension between being led by the client and being more proactive

In conventional counselling, the counsellor needs to be client led. The problem of using this way of working with people with dementia is that the nature of the illness means that they often find it hard to recall, or to express aspects of, their experience that are causing them difficulty or distress. For many people with dementia, the implications of this illness are so profound that many of their worst fears about the future may, during the initial sessions of work at least, be too painful to bear.

Counsellors therefore usually need to be more proactive in their relationship with clients, perhaps by introducing issues related to the process of assessment and diagnosis. At the same time, when they are taking more initiative within sessions, counsellors risk placing their own concerns into the mouths of their clients.

In balancing this tension, counsellors need to offer reflections tentatively and to be sensitive to their clients' reactions. Counsellors also need to recognize that clients may not be ready to discuss some issues; indeed, there may be some painful areas that they may never wish to explore. The aim of counsellors must be to support rather than delve unnecessarily.

Tension between concentrating exclusively on what the client says and taking into account the views of those who are close to the client

A fundamental part of the counselling relationship is the importance of bound-aries, including those of confidentiality around the session, yet people with dementia frequently live in contexts in which they are disempowered and in which their actions are often misinterpreted. Moreover, counsellors often need to interact with those who are close to the person with dementia – especially any family carers – because such people can give counsellors vital background information that the client may no longer be able to provide.

Although counsellors need to be careful that they continue to listen to what clients themselves are saying and are not misled by assumptions picked up from those around them, it is important to be able to place the work within the context of the client's life. Indeed, if counsellors are, by providing some feedback to carers, especially family carers, able to correct misinterpretations, this may help to bring carer and client together. It may be, then, that counsellors should negotiate with clients about what issues from the sessions are discussed with carers and how such discussions should take place. In this respect, counsellors may have a role to play as translators of the client's feelings to those around him or her, a role that we will discuss more fully later in the chapter.

Difficulty in deciding when to terminate a counselling relationship

In a conventional counselling relationship, the process of agreeing an end to the work is usually relatively straightforward. In the case of people with dementia, however, it is much more difficult to determine the end point because of the ongoing and changing needs of the client and the danger that clients will see termination as another failure on their part.

At the same time, because the context in which this work takes place often involves such an unbalanced power relationship, counsellors should be sensitive to signs that consent for the work is being withdrawn. There is therefore a tension for counsellors to continue their relationship with the client while being aware of signs that he or she may have withdrawn consent for this work. At the same time, there is a clear need for dementia counsellors to use their time effectively and to support as many clients as possible.

The difference between the integrated counselling approach for a typical person with dementia who has a close family carer – usually a husband or wife – and the more conventional model of counselling for people who do not have dementia is shown schematically in Figures 6.1 and 6.2.

THE COUNSELLING PROCESS

Building a therapeutic engagement

A vital first stage in any counselling relationship is to build a therapeutic engagement based on trust. In the case of work with people with dementia, this process of therapeutic engagement needs to be more explicit. This is partly because the person with dementia may have difficulty in understanding the counsellor's role simply on the basis of written statements about his or her position. More significantly, the process through which people often receive a diagnosis of dementia

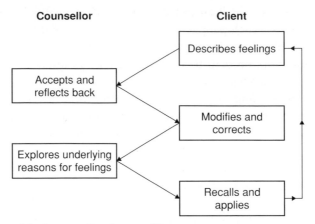

Figure 6.1 A model of conventional counselling

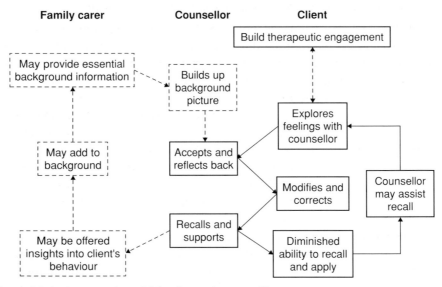

Figure 6.2 An integrated model for dementia counselling

may have sensitized them to contact with other professionals. Keady and Bender (1998) report a series of interviews with people who had been assessed at a memory clinic. Comments on this process typically described it as an intimidating and frightening one. For example, a 67-year-old man with a very mild level of dementia said (p. 134):

They kept putting me in a room and asking me to do all these things ... counting and things. I never knew why I had to do it and I didn't want to go back. I got frightened and worried because I knew I couldn't do what they wanted.

In the Learning to Live with Dementia project, a typical question from a client on a first encounter was 'Have you come to test me?' Another client remarked, 'I feel bad about having to answer lots of questions that I should know and can't always remember.' It is therefore essential to get the atmosphere and tone for the relationship right from the beginning. In setting that tone and establishing a good therapeutic engagement:

- Be clear about the purposes of the work.
- Be prepared to listen to both verbal and non-verbal communication.
- Listen out for metaphorical and other indirect ways in which people may be beginning to explore what has happened to them (Cheston 1996, 1998).
- Let individuals with dementia know that what they are trying to say is really being understood – check carefully any interpretation of their statements and, when necessary, acknowledge their pain.
- Remind them of their achievements, both recent and earlier in life.
- Reassure them that the effort they are putting into coping with the experience of dementia has been recognized.
- Encourage those with dementia to express their feelings and anxieties – some of which may be very painful – about their experience of dementia.
- Let them know that there are other people with dementia who are experiencing some of the same difficulties and fears, and thus reduce their sense of isolation.

Here, the counsellor may wish to talk about aspects of the experience of other people with dementia, while, of course, taking care to protect the confidentiality of individual clients. This can also help to counteract the fear many people have of meeting others with dementia as they imagine that this will confirm anxieties about their illness.

All of this requires workers who try to counsel people with dementia not merely to be active listeners, but also to give positive feedback to clients. If it is also possible for counsellors to provide useful information about local services or other practical issues, this will add to the positive atmosphere.

Although the detailed content of a session may be forgotten, its mood is likely to be retained. As one person put it, 'Even if I forget my facts, I can remember my feelings.'

UNDERSTANDING THE DIAGNOSIS

In this chapter, we are only considering dementia counselling with people who have already been given a clinical diagnosis of dementia. Although there is clearly a role for counselling people who are concerned about their memory problems and also those who are considering having a formal assessment, this issue is beyond the scope of the present chapter. Instead, we will focus on the role of counselling in the time shortly after a diagnosis has been made, when the person with dementia is most likely to be still living in the community.

An important initial step for the counsellor is therefore to find out what the diagnosis is and how it has been understood by the client and those around him or her. This can be done by obtaining information from those professionals responsible for the patient's care (psychiatrist, general practitioner, community psychiatric nurse or social worker), ideally as part of the referral process. This will also be an opportunity to establish the type of dementia and whether the client has other medical conditions.

Early on in working with people with dementia, it is important to ask them about their memory problem, including what they have been told and by whom. If the client's version is significantly different from the diagnosis that professionals believe they have actually given, counsellors will need to make a judgement about the extent to which they should seek to change an incorrect or incomplete understanding on the part of the client. It may be that by subconsciously rejecting part of the information they have received, clients are reducing their distress and making their experience more bearable. The key question is 'Will correcting or amplifying clients' current understanding of their diagnosis be likely to help them to live better with the problems they are experiencing?'

The aim of working with those with dementia is frequently to provide them with the time and space to make sense of what is happening to them. In our experience, most people with dementia know that something is wrong, even if they are often very good at presenting a 'brave face' to the world. The process of working together is one in which people can begin to explore their fears and experience the emotional pain of their losses. Clients' understanding of what has happened often deepens and develops as the work progresses without the counsellor ever having to remind them of their diagnosis. We will return to this issue in the next section, where we consider how to help people to accept the reality of their condition.

THE NEEDS OF PEOPLE WITH DEMENTIA

Self-esteem

People who have recently received a diagnosis of dementia are likely to have a serious sense of loss, even though some have considerable insight into their experience. For example, one person with a professional background who took part in the Learning to Live with Dementia project said:

> I've still got a good analytical brain, but my retentive memory is breaking down. It's not the memory, it's the retention problem. It's like a computer programme. When I go to bed, the tape's wiped out, but it's somewhere on the tape if I get the right prompt.

The sense of loss experienced by individuals with dementia often includes some of the following elements:

- *A loss of intellectual ability*, especially of short-term memory, and in some cases, a reduced ability to make logical connections
- *A reduced ability to communicate*, because of an inability to concentrate and difficulty in finding the correct words
- *Reduced independence*, for example because of a tendency to get lost, or a loss of the ability to judge the passage of time, both of which result in a need for increased supervision and the restriction of activity to well-known and safe spaces.

All of these factors lead to a loss of self-esteem, which is arguably the most important single loss because it has a major impact on the way people with dementia respond to their diagnosis, to their environment and to the people around them. As individuals with dementia lose their ability to keep up activities, such as driving, which are a fundamental part of their sense of identity, they may become at risk of developing a clinically significant level of depression. Similarly, the threat of additional future losses may lead to profound feelings of anxiety about what is to come. Typical comments made by clients in the Learning to Live with Dementia project reflected this loss:

I don't feel good about myself any more.
I feel irritated with myself.
People with dementia try hard to overcome their memory problems, but if they still forget, they feel very dispirited.
Alzheimer's has robbed me of my independence.

The centrality of self-esteem has been clearly recognized by others who have worked with people with dementia. Thus, Kitwood (1990, p. 181) observes:

The maintenance of self-esteem is essential for good learning, efficacy and constructive relationships with others. Conversely, when self-esteem is lacking or damaged, a person is disastrously incapacitated in many ways and easily falls into a cycle of discouragement and failure.

Schematically, the negative cycle that a person with dementia is liable to experience is represented in Figure 6.3. One of the aims of counselling is to help clients to break out of this cycle, as indicated in Figure 6.4.

Many of the approaches suggested in the previous section for enhancing trust are likely to contribute to the process of rebuilding a client's self-esteem. If successful, they will:

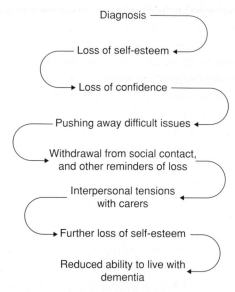

Figure 6.3 Typical experience of a person with dementia

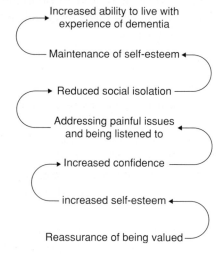

Figure 6.4 Desired outcome with effective counselling

- Demonstrate that the clients' opinions and feelings still matter to other people
- Help clients to recognize their own achievements in coping with the experience of dementia
- Make it clear that, even if clients have difficulties in finding the right words, there are still ways of sharing their experience
- Make it clear that clients are not alone in their experience.

Another very effective way of helping to increase people's self-esteem is the creation of a life history, as shown in Box 6.1 (Tobin 1991; Bender 1994; Mills 1998). When creating a life history for this purpose, it is obviously desirable for it to be a truthful record, but the worker should not be unduly concerned if the person's autobiographical memory (Brewer 1986; Conway 1990) includes subjective impressions and feelings that may not coincide with other people's recollections of the same events. The main aim is to produce a record that is meaningful for the person with dementia themselves.

Working with people with dementia shows that there are a number of other concerns, in addition to individuals' very fundamental need to know they are still valued for themselves, that affect a high proportion of people. The following paragraphs suggest ways of addressing some frequently occurring needs.

Help towards accepting the reality of their condition

Not surprisingly, many people find that the experience of having dementia is itself very disorientating and leaves them uncertain about what is happening to them. In addition, people share the almost universal response of disbelief or denial in the face of a life-changing event and therefore find it hard to accept the implications of a diagnosis of dementia. Typical questions that people are struggling with at this stage include:

- What is happening to me?
- What is wrong with my brain?
- What will be the next thing to go wrong with me?
- How long will it be before I can't do things for myself?

Although superficially, these sound like requests for factual information, it is clear from the way in which the questions are asked that what the person is really seeking is a better understanding of his or her problems.

Externalizing the problem

A particular issue for many people with dementia is a sense of guilt – a feeling that if only they tried hard enough, they would be able to remember more. This feeling

Box 6.1 The value of creating a life history

- Helps those with dementia to retain their sense of personhood
- Reminds people of how much they have achieved in their lives
- Can be a very good co-operative process between the person with dementia and the family carer
- Creates opportunities for individuals with dementia to express their feelings about the present as well as the past
- Can become a valuable resource for reminiscence as the dementia progresses

of guilt and inadequacy is sometimes unintentionally compounded by people close to the person with dementia:

> My husband keeps saying, 'Just try and remember!' I do try – and when I can't remember, I feel even worse.
> My wife plays guessing games which she thinks will stimulate me, but I get self-conscious when I don't remember.
> People look at me to see if I've forgotten.

One of the most important ways in which a counsellor can assist those with dementia to begin to accept the reality of their condition is by emphasizing that they are not responsible for their dementia. We need to be able to communicate the sense that the person is more than his or her illness, that the illness is a separate entity. One person put it thus: 'I don't blame myself any more. I blame my neuro-transmitters!'

By helping people to put their concerns into words, we can give those with dementia a language that they can use to talk about their diagnosis. In finding the words to describe something, we are able to move away from it. In contrast, fears that cannot be put into words seem much worse than those which can be expressed, even if incompletely. This process of finding the words to describe our feelings is one way in which difficult issues can be worked through.

Alleviating a sense of guilt

It is also important to allow people to express any feelings of guilt and to help them to realize that the counsellor will accept what they feel rather than dismiss their feelings as unreasonable or unjustified. Being accepted by a counsellor helps people to accept themselves. In some cases, it is even possible to show that a strategy that a person may feel guilty using is actually a positive way of coping with a difficult situation. For example, when a retired judge confessed, 'When I don't know the answer to a question, I'm afraid that sometimes I make it up!', the counsellor was able to reassure him this was an acceptable way of coping with some socially awkward situations.

The value of directly addressing guilt and blame was illustrated by a client who said to the counsellor at the end of a session, 'When I was told I had dementia it worried me that I had done something wrong, but you helped me to understand it is not my fault.'

Giving information

As pointed out above, people often want to ask questions such as 'How long will it last?' and 'Is there a cure?' as part of the process of coming to terms with their diagnosis. One way of answering such questions openly and honestly is to use written information. In the UK, the Alzheimer's Society (2001) has produced a well-illustrated booklet entitled *I'm Told I Have Dementia,* and similar publications have been produced in other countries. Many clients find it helpful to work through sections of the booklet with the counsellor. In particular, the booklet contains illustrations that clearly demonstrate the physical changes occurring in the brain of a person with dementia. Looking at these pictures can help people to realize what is gradually happening to their own brain, but not everyone is ready to do this, and the counsellor should ensure that the client is not overwhelmed with more information than he or she can absorb, either intellectually or emotionally.

Now that anti-dementia drugs are becoming more readily available, clients may want to ask questions about them. The counsellor again needs to be well informed but should not try to take on the role of a professional medical advisor. It is generally best to check what clients think they have already been told and, if necessary, refer back to the professionals responsible for their care.

Finally, it is important to recognize that a person with dementia may need information to be repeated and the same reassurances to be given many times. Even if this seems very repetitive, counsellors should not allow themselves to become irritated by this need. The dementia counsellor's aim is not so much to impart information as to help individuals to live with their dementia.

Help with social contacts

It often becomes increasingly difficult for a person with dementia to maintain his or her social contacts. There are a number of reasons why this might happen. Individuals may:

- Be embarrassed that they are not able to remember the names of or other basic facts about the people they meet
- Be unsure how to initiate or sustain a conversation
- Feel that other people are judging them or commenting about their failures behind their back
- Feel that they are becoming a burden to other people
- Be uncertain whether they can remember how to conduct themselves in a group, as with a retired vicar who felt he could no longer recall what to do in different parts of a church service.

All of these effects lead to considerable social isolation, and it becomes important for people with dementia to find settings in which they can feel 'safe' and accepted. Work with groups of people with dementia who are aware of their own diagnosis can be one way of helping people (*see* Chapter 9), as can attending appropriate day centres where sensitive staff can create the right environment. Such activities can, however, never fully compensate for the loss of a person's normal social experience.

For many people with dementia there is therefore an increasing sense of being 'taken over' or overwhelmed by their condition. The world around the person with dementia often begins to shrink as a large and complex network of relationships is progressively reduced to a much smaller number of contacts, many of them with very defined roles and relationships – doctor/patient, carer/dependent. The world surrounding a person with dementia can in many cases be reduced to four main elements – health and care, finances, social contacts and daily living – as shown in Figure 6.5.

A very specific difficulty that emerged from conversations with a number of people was how to tell others that they had dementia. One participant in a group for people with dementia that the authors facilitated told the group that they should all 'come out of the closet with Alzheimer's'. However, if individuals do not feel able to find a way of telling other people about their dementia, the counsellor's role may be to help them see that it is permissible to withdraw from some situations that they are finding difficult.

Case 1   Mrs B's grandson was getting married, but she was very anxious about going to the wedding and not knowing how to talk to lots of different people. After talking it over with her husband, they both agreed that 'When you are eighty, you don't have to go to a wedding if you don't want to'.

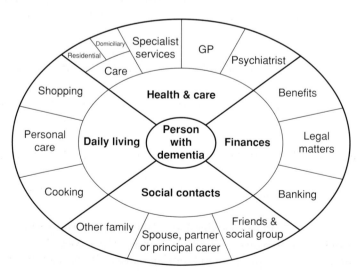

Figure 6.5 A typical view of the world around a person with dementia

Helping people to keep control over their lives and future

As the social world around the person with dementia begins to reduce, there is often an effect of increasing powerlessness. The counsellor can assist in several ways, some of which go beyond the normal counselling role:

- Giving practical advice, which can include informing clients about arrangements they can make, such as an enduring power of attorney, creating advance directives and ensuring that they receive benefits to which they are entitled
- Acting as a facilitator or advocate, for example when individuals are discussing plans for their future care, finances or other matters with professionals
- Helping the client to formulate desires for the future. This is a very skilled task in which counsellors must take great care not to influence decisions by their own preferences. One way to do this is to explore clients' fears (e.g. becoming a burden on their family) and then to consider together practical ways of avoiding such situations (e.g. making sure that their family understands that they are willing to move into residential care when it becomes necessary).

Assistance in finding and using coping strategies

We now know much more about the ways in which people with memory problems can use a variety of strategies to help to compensate for their loss of memory (*see*, e.g., Kapur 2001). Similarly, we are now aware that people with dementia use a very wide range of strategies to cope with different aspects of the experience of dementia (Cheston and Bender 1999). In the group of people who were seen as part of the Learning to Live with Dementia project, the following strategies were noted:

- *Denial*: 'I try not to think about it'; 'I know I'm denying it, but it's one way to deal with it'
- *Humour*: 'I make a joke of it'; 'My goodness! Rita Heyworth, Ronald Reagan, Harold Wilson. How did I manage to get with that group with my brain?'
- *Avoidance*: 'I can't think what the dickens to say, so I don't talk to strangers'; 'I've learned when people ask me questions to say, "I'll remember in a minute"'
- *Dependency*: 'I find it easier to swim along on someone else's memory.'

Or, as one man who was still struggling to find effective ways to cope put it, 'I know there is no cure, but I am trying to develop a *modus vivendi*.'

In this area, the role of the person working with individuals with dementia is likely to be two-fold:

1. Acknowledging the techniques people are already using and thus effectively 'giving them permission' to continue to use them. Even if a particular technique cannot be shown objectively to be enhancing clients' capabilities, it may still be important to them as one way of keeping some control over their own lives.

2. Suggesting other coping strategies that might not have occurred to the individual concerned but which seem appropriate for him or her (*see*, e.g., the IMMEL system; Keady and Nolan 1995a, b).

WORKING WITH FAMILY CARERS

The importance of working with the family carer – if there is one – has been emphasized throughout this chapter. There are two main reasons for this:

1. Counsellors need the background that family carers can provide if they are to understand the significance of statements the client is making, especially if these are related to experiences and events that occurred earlier in the client's life.

2. The counsellor can help family carers to understand what the client is experiencing now and therefore help them to cope better with the effects of their partner's dementia.

Even when there has been a good relationship between the person with dementia and the carer, dementia inevitably places a great strain on that relationship. Carers are frequently exasperated and frustrated by the client's loss of skills and the constant demands made upon them. People often say something like 'He/she is not the person I married.' At the same time, the person with dementia is liable to interpret the carer's impatience as personal rejection.

We have suggested above that one role of a counsellor is to discuss with people with dementia what they should talk about with their carer, and how. The counsellor effectively acts as a conduit between the person with dementia and the carer. This may at times involve joint sessions in which ideas taken from marital or couple counselling can be important. This joint work can sometimes help a couple to appreciate that the pattern of behaviour that they now find frustrating actually stems from aspects of their personalities that originally attracted them to one another.

One approach that can be very helpful when working with a couple is to talk about the beginning of their relationship. The counsellor may try to get each of them to recall the attraction or 'chemistry' they originally felt for each other. This has the effect of helping both of them to focus on positive memories and can be very reassuring. One client commented, 'Nobody else seems to be interested in my past.'

Case 2 One woman with dementia frequently made rude and offensive remarks to her husband, friends and visitors to their home. Her husband was told that the dementia had made her 'disinhibited', probably as a result of damage to the frontal lobes of her brain. During some joint counselling sessions, however, the couple were asked to talk about how they had met and what had initially attracted them to each other. Her husband recalled how he had been entranced by her vivacious and out-going character, and he described how, on their honeymoon, she had defused an argument between two strangers in their hotel by telling them off for their childish behaviour. Although the woman's behaviour continued unchanged, her husband now found it reassuring to see that it was not something completely new but instead an extension of how she often reacted to stress in the past.

Since it is often best to conduct interviews in the client's own home, many people find that having their main carer present at the beginning is reassuring and can help them to express themselves. It also provides reassurance for the carer, who may initially be uncertain about the counsellor's role.

As time passes, however, and the person with dementia gains confidence, it is desirable to arrange for the client to spend time alone with the counsellor. This will give clients an opportunity to express feelings that they do not want their family member to hear, either because they feel they may seem disloyal or because they do not want to cause their carer further pain. It will also make it easier for the counsellor to explore the client's feelings – which might not be the same as those of their carer. If, as a result of such discussions, there are points that it seems desirable to share with the carer, the counsellor will need to proceed with great discretion, negotiating what is to be said and when, and ensuring that the person with dementia agrees with this course of action. When successful, this approach can be warmly received by the carer. As one man put it, 'Nobody else can get my wife to talk like you do.'

In another case, a counsellor worked with a woman with dementia who had agreed that the interviews be taped so that they could listen later to what had been discussed. Unfortunately, the woman died quite suddenly, but after her death her husband listened to the tapes and remarked, 'I enjoy listening to my wife laughing, even though we were talking about her dementia.'

ACKNOWLEDGEMENTS

We would like to thank all those individuals who have contributed to our work with people with dementia over the past years. In particular, we need to acknowledge the important contributions of members of the Salisbury Alzheimer's Society Learning to Live with Dementia steering group, Marie Mills, Rachael Litherland, Kerry Jones, Jane Gilliard, Deirdre Sutton-Smith and Mike Bender.

REFERENCES

Alzheimer's Society. 2001: *I'm told I have dementia.* London: Alzheimer's Society.

Bender, M.P. 1994: An interesting confusion: what can we do with reminiscence group work? In: Bornat, J. ed. *Reminiscence reviewed: perspectives, evaluations, achievements.* Buckingham: Open University Press, 32–45.

Brewer, W.F. 1986: What is autobiographical memory? In: Rubin, D.C. ed. *Autobiographical memory.* Cambridge: Cambridge University Press, 25–49.

Cheston, R. 1996: Stories and metaphors: talking about the past in a psychotherapy group for people with dementia. *Ageing and Society* **16:** 579–602.

Cheston, R. 1998: Psychotherapeutic work with dementia sufferers. *Social Work Practice* **12:** 199–207.

Cheston, R. and Bender, M.P. 1999: *Understanding dementia: the man with the worried eyes.* London: Jessica Kingsley.

Conway, M. 1990: *Autobiographical memory: an introduction.* Milton Keynes: Open University Press.

Department of Health, 2001: *National service framework for older people.* London: Stationery Office.

Gardner, I. 1993: Psychotherapeutic intervention with individuals and families where dementia is present. In: Chapman, A. and Marshall, M eds. *Dementia: new skills for social workers.* London: Jessica Kingsley, 16–39.

Kapur, N. 2001: *Managing your memory.* Southampton: Wessex Neurological Centre.

Keady, J. and Bender, M.P. 1998: Changing faces:the purpose and practice of assessing older adults with cognitive impairment. *Health Care in Later Life* **3:** 129–44.

Keady, J. and Nolan, M. 1995a: IMMEL: assessing coping responses in the early stages of dementia. *British Journal of Nursing* **4:** 309–14.

Keady, J. and Nolan, M. 1995b: IMMEL2: working to augment coping responses in the early dementia. *British Journal of Nursing* **4:** 377–81.

Kitwood, T. 1990: The dialectics of dementia: with particular reference to Alzheimer's disease. *Ageing and Society* **10:** 177–96.

Mills, M. 1998: *Narrative identity and dementia.* Gateshead: Athenaeum Press.

Tobin, S.S. 1991: *Personhood in advanced old age: implications for practice.* New York: Springer.

Addressing the physical care needs of people with dementia

Roger Watson

The physical needs of people with dementia are, essentially, no different from those of any other person. In common with others, a person with dementia requires food, air, warmth and protection from harm. In common with others too, the person with dementia is vulnerable on all these fronts if, for example, illness, disability or a lack of support prevents the fulfilment of physical needs. Individuals with dementia are nevertheless especially vulnerable in physical terms because of reduced cognitive function and other aspects of their particular underlying condition that may reduce their ability to recognize signals such as hunger and cold, and which may lead them to situations in which they are physically at risk, for example, of damage to their skin. The physical needs of a person with dementia are therefore precisely the same as those of any other person and increase with decreasing physical and mental ability. As for others, the physical needs of the person with dementia can be considered under the following headings:

- Safety
- Nutrition and hydration
- Skin care
- Body temperature
- Death and dying.

The final point listed above is considered elsewhere in this volume (*see* Chapter 8), this chapter considering nutrition and hydration, body temperature and skin care. Although the literature quoted will mainly present a nursing perspective (Wykle and Morris 1994), in line with the experience and background of the author, these aspects of the physical care needs of people with dementia will not be presented as purely 'nursing problems'; instead, they will be presented as the potential needs of and risk factors for people with dementia of which everyone – informal carer, care assistant, nurse or individual with early dementia – should be aware.

WHY DO PEOPLE WITH DEMENTIA HAVE PHYSICAL CARE NEEDS?

Dementia, although not a disease but the manifestation of several conditions that reduce a person's ability to understand and communicate, leaves those who suffer it less able to look after themselves. Dementia is a progressive condition from which recovery is not currently possible, and it can be assumed that continuing support will be required for the rest of the person's life for whatever physical care needs arise (Richards 1990).

Although it is not true that all people with dementia are old, dementia is nevertheless an age-related condition (Watson 1997a), and this alone gives rise to a greater level of risk if not necessarily physical care needs. Older people can live perfectly healthy and fulfilled lives but are more vulnerable to the effects of illness and disability. This is the result of several factors, the underlying reason being a reduced ability to keep their body conditions constant, especially in adverse circumstances. In other words, individuals' ability to maintain homeostasis is reduced (Watson 2000), which directly gives rise to a reduced ability to, for example, detect thirst or a changing ambient temperature. This is compounded by a reduced ability to respond physiologically to changing and adverse circumstances. Similarly, older people are at increased risk of skin damage and have reduced skin-healing capacity. Because of the association of age with dementia, it can be seen that the physical care needs of people with dementia are, to some extent, those of the older age group into which people with dementia largely fall (Watson 2001a).

NUTRITION AND HYDRATION

Nutrition and hydration are essential to sustain life. Without fluids, we will die in a few days, and without food in a few weeks. However, although sustaining a reduced fluid intake over a long period can be compatible with survival, albeit with a reduced quality of life, dehydration leads to other physiological disorders and can also exacerbate confusion and increase the risk of skin breakdown.

Similarly, poor nutrition can be sustained but also leads to a reduced quality of life, including exacerbated confusion and an increased risk of skin breakdown.

For reasons that are not fully understood, the process of dementia leads to disturbances in nutrition and hydration (Watson 1997b). Whether these disturbances are related to changes in the mechanisms indicating that we have eaten enough (satiety) or whether they are related to behavioural changes or alterations in energy requirement is not known. It is impossible to consider any aspect of dementia in isolation: wandering, disturbances in the sleep/wake cycle and repetitive activity are, for example, experienced by people with dementia, and these may lead to increased energy expenditure and an increased requirement for food (Coltharp et al. 1996). It is certainly the case, in the middle stages of the process, that many people with dementia apparently have an increased appetite (or a loss of satiety mechanism), which leads them to eat large quantities of food, some also eating inappropriate food and disgusting substances (Hope et al. 1989). It is almost inevitable, in the late and terminal stages, that people with dementia will have a reduced intake of food, caused either by an inability to eat, which may be behavioural or the result of poor psychomotor co-ordination, or by a reduced ability to sense hunger (Watson 1997b). A poor fluid intake usually accompanies this reduced food intake, which exposes the person with dementia to the risk of dehydration and even death.

Clearly, increased and reduced food intake both pose risks to the person with dementia. If the individual is liable to eat large quantities and to eat inappropriate food, there is a risk of choking and also poisoning. The solution to this change in behaviour is not easy. It is simply impossible, at home, to keep an eye on those with dementia all the time; similarly, it is not possible to restrict their movement unduly. One answer may lie in the judicious use of locked cupboards where potentially harmful substances can be kept safely. Another locked cupboard may be used to store food items to which the person with dementia is especially prone to eating in large quantities. Areas where food is stored may eventually have to be locked at night but only if the person with dementia wanders. Any injudicious use of restraint – locking doors being a form of restraint – can be very harmful to a person with dementia by increasing his or her confusion or agitation, and even by causing physical harm (Watson 2001b).

Towards the terminal stages of dementia, it is very common for the person with dementia to lose weight (Wang et al. 1997), and it is also common for the person with dementia to lose interest in food. The relationship between the reduced ability to eat and weight loss is not fully understood, nor are the reasons why people with dementia have a reduced ability to eat (Barrett-Connor et al. 1996). If a person with dementia does not eat, starvation will clearly ensue, but it has been reported that older people with dementia may continue to lose weight even with an adequate dietary intake. One possible explanation for this loss of weight is that older people with dementia have an increased energy requirement and increased energy utilization by the body, which may arise from wandering or even from some metabolic disturbance accompanying the dementia. The evidence in favour of an increased energy requirement in dementia is, however, ambiguous, and there is some evidence that the energy requirement may even be reduced in dementia (Poehlman and Dvorak 2000).

Why people with dementia lose the ability to eat is also poorly understood, the main problem lying in distinguishing between an inability to eat, perhaps based on a lack of hunger, and an unwillingness to eat, perhaps based on a desire to die. There are, however, other reasons, such as poor attention span, ease of distraction, wandering and the inability to recognize food or the utensils with which it is eaten. Whatever the reason, reduced eating is commonly observed and is very difficult to alleviate. In the early stages of reduced eating, it may be sufficient to remind people with dementia to eat or, if they wander, to help them to return them to the dining table. As difficulty with eating progresses, the person with dementia may show signs of refusing to eat and then may actively resist eating and eventually stop swallowing food, simply allowing the food to fall from the mouth. The response to the different stages clearly has to be different, but there is very little research to guide carers in this area. The early stages of difficulty with eating and refusing to eat may take place at home, but the advanced stages, which are related to advanced stages of dementia, may take place in hospital or another residential environment.

Perhaps more than any other feature of dementia, the refusal or inability to eat and the marked weight loss in the terminal stages of dementia are most distressing to carers and relatives (Watson 1990). Weight loss and reduced eating inevitably (and logically) become tied together in the minds of carers and may lead to guilt and accusations that those caring for individuals with dementia are starving them to death. There is really no evidence that older people with dementia are deliberately being starved to death (Alzheimer's Society 2000), but at some point the decision to discontinue efforts to feed the person must be taken to prevent further distress and discomfort for the person with dementia. This is an ethical dilemma and ethics related to dementia are covered in Chapter 8.

It is possible to improve eating in older people with dementia, but only to a point. An older person with dementia may not be able to engage with others for long enough to sit through a meal and may prefer to eat small amounts of food frequently. One way in which this can be accommodated is through the use of finger foods – sausage rolls, chips, samosas, fruit and other items that can be easily picked up and eaten, obviating the need for cutlery, which the person with dementia may find difficult or impossible to use (Copeman 1999). Such finger foods can be made available between meals as the person with dementia may not be able to fit in to the usual routine of mealtimes.

There is some dispute over which meals people with dementia will eat most at – evidence suggests breakfast and lunch (Watson 1997b). Generally speaking, such studies are conducted in formal care environments, and the result may depend upon the pattern of mealtimes, the availability of food between meals and, especially after the evening meal, how hungry an older person with dementia is first thing in the morning. In hospital, it is not unusual for an evening meal to take place at 5 p.m., no further food being available until 9 a.m. – a gap of 16 hours without food – which will make eating at breakfast very important. Conversely, it has been suggested that people with dementia may not function very well in the morning and will be most alert and able at midday (Watson 1993a). Whatever the case, if a person with dementia appears more able to eat at a particular meal, that should be exploited in order to help him or her to eat as much as possible.

There is also a preference for sweet foods among many older people with dementia (Mungas et al. 1990), which can similarly be exploited and be used as a strategy for helping the person to eat high-calorie foods, the number of calories being an important aspect of dietary intake for someone with poor food intake and, possibly, a higher energy requirement. Notions of healthy eating may have to be suspended with older people with dementia in favour of helping them to eat as much of what they need and like when they want to eat it. Another strategy to help with older people being cared for in nursing or residential homes is working in partnership with relatives or friends: the individual with dementia may feel more at ease with them than with care-workers, and they can be asked to visit and assist with eating, especially at mealtimes (Archibald et al. 1994). This will work as long as the older person with dementia continues to recognize the significant other person.

To summarize, older people with dementia experience difficulty with eating and weight loss. Much can be done to alleviate the problem in the short term, but difficulty with eating may ultimately become so severe that individuals with dementia are no longer able to feed themselves. At this point, carers are faced with an ethical dilemma.

Closely linked to nutrition is the issue of fluid intake and dehydration. An older person with dementia who is having difficulty eating is also likely to have difficulty drinking. A reduced fluid intake that is sustained for several days or even weeks will lead to dehydration. Although the body can adjust within certain limits to this – provided that fluid intake does not completely stop – there will be consequences such as increased confusion, urinary incontinence, constipation and an increased risk of skin breakdown. Dehydration leads to confusion in older people (Watson 1993b) because of the ensuing electrolyte imbalance – the older person's brain is less able to cope with this, and confusion is remarkably common in older people with acute illness, not just those with dementia. A low fluid intake leads to a reduced production of urine and a reduced urinary output. Urine becomes more concentrated in the bladder, leading to irritation of the urinary tract, and the reduced production of urine predisposes the person to urinary tract infection. These factors, combined with the decreasing cognitive function of the older person with dementia, which means they may no longer be able to sense the signs of the bladder-filling and the need to pass urine, will lead to urinary incontinence.

In older people with dementia, a great deal can be done to alleviate the problems caused by urinary incontinence even though the urinary incontinence itself cannot usually be treated. One way to help is to encourage an adequate fluid intake of approximately 1500 mL daily. As with eating, all that may be required in the early stages of the process to ensure an adequate intake of fluids in a person with dementia is encouragement and the opportunity to have drinks. Although care should – because of an increased risk of choking – be taken with presenting food and fluids together to a person with dementia who is having difficulty eating, the opportunity to have a drink should be available at every mealtime as well as in between meals. Drinks should be varied – hot and cold – with a choice of flavours, tastes and types.

The challenge of helping a person with dementia to take in adequate fluids should not be overestimated: if food intake is low, this will also adversely affect fluid intake because part of our normal intake of fluids derives from the food we eat. Using a recommended intake of 1500 mL daily and estimating that the average drink container holds 150 mL, the person with dementia should be taking 10 drinks per day (Watson 1993b). If there is one drink with each meal and one between each pair of meals, only five drinks are accounted for, so other opportunities must be created, especially if the person with dementia is unable to get his or her own drinks.

If the person with dementia is at a more advanced stage and is having profound difficulty drinking, a greater degree of assistance will be required. The person with dementia will require help with drinking, which may require a carer holding a cup to the mouth, being careful not to induce choking, or providing the person with dementia with a straw to drink through or with specially adapted cups with spouts. It is not correct to tip someone's head back in order to help them to swallow; in fact, swallowing is easier if the head is tipped slightly forwards, and tipping the head back encourages choking. When the person is no longer able to drink, it is unusual in the UK to institute any kind of tube-feeding, although this is relatively common in the USA (Grimley Evans 1992). The ethical issues surrounding the use of tube feeding are covered elsewhere (*see* Chapter 8). It is, however, worth pointing to research showing that tube-feeding does not necessarily prolong the life of older people with dementia (Kim 2001), and it may indeed prolong their misery.

SKIN CARE

Older people who are ill have an increased risk of skin breakdown, the additional risk factors including dehydration, immobility, undernutrition and incontinence. It will be clear that all of these risk factors are increased in people with dementia,

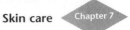

especially in the later stages of the condition. Skin damage may occur as a result of injury, the damaging effects of incontinence on the skin, and pressure ulcers. The issue of damage is related to safety, and the issue of incontinence and pressure ulcers will be considered in this chapter.

Incontinence damages the skin, especially the groins of the person who is incontinent, because of the caustic nature of urine and faeces. Urine is slightly acidic and will be more so if a person is dehydrated and passing concentrated urine. Faeces contain digestive enzymes that will digest the protein in the skin. Incontinence is usually intractable in older people with dementia because of the loss of the usual signals indicating the need to use the toilet and also the loss of social inhibition. Figures for the extent of urinary incontinence among older people with dementia range from 10 to 90 per cent (Skelly and Flint 1995).

Although moderate success may be attained in the early stages in retaining the continence of the person with dementia, it is more usual for the problem to become one that has to be managed (Watson 1997c). The management of incontinence may involve the use of appliances that either collect urine (especially useful for men) or absorb urine and faeces, thereby preventing skin damage. Such appliances are, however, insufficient in themselves, good skin hygiene also being required, with regular bathing or showering and the limited use of creams to prevent skin breakdown and infection (Jenkins 1999). It will also, as indicated above, help if the person has an adequate fluid intake – urinary incontinence should never be managed in a person with dementia by restricting fluid intake.

Older people with dementia are at particular risk of developing pressure ulcers, breaks in the skin that can be superficial or deep and result from prolonged pressure, especially in the late stages of dementia, in which nutrition may be poor and body weight low. Dehydration, as well as incontinence, may be present (Nixon 2001). In addition, the person with dementia may, in the later stages of the condition, have become relatively immobile instead of wandering, which will lead to prolonged periods sitting in a chair; this is a prime risk factor for the development of pressure ulcers. Because of reduced brain function, the older person with dementia may not be able to interpret the usual signals, such as pain and numbness, that indicate that an area is suffering from prolonged pressure, which prevents blood flowing into the skin (occlusion) and causes oxygen deprivation. The person with dementia may also be unable to perform the small reflex movements that are normal while sitting and help to prevent pressure ulcer formation. Pressure ulcer formation should be avoided because the skin breakdown is painful and unsightly, infection may result, and the ulcers can be malodorous. In addition, a pressure ulcer from which fluid is being lost may exacerbate dehydration, and inflammation will lead to a depletion of much-needed protein from the body.

Pressure ulcers can be avoided (Clark 2001). Attention to all of the risk factors is clearly paramount, and addressing factors such as nutrition, fluid intake and incontinence will help. Ultimately, however, pressure ulcers develop because of prolonged pressure on a part of the body, leading, as described above, to occlusion of the blood supply and oxygen deprivation. This can only be avoided by relieving pressure on areas that are at risk, such as the base of the spine (sacrum). The person with dementia should be discouraged from sitting for prolonged periods. Two hours is certainly the maximum, but a person who is frail because of a combination of factors such as loss of weight and dehydration may not be able to endure even that length of time without damage. The key test is whether or not the skin is reddened after sitting and whether or not it blanches when light pressure is applied to the reddened area – if the area does not blanch, the person is at risk of further skin damage.

Pressure can be relieved by helping the person with dementia to take short walks or, if he or she is unable to do this, to lie down for a while, which distributes the pressure over a larger surface area. When lying down, further positional change can prevent damage to any areas still at risk, such as the hips. Pressure-relieving devices such as alternating pressure mattresses, and surfaces such as pressure-distributing cushions, are available for purchase from commercial organizations as well as the health services, but these are only adjuncts to the other aspects of skin care recommended above and should never be relied upon in isolation. If a pressure ulcer does develop – the removal of the surface layer of skin being evidence of pressure ulceration – expert nursing care is required; this is covered more fully elsewhere (Morison 2001).

BODY TEMPERATURE

The regulation of body temperature is rarely a problem for young, fit people, only extremes of ambient temperature being dangerous. Older people are, however, more at risk from variations in temperature, leading to dangerous changes in body temperature and even death (Watson 1995). As we age, we are less able to recognize alterations in ambient temperature and our bodies are less able, through homeostasis, to respond to changes in body temperature. If body weight is reduced – as is often the case in the advanced stages of dementia – heat is lost from the body more quickly, partly because of the loss of the insulating fat layers and partly because fat is one of the fuels the body uses to increase its temperature.

The body raises body temperature by changing the distribution of heat between the core and the periphery. This is achieved by the vascular system and is exemplified in Caucasian people by the skin's being paler when it is cold – this mechanism redistributes heat away from the skin to the core, thereby preserving it. The opposite is seen in flushing, in which the heat is distributed mainly to the surface of the body, from which it is lost by evaporation and convection. Other ways in which the body can maintain temperature are metabolically, by creating heat from the breakdown of carbohydrates and fats in the liver, and also by shivering. This is a reflex response to reduced body temperature whereby the skeletal muscles make small, uncontrolled contractions that metabolize carbohydrates and fat, generating heat as a byproduct. Body heat can also be generated behaviourally by taking some exercise, which creates heat metabolically, by moving to a warmer environment or by putting on more clothes.

Older people with dementia, particularly in the advanced stages, will be especially at risk of low body temperature, or hypothermia, because they will have lost body weight and body fat; their shivering reflex may also be impaired. Individuals may also be immobile and unable to alter their environment or clothing to adapt to changes in ambient temperature. Although this is less of a risk, they may be in danger of hyperthermia, for example from sitting next to a radiator or even sitting out in the sun; combined with a predisposition to dehydration, this could be very dangerous.

In order to avoid problems arising from such risk factors, the best strategy is to maintain a carefully controlled environment with regard to temperature and to avoid exposure to extremes of heat and cold. This can be more easily said than done if the person with dementia is living at home, where financial circumstances may be poor, but standard advice to older people on avoiding hypothermia should be followed (Watson 1996). It would clearly be restraining to prevent an older person going outside in extreme weather conditions, but there is no reason why he or she cannot be dressed appropriately for cold weather and, with the use of sun-blocking agents, be enabled to sit in the sun for short periods.

CONCLUSION

As emphasized at the start of this chapter, the physical needs of people with dementia are really no different from those of other people. Certain aspects, however, require special attention because of additional risk factors to which the person with dementia will be subject, and also because many people with dementia will be older and some risk factors are heightened with age – especially in older people who are also frail. This chapter has outlined some of the main physical care needs of people with dementia but is by no means exhaustive. Nor has the treatment of each been exhaustive in terms of meeting these physical care needs. More specialized texts, for example on nursing care or the care of older people, should be consulted for this.

Caring for older people with dementia takes its toll, both physically and mentally, on those involved, especially family care-givers (Baumgarten et al. 1994; Briggs and Askham 1999), and nurses and family care-givers should work in partnership in the physical care of those with dementia – whether in the community or in hospital. Community nursing staff have a role to play in advising family care-givers about aspects of physical care such as eating, drinking and skin care. If necessary, nurses can ensure that the help of other experts is available, for example that of speech and language therapists, who may be able to advise on how to deal with choking so a person can eat safely at home. Without such assistance, family care-givers may be reluctant to assist for fear of causing harm or even death. We have already mentioned how family care-givers can – if they wish to – help in hospital and residential homes at mealtimes by providing a familiar face and advice on the likes and dislikes of the person with dementia. Older people living in the community who remain under the care of their general practitioner are entitled to annual health checks by the general practitioner or practice nurse, and any problems uncovered during such checks should be addressed: dementia may not be curable, but there is no reason why the person with dementia should suffer pain, discomfort or ill-health for other reasons.

People with dementia, in many ways, leave aspects of the world behind them in terms of their declining mental function. They do not, however, leave behind the physical aspects of their survival, and as they inevitably become less able to look after their own needs, others are required to provide help. It is hoped that this chapter will provide some guidance on this aspect of the needs of people with dementia.

REFERENCES

Alzheimer's Society. 2000: *Food for thought*. London: Alzheimer's Society.

Archibald, C., Carver, A., Keene, J. and Watson, R. 1994: *Food and nutrition in the care of older people with dementia*. Stirling: Dementia Services Development Centre.

Barrett-Connor, E., Edelstien, S.L., Corey-Bloom, J. and Wiederholt, W.C. 1996: Weight loss precedes dementia in community-dwelling older adults. *Journal of the American Geriatrics Society* **44:** 1147–52.

Baumgarten, M., Hanley, J.A., Infaante-Rivard, C., Battista, R.N., Becker, R. and Gauthier, S. 1994: Health of family members caring for elderly persons with dementia. *Annals of Internal Medicine* **120:** 126–32.

Briggs, K., and Askham, J. 1999: *The needs of people with dementia and those who care for them: a review of the literature*. London: Alzheimer's Society.

Clark, M. 2001: Pressure sore prevention. In: Morison, M. ed. *The prevention and treatment of pressure sores*. London: Mosby, 75–98.

Coltharp, W., Richie, M.F. and Kaas, M.J. 1996: Wandering. *Journal of Gerontological Nursing* **22:** 5–10.

Copeman, J. 1999: *Nutritional care for older people*. London: Age Concern.

Grimley Evans, J. 1992: From plaque to placement. *Age and Ageing* **21:** 77–80.

Hope, R.A., Fairburn, C.G. and Goodwin, G.M. 1989: Increased eating in dementia. *International Journal of Eating Disorders* **8:** 111–15.

Jenkins, D.A.L. 1999: *Urinary and faecal incontinence: a heightened problem when dementia is a factor*. Stirling: Dementia Services Development Centre.

Kim, Y.-I. 2001: To feed or not to feed: tube feeding in patients with advanced dementia. *Nutrition Reviews* **59:** 86–8.

Morison, M. ed. 2001: *The prevention and treatment of pressure sores*. London: Mosby.

Mungas, D., Cooper, J.K., Weler, P.G., Gietzen, D., Franzi, C. and Bernick, C. 1990: Dietary preference for sweet foods in patients with dementia. *Journal of the American Geriatrics Society* **38:** 999–1007.

Nixon, J. 2001: The pathophysiology and aetiology of pressure ulcers. In: Morison, M. ed. *The prevention and treatment of pressure sores*. London: Mosby, 17–36.

Poelhman, E.T. and Dvorak, R.V. 2000: Energy expenditure, energy intake, and weight loss in Alzheimer disease. *American Journal of Clinical Nutrition* **71**(S): 650S–655S.

Richards, B.S. 1990: Alzheimer's disease: a disabling neurophysiological disorder with complex nursing implications. *Archives of Psychiatric Nursing* **4:** 39–42.

Skelly, J. and Flint, A., 1995: Urinary incontinence associated with dementia. *Journal of the American Geriatrics Society* **43:** 286–94.

Wang, S.Y., Fukagawa, N., Hossain, M. and Ooi, W.L. 1997: Longitudinal weight changes, length of survival, and energy requirements of long-term care residents with dementia. *Journal of the American Geriatrics Society* **45:** 1189–95.

Watson, R. 1990: Feeding patients who are demented. *Nursing Standard* **25**(4): 28–30.

Watson, R. 1993a: Measuring feeding difficulty in patients with dementia: perspectives and problems. *Journal of Advanced Nursing* **18:** 25–31.

Watson, R. 1993b: Thirst and dehydration in the elderly. *Elderly Care* **5:** 41–6.

Watson, R. 1995: Hypothermia in the elderly. *Elderly Care* **8:** 25–30.

Watson, R. 1996: Hypothermia. *Emergency Nurse* **3:** 10–15.

Watson, R. 1997a: Is dementia a challenge to the identity of the mental health nurse? In: Tilley, S. ed. *The mental health nurse: views of practice and education*. Oxford: Blackwell, 186–202.

Watson, R. 1997b: Undernutrition, weight loss and feeding difficulty in elderly patients with dementia: a nursing perspective. *Reviews in Clinical Gerontology* **7:** 317–26.

Watson, R. 1997c: Mostly male. In: Getliffe, K. and Dolman, M. eds. *Promoting continence*. London: Baillière Tindall, 107–37.

Watson, R. 2000a: Normal ageing. *Elderly Care* **12:** 23–4.

Watson, R. 2001a: Old age: mind, body and spirit – the biological stages of ageing. *Journal of Community Nursing* **15:** 24–8.

Watson, R. 2001b: Restraint: its use and misuse in the care of older people. *Nursing Older People* **13:** 21–5.

Wykle, M.L. and Morris, D.L. 1994: Nursing care in Alzheimer's disease. *Clinics in Geriatric Medicine* **10:** 351–65.

Palliative care for people with dementia

Kay de Vries

Only within the past 10 years has it been generally acknowledged within the palliative care literature in the UK that diseases manifesting a dementia syndrome are terminal illnesses (Black and Jolley 1990, 1991; Jolley and Baxter 1997; McCarthy *et al* 1997; Addington-Hall 2000). The admission of people with dementia into a hospice programme of care has been promoted in the USA since the early 1980s (Volicer 1986, 1997; Brechling and Kuhn 1989; Luchins and Hanrahan 1993; Hanrahan and Luchins 1995a, b; Luchins et al. 1997; Hanrahan et al. 1999). In the USA, however, if they are admitted to an acute unit, these people will often receive aggressive treatment for their illnesses (Ahronheim et al. 1996). The claim by Luchins and Hanrahan (1993), that older people who receive hospice care rarely have a primary diagnosis of a dementia syndrome, is equally true for the provision of palliative care in the UK. In the UK, the majority of palliative care teams do not include people with end-stage dementia in their remit (Lloyd-Williams 1996).

The hospice movement has had a major impact on the standard of care provided for dying people across the entire health care spectrum. This influence has infiltrated all parts of the health care system, and palliative care is no longer confined to the hospice environment. As early as 1990, Black and Jolley suggested that the management of dying of psychogeriatric patients could be improved if lessons learned from hospice practices were adopted, but changes have been slow to develop. The National Council for Hospice and Specialist Palliative Care Services (NCHSPCS) now recognizes the palliative care needs of this group of people.

Initiatives began following research into the palliative care needs of people who die from causes other than cancer (McCarthy et al. 1997; Addington-Hall et al. 1998). This led to recommendations from the NCHSPCS for specialist palliative care for non-malignant diseases (Addington-Hall 1998) and has more recently extended to psychiatric services (Addington-Hall 2000). The Council makes several recommendations for initiatives aimed at developing partnerships between palliative care services, nursing homes and psychogeriatric specialists, particularly in relation to education. They recommend that local care of the elderly and palliative care services develop joint training programmes and promote a close collaboration between psychogeriatricians and palliative care specialists (Addington-Hall 2000).

Although specialist palliative care services tend to cater specifically for difficult end-of-life situations, palliative care is a philosophical approach to the care of any person suffering from a disease for which there is no cure in which the person may be nearing the end of life. The palliative care philosophy aims neither to prolong nor to shorten life but to maintain the physical, psychological and spiritual comfort of the individual until death. This approach uses a partnership model in which the multidisciplinary team, patient and family are closely involved in the decision-making processes. Volicer (1986) suggests that, within this framework, the treatment of end-stage dementia, using a hospice approach to address some of the ethical issues, such as hydration and percutaneous endoscopic gastrostomy feeding for people with dementia, would be considered differently. (Ethical issues in relation to the provision of care for people with dementia are dealt with in Chapter 13).

The final cause of death for a person with dementia is not easily distinguished as death certificates rarely record the death as being caused by dementia, particularly dementia of the Alzheimer type (DAT), and an autopsy is not routinely carried out in the event of the death of an individual from this group. Dementia may, however, be mentioned as a secondary illness (Burns et al. 1990). The most commonly recorded cause of death is bronchopneumonia (Burns et al. 1990; Black and Jolley 1991; Jolley and Baxter 1997). These people will die in a variety of settings, usually a residential or nursing home, or a hospital ward. This chapter will focus on the use of palliative care principles in the management of people with an end-stage dementia syndrome or those who have a terminal illness, such as cancer, superimposed on an existing dementia syndrome.

The following areas will be covered:

- The symptoms that may occur in end-stage dementia
- The assessment processes for managing the palliative care of those with advanced dementia
- The management of key symptoms using a palliative care approach
- The bereavement issues that arise for people with advanced dementia and their families.

CAUSE OF DEATH IN DEMENTIA SYNDROMES

The most common underlying causes of organic brain disease identified in population studies are the degenerative dementias, particularly DAT, multi-infarct dementia and Lewy body disease (Black and Jolley 1991; Jolley and Baxter 1997). Research in the 1950s showed that the death rate of this group was raised compared with that of the general old age population (Roth 1955, cited Jolley and Baxter 1997), and the generation of studies since the 1950s has tended to concentrate on the DAT population (Jolley and Baxter 1997).

Jolley and Baxter (1997) provide a comprehensive overview of the life expectation of people with organic brain disease, identifying factors associated with increased mortality. These include age, a later age of onset being associated with a shorter life expectancy, gender, an increased risk being seen in males, and social class, for which there is longer survival of individuals in social class I. Eagles et al. (1990) further suggest that care in a residential home may increase survival time.

The factors usually associated with a shorter survival include severe cognitive impairment, parietal lobe dysfunction, dysphasia, psychotic symptoms, behavioural abnormalities, physical incapacity and illness and poor nutrition (Jolley and Baxter 1997). Mortality and co-morbidity are significantly increased in the presence of other diseases, particularly atrial fibrillation, heart failure and myocardial infarction (Jolley and Baxter 1997). The cause of death of a significant number of people with a dementia syndrome will consequently be a physical illness (Burns et al. 1990; Jolley and Baxter 1997). There are as yet no reliable statistics on the number of people with a dementia who die with a superimposed terminal illness such as cancer.

CARE ENVIRONMENT

Field and James (1993) comment that British society finds it easier to accept the deaths of older people than those of young people. In an ageist society, the deaths of older individuals are viewed as acceptable and inevitable, the death of a person with dementia often being referred to as a relief (Sweeting 1997; Gessert et al. 2001).

People with end-stage dementia will die in a variety of settings. It is estimated that 80 per cent of people with dementia live in the community (Dementia Services Development Centre 1995), but it is not certain that this is the most probable place in which they will die, and there are no reliable statistics on the place of death for this group. The most likely place will be a residential or nursing home environment, where Ineichen (1990, 1992) has estimated that over 50 per cent of residents have dementia. No figures have, however, recently been published on the number of people with dementia in residential and nursing homes. A proportion of older people with dementia may die in a hospital ward following admission resulting from an acute illness. People with dementia and a superimposed terminal illness may also die in these settings. If they have cancer, it is more likely that their needs will be brought to the attention of specialist palliative care services.

The most common reason for the admission to hospital of a person with dementia is an acute episode of physical illness (Hermans et al. 1989; Ahronheim et al. 1996; Luchins et al. 1997). Another frequent reason for hospitalization relates to fractures, which are difficult to avoid as the dementia progresses (Hermans et al. 1989). Fractures contribute to the mortality and morbidity risk for this patient group, but, as reported above, the main cause of death of people with dementia recorded on death certificates is bronchopneumonia (Burns et al. 1990; Black and Jolley 1991; Jolley and Baxter 1997). If admission has been from home, individuals often stay on a medical ward until a place in a residential or nursing home can be arranged, or alternatively they may die in the hospital. Common problems identified among people with dementia in hospital by nurses and doctors include swallowing difficulties, decubitus ulcers, aspiration pneumonia, dehydration, malnutrition, incontinence and urinary tract infections, constipation, low mood, pain, osteoarthritis and cardiovascular problems (Luchins et al. 1997).

Following a regional, retrospective survey of the experience of carers of 3696 dying people during their last year of life, McCarthy et al. (1997) carried out a comparative analysis of people with cancer and those with dementia identified within the survey. The authors found that the most commonly reported symptoms of individuals with dementia were mental confusion, urinary incontinence, pain, low mood, constipation and loss of appetite. The researchers also found that the carers of people with dementia needed more help and required more social services at home than did those of cancer patients. As well as physical problems, staff and carers need to help with a wide range of other difficulties associated with dementia; these are discussed in Chapter 12.

PALLIATIVE CARE APPROACH

Hermans et al. (1989) found that admission to hospital can cause unnecessary discomfort and confusion for the older person with dementia and advocated a conservative or palliative approach to care. Such an approach weighs the discomfort resulting from the experience of being taken from one's familiar surroundings to receive what may be invasive technical medical interventions against the probable benefits. Previous to the work carried out in USA and the establishment of a hospice approach to the care of people with advanced dementia, the possibility of people with dementia being moved from a familiar environment to a hospice was not considered. The need for those with dementia to be cared for and supported in a familiar environment by people, family or supporters they are familiar with is discussed elsewhere in this volume (*see* Chapter 16). In relation to the specific

needs of this group, the NCHSPCS has recommended the development of protocols to ensure that individuals with advanced dementia who are admitted to acute
units do not receive aggressive, life-sustaining treatments inappropriately
(Addington-Hall 2000).

Assessment

Difficulties with communication present one of the most challenging problems in
providing care for those with dementia. There is, for carers and staff, always the
difficulty of striking a balance between the ability to understand cues from the
person and ignoring the possibility that some meaning exists that needs to be
interpreted. The difficulty that people with dementia have in communicating
information about symptoms of pain, fever or discomfort associated with, for
example, infection impedes symptom reporting and delays prompt treatment.
Illnesses such as cancer and heart disease may go undiagnosed until they are at an
advanced stage.

The palliative care approach identifies the importance of individual assessment
for the appropriateness of treatment-planning. It also emphasizes the need for
well-validated assessment procedures, sound communication and facilitation
skills, and a consideration of environmental factors, tone of voice, touch and other
body language cues expressed by the nurse or doctor when carrying out an assessment (Buckman 1993). When making decisions regarding medical or nursing
interventions, individuals' own views and their wishes prior to dementia should,
if they are known, be considered, and the wishes of the family and recommendations of the multidisciplinary team should be taken into account (Twycross and
Lichter 1993).

Pain/discomfort

Pain in older, cognitively impaired people has been consistently untreated or
undertreated (Marzinski 1991; Ferrell et al. 1995: Kovach et al. 1999). In any assessment of pain, it is helpful to use a pain assessment tool. Assessing pain in cognitively impaired people poses an enormous challenge to anyone, be they nurse,
doctor or family member. There is a plethora of literature on the subject of pain
and a steadily growing body of research on the pain experiences of cognitively
impaired people. Original definitions of pain focused on the individual's subjective judgement of the pain, which has not been a helpful starting point for
assessing pain in those who have difficulty expressing themselves. Visual
analogue scales are ineffective when assessing pain in a person who is severely
cognitively impaired and unable to communicate verbally (Radbruch et al. 2000),
although they may be of use in the early stages of dementia. The adaptation of
scales used in the assessment of children's pain has been attempted, but paediatric

scales are used for measuring acute pain and may not be appropriate for assessing chronic or acute-on-chronic pain (Stein 2001).

There is evidence that cognitively impaired older people are able to communicate their pain experience and intensity but that they do not retain any pain memory (Ferrell et al. 1995). There is also evidence that people with dementia experience the same degree and type of pain as everyone else (Porter et al. 1996), although limited research on this subject exists.

Porter et al. (1996) carried out a comparison study of 51 cognitively intact, community-dwelling individuals, aged 65 years or older, and 44 community- or nursing home-dwelling individuals with different severities of dementia who were in the same age range. The authors used a variety of tests for assessing the pain response after a standard venepuncture procedure. The parameters measured were heart rate, the amplitude of respiratory sinus arrhythmia, self-reported anxiety and pain, and videotaped facial expression. The researchers concluded that both cognitively impaired and cognitively intact people experience the same degree of pain and that facial expression was the most effective indicator of the pain responses by the individuals who had cognitive impairment.

Facial expression was also identified as an important indicator of the pain or discomfort response in other studies aiming to develop pain assessment tools and protocols for use in the assessment of cognitively impaired individuals (Hurley et al. 1992; Simons and Malabar 1995; Parke 1998; Galloway and Turner 1999; Kovach et al. 1999; McLean 2000; Lefebvre-Chapiro et al. 2001). The DOLOPLUS 2 pain assessment scale (Lefebvre-Chapiro et al. 2001) was developed by palliative care practitioners and has been well validated and systematically applied by teams already trained in palliative care. Diagnosis, followed by the successful treatment of pain, was demonstrated in 20 per cent of people with dementia (Lefebvre-Chapiro et al. 2001).

All the studies conclude that assessment needs to be individualized using a systematic approach. It is also important that a comprehensive history of the usual or baseline physical and behavioural responses of the person with dementia is taken from a carer who is familiar with his or her behaviour pattern. This approach assumes that a person with dementia experiences the same or similar pain or discomfort as someone who is able to express this, and analgesia or pain relief should be administered appropriately to meet this need (Morrison et al. 1998).

World Health Organization analgesic ladder

When providing pain relief, the World Health Organization (1996) analgesic ladder is a useful guide to controlling pain. It was developed specifically in relation to cancer pain, but can be used as a principle in the assessment and treatment of other pain needs. Drug treatment is the main approach employed. A detailed assessment must first be carried out, adherence to the following three principles

(World Health Organization 1996) being recommended. Analgesics should, when possible:

- Be given by the oral route
- Be given at a fixed time (by the clock)
- Be prescribed and administered according to the severity of pain and the response to the drug prescribed.

Step one of the ladder involves the use of non-opioid analgesics such as para-cetamol along with an adjuvant such as a non-steroidal anti-inflammatory agent (e.g. brufen) if needed. This regime is appropriate for people with mild pain. If this fails to relieve the pain when given regularly (by the clock), the second step of the ladder should be considered; this involves the use of weak opioids such as dihy-drocodeine. If pain is still not relieved, step three should be discussed. This employs the opioid drugs that are most commonly associated with cancer pain management. The effective dose is whatever relieves the pain, but the dose must be gradually increased until pain relief is achieved or side-effects are experienced. These must then be dealt with appropriately. A laxative should always be prescribed with the opioid as constipation is a side-effect of opioid use.

Infections and general care at the end of life

End-stage dementia is a period during which the person is particularly vulnerable to infection. Prolonged physical immobility increases the risk of pressure sores, leads to reduced coughing and deep breathing, and increases the susceptibility to bronchopneumonia; incontinence and catheterization similarly increase the risk of urinary tract infection. It is not easy to identify the cause of infection in cognitively impaired patients as fever can also be caused by conditions such as constipation or transient dehydration (Fabiszewski et al. 1990). Fever is, however, often the only symptom of infection in the person who is unable to communicate and is, in a vulnerable, non-communicative patient, a threat to survival. In a long-term care setting, the temperature would normally only be measured when signs of poten-tial temperature elevation were observed by carers or staff; it can therefore easily be overlooked. Fabiszewski et al. (1990) suggest that the higher mortality rate encountered in this patient group may be associated with fevers of longer compared with fevers of shorter duration. They suggest that the management of fevers in institutionalized patients with DAT should take into consideration the indication that the progression of DAT increases the susceptibility to infection.

Treatment for infection should ideally be based on diagnostic procedures that may include the use of venepuncture to obtain blood cultures as well as methods such as suctioning to obtain upper respiratory tract sputum. These procedures inflict physical and emotional distress on people with dementia. The palliative care approach to managing episodes of fever in this group of people includes avoiding admission to an acute unit and administering an antipyretic/analgesic such as paracetamol to reduce the temperatures and provide pain relief. The burden of other treatment needs to be weighed against the possible benefits, and the decision to administer antibiotics must be based on individual patient assessment: it will depend on the clinical situation and whether it is felt that this will result in a prolongation of the process of dying (Morant and Senn 1993). The management of bronchopneumonia and other infections will depend on the previous wishes of the person and on discussion with the family. Nursing management should include careful regard to positioning to minimize respiratory distress, reduce bouts of coughing and lessen pulmonary secretions, preferably helping the person to sit in a propped-up position. Nurses and carers should also provide a comforting presence by their tone of voice and a careful and gentle touch when carrying out any nursing interventions.

Poor nutritional status and becoming bed-bound are significant risk factors for pressure sores for people with end-stage dementia. As the person becomes more debilitated, and fatigue and weakness become profound, the correction of malnutrition is impossible, and healing ability is limited. The use of specialist mattresses, along with careful and gentle handling of the patient at all times, is essential. Ongoing risk assessment with a detailed documentation of care plans and day-to-day changes in condition communicated between carers and staff is essential in maintaining the comfort of those who are dying, with particular awareness of the reduced ability of people with dementia to communicate their possible discomfort. In the terminal stage, obsessive turning is not required as healing is not an issue (Twycross and Lichter 1993). At this stage, the person's comfort is an essential consideration, and pain and discomfort assessment tools, as discussed earlier, should be used to ensure that comfort is maintained.

Mouth care

Dysphagia, or difficulty in swallowing, which can be a feature of end-stage dementia, increases the risk of oral conditions. Mouth care becomes essential at the terminal stage, and nurses or carers must aim to keep lips and internal lining of the mouth as far as possible clean, soft and intact. Key areas for oral care assessment, as identified by Krishanasamy (1995), are as follows:

- The lips may be dry or cracked, or show evidence of ulceration.
- The tongue may be coated, with a loss of tongue surface tissue, bleeding or blisters.
- The saliva may be thick or ropy.
- The internal lining of the mouth may be coated, red, ulcerated or bleeding.
- The gums may be red or swollen, and bleeding may occur under pressure.

- The teeth or dentures may be contaminated with plaque or debris.
- The voice may be rasping.
- The person may find it difficult to swallow.

It is crucial to be aware that the person might experience oral pain as a result of a number of conditions that occur in advanced illness. The most common of these are oral pain, xerostomia (a dry mouth), a coated tongue and mouth lining, oral fungal infections (*Candida*), ulceration and denture problems (among those patients who wear them) (Jobbin et al. 1992; Milligan et al. 2001). Regular (daily) examination of the condition of the mouth of terminally ill individuals is essential, and measures that prevent the above conditions need to be in place as part of their care plan. Dentures should be kept scrupulously clean and not left in for 24 hours at a time as they can harbour *Candida* species, as can toothbrushes.

There are several reasons why a dying person may develop oral fungal infection (candidiasis): poor oral hygiene, xerostomia, a suppressed immune system, steroid medication, broad-spectrum antibiotics, poor nutritional status and systemic diseases. The *Candida* infection may not be confined to the mouth but may extend into the upper gastrointestinal tract and throughout the gut. Nystatin is the most commonly prescribed treatment, but there are several species of *Candida*, not all of which are sensitive to the drug. As testing for different species and resistance to antifungal agents is not routinely carried out, Finlay (1995) suggests that systemic antifungal treatment should be considered rather than waiting to see whether the nystatin has been effective.

Xerostomia can be caused by several medications that are used in palliative care and may be prescribed for people with dementia. These include antidepressants, neuroleptics, antihistamines, anticholinergic agents, opioids and antihypertensives (Atkinson and Fox 1992). Apart from stopping unnecessary medications, palliative care for xerostomia involves simple measures such as keeping the dying person's mouth moist and stimulating salivary flow. A range of methods may be employed, for example using mouth sponges or giving small sips of water or citrus fruit juices, sucking ice chips and frozen fruit juice, and giving sips of tonic water, with or without gin. Cider and soda water is also effective, with a pleasant taste, and pineapple juice has been anecdotally reported to be an effective treatment. It is also important to keep the dying person's lips moist with a moisturising lotion or petroleum jelly.

Dehydration/starvation

The issue of starvation and dehydration may arise when it becomes obvious that the person with dementia can no longer swallow and starvation and dehydration may be the final cause of death. Swallowing difficulties may, however, have been reported earlier by observant carers, and a swallowing assessment by a speech therapist is an essential part of preparing and anticipating the future care needs of patients with progressive dementia, as well as helping to prevent the risk of aspiration pneumonia.

No studies specifically deal with death in relation to malnutrition in older people with cognitive impairment, and malnutrition is a largely unrecognized problem in hospitals (Dickerson 1995; Holmes 1998; McLaren and Green 1998). Malnutrition is a cause of increased morbidity and mortality for all people, particularly in the presence of illness (McLaren and Green 1998). The insertion of a nasogastric tube for the purpose of feeding at the end of life is not generally carried out in palliative care units in the UK. Issues related to help with eating and drinking are addressed elsewhere in this volume (*see* Chapter 7).

Cancer induced anorexia–cachexia syndrome may be a feature in the person with dementia who also has cancer. It results from abnormal metabolism secondary to substances released from a cancer and/or the immune system. The condition results in anorexia, weight loss and chronic nausea (Walker and Bruera 1998). Cancer cachexia is difficult to treat, and priority should be given to improving patient comfort (Walker and Bruera 1998).

Hydration, or providing fluids intravenously or subcutaneously for people who can no longer swallow, remains one of the most challenging issues when caring for the dying person (Craig 1994; Roberts 1997). Research evidence is confusing and inconclusive, and there is no firm knowledge base in relation to the practice (Meares 2000). Artificial hydration is rarely used in hospice practice (Ellershaw et al. 1995), but, in the acute setting of the hospital, terminally ill patients who are unable to swallow and maintain an adequate oral intake are regularly artificially rehydrated via either intravenous or subcutaneous infusions (House 1992; Ahronheim et al. 1996).

A number of controversies surround the rehydration of terminally ill patients, MacDonald (1998) and Fainsinger (1998) summarizing the arguments for and against this practice within a palliative care context. The arguments against rehydration include the beliefs that fluids may prolong the dying process, that comatose patients do not experience pain or thirst, and that a lower urine output means less need for catheterization, less gastrointestinal fluid and less vomiting, as well as reduced fluid retention. Decreased fluid level and electrolyte imbalance may act as a natural anaesthetic for the central nervous system. With a decreased level of consciousness and reduced suffering, any thirst experienced is readily controlled with minimal oral fluids and good mouth care. With reduced pulmonary secretion and less cough, there is less choking and congestion, which may reduce the bubbly excretions that produce the 'death rattle'.

The arguments for rehydration summarized by the above authors include evidence that dehydration is recognized as a cause of confusion, agitation and delirium, and that it is a risk factor for pressure sores and renal failure, which may result in an accumulation of medications. A number of ethical issues regarding quality and standards of care are also used as arguments to promote rehydration, particularly in relation to sedation (Craig 1994). Bruera et al. (1995) suggest that a more vigorous approach to hydration has been responsible for the diminished incidence of delirium, particularly in relation to drug toxicity. Craig (1994) maintains that any decision to sedate a terminally ill person must seriously consider maintaining hydration at the same time. Relatives frequently express concern about the lack of fluids or nutrients being provided for the dying patient, and it is important that health care professionals strive to address these anxieties while not compromising the interests of the patient.

When dying patients become unable to swallow, are vomiting, have severe weakness or are unconscious, medications that are essential to maintain their comfort may be administered via a subcutaneous syringe driver or via the rectal route. This is of particular importance if the person with dementia had, before losing the ability to swallow or becoming unconscious, needed certain medications to control distressing symptoms such as pain. Medications that are not essential to the comfort of the patient at the end of life should be discontinued (Twycross and Lichter 1993).

In the final hours of life, patients may be semiconscious or deeply unconscious and unable to swallow secretions from the lungs and throat or to cough. Breathing with partially loose obstructions in the central airway produces noisy respiration that is referred to as the 'death rattle'. This is reported to occur in 56–92 per cent of people who are dying (Bennett 1996; Watts et al. 1997). Witnessing the 'death rattle' can be a distressing experience for family members as the person nears the end of life, and they may believe that the dying person is suffering. There has been little research on the subject, and it is not known how much distress this causes the dying person. It is important that family members and carers are reassured and that the cause of the condition is explained.

Management includes positioning to allow postural drainage of the secretions and possibly suctioning with a very soft catheter, although suctioning the secretions can also be distressing to the person and for the family to witness. The drugs scopolamine (hyoscine hydrobromide) or glycopyrronium bromide as a single parenteral (non-oral) dose or a subcutaneous infusion via a syringe driver may be administered as these are effective in drying up secretions (Ahmedzai 1993; Twycross and Lichter 1993; Bennett 1996). Care needs to be taken when using these drugs in older people as hyoscine can cause agitation (*British National Formulary* 2001).

Sedation

The practice of using sedation in the hospice environment has become a controversial topic (Balfour Mount 1996; Chater et al. 1998; Fainsinger 1998; Morita et al. 1999; Fainsinger et al. 2000). The controversial aspect of this practice has been related to the ethical issues of euthanasia, particularly the doctrine or principle of double effect and the implications to hospice practice of using medications that are deemed to shorten life. The doctrine of double effect is one attempt to specify conditions of the principle of non-maleficence, or doing no harm in situations in which a person cannot avoid all harms and still achieve important goods (Beachamp and Childress 1994).

It is important that care staff who are experienced in palliative care but less experienced in dementia care understand the difference between dementia behaviour and delirium. In the older population, a mixed syndrome may present, with delirium superimposed on a pre-existing dementia (Fraser 1998). A comprehensive history from family or friends will help health care professionals to arrive at a correct diagnosis. Delirium generally develops as an acute event, at least until the last days of life, whereas a dementia will have been present for some time prior to the terminal stage (Fraser 1998). In the field of palliative care, the most common problem requiring sedation is delirium (Fainsinger et al. 2000), or physical restlessness with or without delirium (Morita et al. 1999).

Chater et al. (1998), having carried out a postal survey of 61 selected palliative care experts, provided a scale of reasons for 'terminal sedation'. They identified pain as the most common reason for using 'terminal sedation', followed by anguish, with agitation, delirium, confusion and hallucinations identified as the third most common reason, in equal place with fear, panic, anxiety and terror. In identifying the limitations of this study, Morita et al. (1999) note the lack of an internationally accepted definition of sedation. It is evident within the literature that there is no firm agreement on what sedation or even 'terminal sedation' means.

The sedatives cited as the first-line approach were the opioids (Morita et al. 1999), midazolam being the second most frequently used agent. Chater et al. (1998) and Fainsinger et al. (2000), however, identify the administration of midazalom as the first-line approach to sedation. A range of other sedating agents were identified and were sometimes administered in conjunction with both opioids and midazalom. Descriptions vary in terms of what criteria should be used in the identification of 'intractable distress' in a person who is dying, and personal judgements to administer these are made by palliative care medical and nursing staff.

Research on this subject has focused on the cancer patient rather than on those with dementia. The anecdotal evidence of an episode of lucidity occurring immediately prior to death in patients with advanced dementia is an argument in favour of a non-sedating approach to the care of people with advanced dementia. The experience of family and care staff witnessing this lucidity may have a positive and profound impact on their bereavement.

End Stage

The question that is often asked by relatives during the terminal stage is how long it will be before the person dies. Family members often want to be at the bedside of the dying person, and one concern for staff is when to call the family so that they can be with the dying person at the end. Accuracy of prediction of survival by different professional groups in a hospice found that nursing auxiliaries could predict the imminent death more accurately than other health professionals (Oxenham and Cornbleet 1998). Some of the physical changes that can occur and that indicate that death may be imminent are the altered appearance of the dying person. The dying person's skin will be cool to touch, and there may changes in pulse rate and breathing pattern. Allowing and supporting family members to stay with the dying person is an important contribution to managing bereavement. Making provision for family to stay overnight needs to be considered if this is important for them. The opportunity for family and friends to be able to spend quality time with their terminally ill relative and to be able to say their good-byes has a significant impact on their ability to cope with the loss when it does occur (Parkes 1996).

Bereavement

Bereavement experiences and responses are highly influenced by the manner in which people came to know of their illness and how the time between diagnosis and death was spent (Shuchter and Zisook 1993; Parkes 1996). Breaking bad news is a skill that has a high profile in oncology and palliative care, and there is an extensive literature on ethical discussions regarding truth-telling within these specialities. The general indication is that, within the Western world, patients should be informed of a diagnosis of a terminal illness.

Surveys on the practice of telling patients that they have a diagnosis of dementia show a wide variation in what occurs (Erde et al. 1988; Rice and Warner 1994; Maguire et al. 1996). Carers are invariably told the diagnosis, whereas there is considerable variation in the practice of informing the individual concerned of the diagnosis. At a stage at which the dementia is mild or even moderate, the person with dementia is often told the diagnosis but rarely the prognosis (Rice and Warner 1994). Maguire et al. (1996) found that 83 per cent of the relatives of sufferers of DAT did not want the person to be told of the diagnosis, although 71 per cent of them would want to be told if they themselves were diagnosed with DAT. Dementia syndromes are terminal illnesses and therefore need to be considered in the same manner as any other life-threatening illness. There are, however, considerations related to the stage of dementia and the ability of those with dementia to take part in discussions related to diagnosis and prognosis, as well as to the impact that such a discussion may have on them psychologically.

Pitt (1997) lists a number of reasons why people should be told the diagnosis, these being similar to the reasons given to support telling other terminally ill people their diagnosis and prognosis. These include providing time to make a will, make an advance directive, arrange power of attorney, settle business affairs and make plans regarding living arrangements. It also allows the opportunity to consider taking medications offered in the treatment of DAT and to be involved in drug trials and new investigations into the treatment of dementia syndromes. Other reasons listed are that unsafe activities such as driving may be more readily stopped, opportunities to develop memory strategies gained, counselling more readily accepted and family issues addressed more freely. Alzheimer Scotland, Action on Dementia (Fearnley et al. 1997) have developed a comprehensive publication, *The right to know? Sharing the diagnosis of dementia*, for the patients and carers of those with a dementia syndrome; this discusses the many issues that impact on informing people of the diagnosis and is a useful resource book for both the families of people with dementia and professionals.

The death of a person with dementia may, for a number of reasons, be viewed with relief by the relatives. The family may believe that the patient does not have a good quality of life and that their misery is prolonged as long as they stay alive (Gessert et al. 2001). Gessert et al. (2001) found that many of the participants of their study were ambivalent about the anticipated death of their relatives, and whereas they believed that death would be a blessing, they did not want to appear overly receptive to death or be seen to be unseemly in advocating death. The researchers identified common challenges faced by the families of people with late-stage dementia. These were guilt associated with the institutionalization of the family member, unfamiliarity with death in general and death caused by advancing dementia in particular, and limited understanding of the natural cause of late-stage dementia. They also found that family members were unfamiliar with setting goals and making decisions on behalf of another and confused about what actions, or inactions, might 'cause' the death of their relative. Lack of contact and communication with health professionals was also identified as a barrier, as was the fact that family members did not understand the physical changes that were taking place, and care needs of the person with end-stage dementia.

The response of relief on the part of the relative at the death of the person with dementia may result in a conflicted grief response in the family member (Parkes 1996). Bereaved relatives may not experience the anxiety or numbness and blunting that are often felt in the phases of grief. They may not expect to miss the dead person at all, and over time it will become clear that there is unfinished business, particularly if there was no opportunity before the cognitive deterioration of the dead person to address family and relationship issues. Those who are bereaved may find themselves haunted by memories and experience feelings of anger and guilt (Parkes 1996). The most intense and lasting form of guilt is associated with 'betrayal' of the spouse and the perception that they may have contributed to the death by improper feeding and deprivation of affection or support (Shuchter and Zisook 1993). An example of this is admission to a care facility even though the relatives may have promised the person with dementia that this would never be allowed. Gessert et al. (2001) recommend that advance care planning would both improve end-of-life care for dying people with dementia and improve the experience of family members involved in end-of-life decision-making and bereavement experiences.

The person with dementia may also experience bereavement, both as a manifestation of the illness and as a result of the move from home. Miesen (1997) states that his clinical observations and research have proved that people with DAT still respond to their illness even after their 'illness-insight' has disappeared. The person with dementia experiences a chronic trauma related to separation, loss, powerlessness, displacement and homelessness (Miesen 1997), symptoms that are also experienced by the bereaved.

Hospices have a long history of providing comprehensive bereavement services for patients, their families and staff, but this is not the situation in relation to residential and nursing homes (Field and James 1993; Katz et al. 2000). Most staff in nursing and residential homes do not have the resources and do not feel able to provide a bereavement service for their residents, and there is a lack of training in communication skills and bereavement care for staff in these environments (Katz et al. 2000). A number of bereavement services in the community may be accessed, but relatives are left to access these through their own efforts or via their general practitioner. Katz et al. (2000) have also identified a need for bereavement support for staff in residential and nursing homes as staff often became very closely involved with the residents in their care, frequently over a number of years.

The events of the last days of life are what relatives are most likely to remember after the death of the patient. Care that maintains the dignity of the dying person during the terminal phase is essential. It is important that relevant discussion is initiated and clear explanations given in relation to care so that no stress is produced from a lack of understanding of the dying process. It is also good practice to reassure relatives that they have made the right decisions regarding any intervention or non-intervention related to care.

CASE STUDIES

Using the principles outlined in this chapter, we can see in the following case illustrations how it is possible to assess and plan high-quality care for individuals with dementia.

The following course of action will be adopted:

Case 1   Mrs M is 81 years old and has been resident for 3 years in a nursing home that caters for a small number of people with dementia. She has a 57-year-old married daughter and three grandchildren who are all regular visitors and are actively interested in her care. Six years before her admission, Mrs M had a right mastectomy for breast cancer. Mrs M's behaviour is usually happy and vivacious, and although her cognitive impairment is very advanced and she is incontinent, she has remained mobile and active. Over the past few weeks, however, she has become more and more withdrawn, spending a lot of time lying on her bed reluctant or unable to get up to walk. The night staff have reported that she is not sleeping much and that she has begun to moan and rock in the night. The care assistants say that her behaviour, particularly when they touch her, indicates that she is experiencing some pain, particularly back pain. She has been taking regular paracetamol for the last week, but this has had no impact on her pain behaviour.

- Using appropriate pain assessment scales and after discussion, the primary care staff will carry out a comprehensive assessment of Mrs M's pain, identifying the site and pain triggers based on a range of responses. All possible causes – urinary tract infection, constipation, muscular pain and osteoarthritis – will be considered.
- Staff will investigate the possibility of bone metastases as a result of Mrs M's history and also consider possible cord compression as she has stopped walking. (Cord compression is a palliative care emergency in which paralysis occurs because of collapse of the spinal vertebrae.)
- A neurological assessment will be carried out by either the general practitioner or the palliative care consultant to assess for possible neurological damage and the possibility of bone disease. If findings are positive, negotiations will take place with the family and care team to decide what further investigations or interventions – hospitalization, bone scan, radiotherapy treatment or a move from her familiar environment – should be undertaken and what impact this will have on Mrs M. If there is no cord compression, a bone scan in should be considered in joint discussion. As Mrs M. was fully mobile before this episode, all efforts should be made to regain her mobility. Future palliative management should be discussed with the family and primary carers if bone metastases are confirmed.
- Referral should be made to the specialist palliative care team in view of Mrs M's previous history of cancer and that the fact that there are now signs of metatastic disease and potential symptom control issues.
- Although Mrs M has been having regular paracetamol (the first step of analgesic ladder), this has not relieved her pain, so a move should be made to the second step of the ladder and a weak opioid such as dihydocodeine commenced, along with a non-steroidal agent (e.g. Arthrotec) possibly with stomach protection.
- If there is incomplete relief, opioid analgesia (along with a laxative; the third step of the ladder) will be started at a low dose but not one below the analgesic level reached at second step.
- If poor pain relief is obtained from opioids, the palliative care team can be asked to examine Mrs M for neuropathic (nerve) pain and add adjuvant medication (e.g. an antidepressant or anticonvulsant) to try to relieve this.
- Staff will continue to monitor the effect of analgesia and watch for side-effects.

- As pain has an impact on mood, psychological interventions to enhance Mrs M's mood will be explored.
- The emphasis of care will be on maintaining comfort and supporting the family.

Case 2   Mr T, aged 76 years, was admitted to a nursing home following the death of his wife. The couple had no children, the only living relative being his sister-in-law, who was in her 80s and physically unable to visit him at the home. He had been diagnosed as having DAT 3 years earlier, and his wife had managed his care at home. Mr T appeared to become very depressed shortly after his admission, and his physical condition deteriorated rapidly. He was prescribed an antidepressant, but this had not had any significant effect on his deterioration, and within 3 months he was unable, or at least refusing, even to walk. He began to refuse to eat or take any fluids, although there is no clear evidence that he could not chew and swallow food or fluids; he becomes aggressive when attempts are made to persuade him to eat. Mr T had been a heavy smoker previous to his admission to the home, and he has developed a persistent and loose cough with green sputum since becoming bed-bound.

Bereavement is a major issue here – Mr T may no longer want to live after losing his wife. The following plan will be implemented:

- Mr T will be referred to a bereavement service experienced in working with people with dementia. Reminiscence techniques can be used to allow him to discuss his wife, photos of his wife can be placed near him, staff can investigate whether he wants to go to her grave but is unable to express this.
- A change of antidepressant may be beneficial if this has not been tried already. Referral will preferably be made to the psychogeriatric services.
- As Mr T was a heavy smoker, he may have nicotine withdrawal so nicotine patches should be considered.
- A chest infection may be present. Mr T should be assessed and treated with a broad-spectrum antibiotic rather than being taken to hospital for an X-ray. Mr T's temperature will be monitored.
- Staff will check that he does not have any mouth or denture problems such as candidiasis or poorly fitting dentures.
- Different foods can be offered – Mr T's sister-in-law may be able to identify his preferences. Above all, Mr T must not be force fed.
- Undiagnosed pain or discomfort related to undiagnosed underlying disease or infection (including oral infection) may be present, which can be assessed using appropriate scales and a detailed history.
- If swallowing remains a problem, non-oral methods of delivering analgesia (i.e. suppositories or the subcutaneous route) can be employed.
- If Mr T is not able resume eating and drinking, the primary carers should discuss a palliative care plan, for example related to managing care and support.
- The emphasis of care will be on maintaining Mr T's comfort.

REFERENCES

Addington-Hall, J.M. 1998: *Reaching out: specialist palliative care for adults with non-malignant disease*. National Council for Hospice and Specialist Palliative Care Services and Scottish Partnership Agency for Palliative and Cancer Care. Occasional Paper no. 14. London: Department of Palliative Care and Policy.

Addington-Hall, J.M. 2000: *Positive partnerships: palliative care for adults with severe mental health problems*. National Council for Hospice and Specialist Palliative Care Services and Scottish Partnership Agency for Palliative and Cancer Care. Occasional Paper no. 17. London: Department of Palliative Care and Policy.

Addington-Hall, J.M., Fakhoury, W. and McCarthy, M. 1998: Specialist palliative care in non-malignant disease. *Palliative Medicine* **12:** 417–27.

Ahmedzai, S. 1993. Palliation of respiratory symptoms. In: Doyle, D., Hanks, G.W.C. and MacDonald, N. eds. *Oxford textbook of palliative medicine*. Oxford: Oxford University Press, 349–78.

Ahronheim, J.C., Morrison, R.S., Baskin, S.A., Morris, J. and Meier, D.E. 1996: Treatment of the dying in the acute care hospital. *Archives of Internal Medicine* **156:** 2094–100.

Atkinson, J.C. and Fox, P. 1992: Salivary gland dysfunction. *Clinical Geriatric Medicine* **8:** 499–511.

Balfour Mount, E.M. 1996: Morphine drips, terminal sedation, and slow euthanasia: definitions and facts, not anecdotes. *Journal of Palliative Care* **12:** 31–7.

Beauchamp, T.L. and Childress, J.F. 1994: *Principles of biomedical ethics*, 4th edn. Oxford: Oxford University Press.

Bennett, M. 1996: Death rattle: an audit of hyoscine (scopolamine) use and review of management. *Journal of Pain and Symptom Management* **12:** 229–33.

Black, D. and Jolley, D. 1990: Slow euthanasia? The deaths of psychogeriatric patients. *British Medical Journal* **300:** 1321–3.

Black, D. and Jolley, D. 1991: Deaths in psychiatric care. *International Journal of Geriatric Psychiatry* **6:** 489–95.

Brechling, B.G. and Kuhn, D. 1989: A specialized hospice for dementia patients and their families. *American Journal of Hospice Care* May/June: 27–30.

British National Formulary. 2001. London: British Medical Association and Royal Pharmaceutical Society of Great Britain.

Bruera, E., Franco, J.J., Maltoni, M., Watanabe, S. and Suarez-Almazor, M. 1995: Changing pattern of agitated impaired mental status in patients with advanced cancer: association with cognitive monitoring, hydration, and opioid rotation. *Journal of Pain and Symptom Management* **10:** 287–91.

Buckman, R. 1993: Communication in palliative care: a practical guide. In: Doyle, D., Hanks, G.W.C. and MacDonald, N. eds. *Oxford textbook of palliative medicine*. Oxford: Oxford University Press, 47–61.

Burns, A., Jacoby, R., Luthert, P. and Levy, R. 1990: Causes of death in Alzheimer's disease. *Age and Ageing* **19:** 341–4.

Chater, S., Viola, R., Paterson, J. and Jarvis, V. 1998: Sedation for intractable distress in the dying – a survey of experts. *Palliative Medicine* **12:** 255–69.

Craig, G.M. 1994: On withholding nutrition and hydration in the terminally ill: has palliative medicine gone too far? *Journal of Medical Ethics* **20:** 139–43.

Dementia Services Development Centre. 1995: *Dementia in the community: management strategies for general practice*. Stirling: DSDC.

Dickerson, J. 1995: The problem of hospital-induced malnutrition. *Nursing Times* 25(91): 44–5.

Eagles, J.M., Beattie, J.A.G., Restall, D.B., Rawlinson, F., Hagen, S. and Ashcroft, G.W. 1990: Relations between cognitive impairment and early death in the elderly. *British Medical Journal* **300**: 239–40.

Ellershaw, J.E., Sutcliffe, J.M. and Saunders, C.M. 1995: Dehydration in the dying patient. *Journal of Pain and Symptom Management* **10**: 192–7.

Erde, E.L., Nadal, E.C. and Scholl, T.O. 1988: On truth telling and the diagnosis of Alzheimer's disease. *Journal of Family Practice* **26**: 401–6.

Fabiszewski, K.J., Volicer, B.J. and Volicer, L. 1990: Effect of antibiotic treatment on outcome of fevers in institutionalized Alzheimer patients. *Journal of the American Medical Association* **263**: 3168–72.

Fainsinger, R.L. 1998: Dehydration. In: MacDonald, N. ed. *Palliative medicine: a case-based manual*. Oxford: Oxford University Press, 91–9.

Fainsinger, R.L., Waller, A., Bercovici, M. et al. 2000: A multicentre international study of sedation for uncontrolled symptoms of terminally ill patients. *Palliative Medicine* **14**: 257–65.

Fearnley, K., McLennan, J. and Weaks, D. 1997: *The right to know? Sharing the diagnosis of dementia*. Edinburgh: Alzheimer Scotland, Action on Dementia.

Ferrell, B.A., Ferrell, B.R. and Rivera, L. 1995: Pain in cognitively impaired nursing home patients. *Journal of Pain and Symptom Management* **10**: 591–8.

Field, D. and James, N. 1993: Where and how people die. In: Clark, D. ed. *The future for palliative care*. Buckingham: Open University Press, 6–29.

Finlay, I. 1995: Oral fungal infections. *European Journal of Palliative Care* 2(2 suppl. 1): 4–7.

Fraser, J. 1998: Cognitive impairment. In: MacDonald N. ed. *Palliative medicine: a case-based manual*. Oxford: Oxford University Press, 48–58.

Galloway, S. and Turner, L. 1999: Pain assessment in older adults who are cognitively impaired. *Journal of Gerontological Nursing* July: 34–9.

Gessert, C.E., Forbes, S. and Bern-Klug, M. 2001: Planning end-of-life care for patients with dementia: roles of families and health professionals. *Omega* **42**: 273–91.

Hanrahan, P. and Luchins, D. 1995a: Feasibility criteria for enrolling end-stage dementia patients in home hospice care. *Hospice Journal* **10**: 47–54.

Hanrahan, P. and Luchins, D.J. 1995b: Access to hospice care for end-stage dementia patients: a national survey of hospice programmes. *Journal of the American Geriatric Society* **43**: 56–9.

Hanrahan, P., Raymond, M., McGowan, E. and Luchins, D.J. 1999: Criteria for enrolling dementia patients in hospice: a replication. *American Journal of Hospice and Palliative Care* **16**: 395–400.

Hermans, D., Lisaerde, J. and Triau, E. 1989: Sense and non-sense of a technological health care model in terminally ill demented patients. The first international conference on the palliative care of the elderly: an overview. *Journal of Palliative Care* **5**: 39–42.

Holmes, S. 1998: The aetiology of malnutrition in hospital. *Professional Nurse Study Supplement* **13**: S5–S8.

House, N. 1992: The hydration question: hydration or dehydration of terminally ill patients. *Professional Nurse* **8**: 44–8.

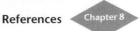

Hurley, A.C., Volicer, B.J., Hanrahan, S.H. and Volicer, L. 1992: Assessment of discomfort in advanced Alzheimer patients. *Research in Nursing and Health* **15:** 369–77.

Ineichen, B. 1990: The extent of dementia among old people in residential care. *International Journal of Geriatric Psychiatry* **5:** 327–35.

Ineichen, B. 1992: Home facts. *Nursing the Elderly* March/April: 24–5.

Jobbin, J., Bagg, J., Finlay, I.G., Addy, M. and Newcombe, G.G. 1992: Oral and dental disease in terminally ill cancer patients. *British Medical Journal* **304:** 1612.

Jolley, D. and Baxter, D. 1997: Life expectation in organic brain disease. *Advances in Psychiatric Treatment* **3:** 211–18.

Katz, J., Sidell, M. and Komaromy, C. 2000: Death in homes: bereavement needs of residents, relatives and staff. *International Journal of Palliative Nursing* **6:** 274–9.

Kovach, C.R., Weissman, D.E., Griffie, J., Matson, S. and Muchka, S. 1999: Assessment and treatment of discomfort for people with late-stage dementia. *Pain and Symptom Management* **18:** 412–19.

Krishanasamy, M. 1995: The nurse's role in oral care. *European Journal of Palliative Care* **2**(suppl. 1): 8–9.

Lefebvre-Chapiro, S. and the DOPOLUS group. 2001: The DOLOPLUS 2 scale – evaluating pain in the elderly. *European Journal of Palliative Care* **8:** 191–3.

Lloyd-Williams, M. 1996: An audit of palliative care in dementia. *European Journal of Cancer Care* **5:** 53–5.

Luchins, D.J. and Hanrahan, P. 1993: What is appropriate health care for end-stage dementia? *Journal of the American Geriatric Society* **41:** 25–30.

Luchins, D.J., Hanrahan, P. and Murphy, K. 1997: Criteria for enrolling dementia patients in hospice. *Journal of the American Geriatrics Society* **45:** 1054–9.

McCarthy, M., Addington-Hall, J.M. and Altman, D. 1997: The experience of dying with dementia a retrospective study. *International Journal of Geriatric Psychiatry* **12:** 404–9.

MacDonald, N. 1998: Ethical issues in hydration and nutrition. In: Bruera, E. and Portenoy, R.K. eds. *Topic in palliative care*, volume 2. Oxford: Oxford University Press, 153–63.

McLaren, S. and Green, S. 1998: Nutritional screening and assessment. *Professional Nurse Study Supplement* **13:** S9–S15.

McLean, W. 2000: *Facilitator's book for pain management in people with dementia in institutional care*. Stirling: Dementia Service Development Centre.

Maguire, C.P., Kirby, M., Coen, R., Coakley, D., Lawlor, B.A. and O'Neill, D. 1996: Family members' attitudes toward telling the patient with Alzheimer's disease their diagnosis. *British Medical Journal* **313:** 529–30.

Marzinski, L.R. 1991: The tragedy of dementia: clinically assessing pain in the confused, non-verbal elderly. *Journal of Gerontology Nursing* **17:** 25–8.

Meares, C.J. 1994: Terminal dehydration: a review. *American Journal of Hospice and Palliative Care* **11:** 10–14.

Meares, C.J. 2000: Nutritional issues in palliative care. *Seminars in Oncology Nursing* **16:** 135–45.

Miesen, B.M.L. 1997: Awareness in dementia patients and family grieving: a practical perspective. In: Miesen, B.M.L. and Jones, G.M.M. eds. *Care giving in dementia: research and applications*, volume 2. Routledge: London, 67–79.

Milligan, S., McGill, M., Sweeney, M.P. and Malarkey, C. 2001: Oral care for people with advanced cancer: an evidence-based protocol. *International Journal of Palliative Nursing* **7:** 418–26.

Morant, R. and Senn, H. 1993: The management of infections in palliative care. In: Doyle, D., Hanks, G.W.C. and MacDonald, N. eds. *Oxford textbook of palliative medicine*. Oxford: Oxford University Press, 378–84.

Morita, T., Tsunoda, J., Inque, S. and Chihara, S. 1999: Do hospice clinicians sedate patients intending to hasten death? *Journal of Palliative Care* **15:** 20–3.

Morrison, R.S., Ahronheim, J.C., Morrison, G.R. et al. 1998: Pain and discomfort associated with common hospital procedures and experiences. *Journal of Pain and Symptom Management* **15:** 91–101.

Oxenham, D. and Cornbleet, M. 1998: Accuracy of prediction of survival by different professional groups in a hospice. *Palliative Medicine* **12:** 117–18.

Parke, B. 1998: Realizing the presence of pain in cognitively impaired older adults. *Journal of Gerontological Nursing* June: 21–30.

Parkes, C.M. 1996: *Bereavement: studies of grief in adult life*, 3rd edn. London: Routledge.

Pitt, B. 1997: 'You've got Alzheimer's disease': telling the patient. *Current Opinion in Psychiatry* **10:** 307–8.

Porter, F.L., Malhotra, K.M., Wolf, C.M., Morris, J.C., Miller, J.P. and Smith, M.C. 1996: Dementia and response to pain in the elderly. *Pain* **68:** 413–21.

Radbruch, L., Sabatowski, R., Loick, G. et al. 2000: Cognitive impairment and its influence on pain and symptom assessment in a palliative care unit: development of a minimal documentation system. *Palliative Medicine* **14:** 266–76.

Rice, K. and Warner, N. 1994: Breaking the bad news: what do psychiatrists tell patients with dementia about their illness? *International Journal of Geriatric Psychiatry* **9:** 467–71.

Roberts, A.L. 1997: Dehydration and the dying patient. *International Journal of Palliative Nursing* **3:** 156–60.

Shuchter, S.R. and Zisook, S. 1993: The course of normal grief. In: Stroebe M.S., Stroebe, W. and Hansson, R.O. eds. *Handbook of bereavement*. Cambridge: Cambridge University Press, 23–43.

Simons, W. and Malabar, R. 1995: Assessing pain in elderly patients who cannot respond verbally. *Journal of Advanced Nursing* **22:** 663–9.

Stein, W.M. 2001: Assessment of symptoms in the cognitively impaired. In: Bruera, E. and Portenoy, R.K. eds. *Topics in palliative care*, volume 5. Oxford: Oxford University Press, 123–33.

Sweeting, H. 1997: Keynote address: Dying and dementia. In: Cox, S., Gilhooly, M. and McLennan, J. eds. *Dying and dementia*. Report of a conference jointly organised by the Centre for Gerontology and Health Studies, Paisley University and the Dementia Services Development Centre, Department of Applied Social Science, University of Stirling. Stirling: University of Stirling.

Twycross, R.G. and Lichter, I. 1993: The terminal phase. In: Doyle, D., Hanks, G.W.C. and MacDonald, N. eds. *Oxford textbook of palliative medicine*. Oxford: Oxford University Press, 649–61.

Volicer, L. 1986: Need for hospice approach to treatment of patients with advanced progressive dementia. *Journal of the American Geriatrics Society* **34:** 655–8.

Volicer, L. 1997: Hospice care for dementia patients. *Journal of the American Geriatric Society* **45:** 1147–9.

Walker, P. and Bruera, E. 1998: Anorexia–cachexia syndrome. In: MacDonald, N. ed. *Palliative medicine: a case based manual*. Oxford: Oxford University Press, 1–14.

Watts, T., Jenkins, K. and Back, I. 1997: Problem and management of noisy rattling breathing in dying patients. *International Journal of Palliative Nursing* **3:** 245–52.

World Health Organization. 1996: *Cancer pain relief*. Geneva: WHO.

Remembering and forgetting: group work with people who have dementia

Richard Cheston, Kerry Jones and Jane Gilliard

In Chapter 6, Bartlett and Cheston set out some of the key elements of individual counselling or psychotherapy with people with dementia. They described how many people with dementia have a sense of personal responsibility for their illness, and how meeting others who are going through a similar experience can have a positive therapeutic effect. An obvious way to help people with dementia to meet others going through a similar process is to bring them together as a group.

BACKGROUND TO GROUP PSYCHOTHERAPY

Group work with older people with a cognitive impairment has been described since the early 1950s. Of particular importance has been the work of Naomi Feil (1990, 1992, 1993), whose development of validation therapy effectively established the first legitimate way of working with and addressing the emotional concerns of older people with a cognitive impairment. Feil suggested that, in many cases, neurological damage interacted with unresolved issues from a person's past so that those psychological defences which had been used up to that point were no longer effective. This precipitated a situation in which the person with dementia returned to the past in order to work through these unresolved issues, the task of the validation therapist being to validate this inward journey back through time. In order to do this, Feil stressed the importance of therapists listening with empathy, using non-threatening questions in order to build up trust and by not confronting people with the loss of their abilities.

Feil's work has proved to be influential – in part because she has been one of the strongest voices urging dementia care workers to take the emotional needs of people with dementia seriously. Two criticisms can, however, be made of this way of working. First, there is the danger that, in associating the apparent 'confusion' of some older people with unresolved psychological issues, we risk attributing the presence of dementia to personal rather than organic factors. Second, although we are all influenced by our past, there is a danger that, in looking backwards, we forget how awful the current reality can be for people with dementia.

One of the most significant clinical developments over the past 10 years has been a growing awareness of how important the perspective of the person with dementia is. This has been a central pillar of the 'new culture of dementia care' (Kitwood and Benson 1995). As researchers and clinicians have grown more aware of the emotional needs of people with dementia, so there has been a concern to find innovative ways of supporting people through this process. This desire to create a supportive context within which people could talk about what was happening to them was stimulated by the publication in 1995 by Robyn Yale of a book setting out how to establish, run and evaluate support groups for those with dementia. This has helped to encourage many clinicians to establish similar support groups within the UK.

THE DEMENTIA VOICE GROUP PSYCHOTHERAPY PROJECT FOR PEOPLE WITH DEMENTIA

Over the 2 years prior to writing this chapter, we have been working on a project funded by the Mental Health Foundation that has involved setting up and evaluating the effectiveness of six psychotherapy groups, each lasting for 10 weeks. Five of the six groups consisted of between six and eight people, the sixth group having 10 par-ticipants. Our referral criteria adapted those that had been set out by Yale (1995). All participants involved in the groups had to have a diagnosis of Alzheimer's disease or another form of dementia; they had to acknowledge, at least occasionally, both that they had a memory problem and that this was caused by more than just the effects of old age; and they had to be willing to attend a support group.

A total of 42 people took part in the groups, all of whom were assessed as having either a mild or a moderate level of dementia. Most people lived at home with their husband or wife, although some lived on their own or in a nursing home. The participants and their carers were interviewed at five different points: about 6 weeks before the groups started; at the start of the groups; after 7 weeks; at the end of the groups; and 10 weeks after the groups had finished. Twenty-seven people finished the groups and the follow-up period, baseline data being available for 19 of these. Overall, our results showed that the levels of anxiety and depression reduced significantly during the groups compared with the baseline and follow-up periods (Cheston, Jones and Gilliard, in review).

In writing about the process of group work with people with dementia in this chapter, we will draw heavily on our experiences of facilitating and evaluating these six groups.

BALANCING THINKING AND DOING

Clare (2001) has described how people with dementia talk about themselves as if caught between two conflicting tendencies: a 'self-protective' tendency, in which individuals wish to deny or minimize the changes that have occurred; and an integrative tendency, in which they begin to acknowledge the full extent of the changes and try to integrate them into their self-concept. In terms of the internal dynamics of the groups, this way of conceptualizing the experience of people with dementia could be viewed in terms of a continuum between two poles (Sutton-Smith, personal communication, 1996): at one end were some people who were concerned with doing things rather than talking about their feelings; at the other were those who were overwhelmed by the awfulness of what was happening and who had difficulty in moving on. Having participants who are able to articulate one or other of the poles of the continuum is vital if a group is to function well. Indeed, it may be that the best groups are composed equally of people who do rather than feel, and people who feel rather than do.

The balancing act of the group facilitators is to hold on to the need of some people to talk about their feelings, and of others to talk about how they will overcome and escape from these feelings. The group needs neither to be overwhelmed with despair, nor to be so busy doing things that they are unable to think, even for a moment, about what is happening to them. The task for the group facilitators is to bring the group back to the central point of the group – the sense of living with these changes – and to do this at a pace and in a way that is sensitive to the needs of the whole group.

THINKING AND FORGETTING ABOUT WHAT HAS HAPPENED

We ask a lot of those who come to our groups: we ask participants to remember what it is like not to be able to remember, and to communicate what it is like when you cannot find the words with which to talk. We ask people to think and to talk together about things that they might otherwise try to forget.

If we are to ask people to do these difficult things, we need to understand something about the psychological processes of 'forgetfulness'. In using this term, we do not mean the process of laying down new memories or the cognitive functions of working memory. What we mean by 'forgetfulness' is both the experience of not being able to remember and the associated wish to forget this experience. We see this as the key theme within group work, indeed within psychotherapeutic work with people with dementia: our task as facilitators is often to remember the forgetfulness.

The theme of 'forgetfulness' is much more than having a poor memory for people's names or a poor memory for the very words with which to describe and to articulate feelings; it is about more than being unable to remember how to solve problems. It is also about how people cope with the emotional consequences of this poor memory – the desire to forget and to be forgotten, the sense of being forgotten about.

UNDERSTANDING GROUP PROCESSES

As human beings, we all screen out and modify disturbing information of all types. The same is true for people with dementia. This forgetfulness is both

Box 9.1 Exercise for group leaders – think about your own forgetfulness

Trying to help others to remember what it is like not to be able to remember is an act of great caring, but it can also be hard and painful. If we expect the people in our groups to talk about difficult feelings, it is important that, as group facilitators, we are able to deal with feelings in our own lives that may be difficult for us. If we are to think about forgetfulness, we also need to hold onto our own forgetfulness – the way in which many of us, as dementia care workers, deal with the tensions and strains of our own work by being forgetful. Perhaps we forget to go back and have that cup of tea we talked about. Perhaps we forget about our own relatives who have died with Alzheimer's disease. We need to have a strategy to allow us to survive; we need to be able to be touched and moved without being overwhelmed ourselves. The danger is that we end up being too forgetful.

Before the group starts, spend time talking together about your own thoughts and concerns for the group:

- What single aspect of dementia do you find most distressing? What are you going to find it hardest to hear people in your group talk about?
- How good are you at working with the anger, tears and despair of others when it may leave you feeling powerless and unable to help?
- Are you someone who finds it easier to be positive than negative? Are you someone who always needs to look on the bright side of life? If so, how will you listen to people for whom life may be very bleak?
- How important is it for you that everyone in the group likes each other? What will you do if group participants seem to take a dislike to each other? What will you do if they become angry with you or with each other?
- How are you going to talk to your colleagues about what you are doing? What are the limits of confidentiality in the group? Who outside the group may be hostile towards and critical of what you are doing?

One place to do this will be through a shared supervision of your clinical work (*see* Chapter 16).

separate from and linked to the neurological process of dementia. It is separate from it in the same way that some people with lung cancer 'forget' to tell their partner that they are receiving treatment or even that they have been diagnosed as having cancer. In other ways, 'forgetfulness' is also linked to the neurological process because this affects the brain and the process of remembering. Moreover, other people around the individual with dementia may attribute all examples of forgetfulness to neurological damage, rather than to the person's fear of neurological damage, as they often find it too painful to think about or to bear. They, too, will be in danger of being forgetful.

If being in a psychotherapy group involves having to think about and remember what is happening, we have to help people to remember so many different things. First, there is the pain of remembering the forgetfulness. There is often fury and sadness when people remember how things have changed for them. For some in our groups, this pain was clear when they remembered how they stopped driving, whereas for others it lay in remembering that they could no longer mend a plug or do the ironing. One woman described it as feeling like falling down a hole, but when the woman next to her said 'Yes, but you climb out of it, don't you?', she replied, 'Yes, but you always climb out in a different place to where you fell in.'

Then there is the pain of remembering that you have been forgotten about. For some, this related to being kept in the dark over important information (e.g. the results of a scan), whereas for others it was about being emotionally neglected. One man, for example, spoke of how his wife forgot that he had feelings too, another saying that his family only ever remembered about him when they asked him to get his cheque book out. Some participants described how friends seemed to know what was wrong but did not know how to share this knowing with them. At other times, group participants talked of how they felt as if they were on their own in a crowd simply because others acted as if a fundamental part of them was just not there. As one group member, Beth, commented: 'I feel like I have a placard around my neck saying "Alzheimer's", as people treat you so differently once they know that you have it.'

Going public with Alzheimer's

As we talked within the groups about the pain of being forgotten, there was a mixture of responses. Whereas some group participants articulated their sense of sadness and despair, others expressed their determination that the world must listen to them. Some felt that the solution lay in direct action by publicly disclosing that they had Alzheimer's disease, so that others could understand them better – as one lady put it, 'We must come out of the closet with Alzheimer's.'

This assertiveness was a strong theme but difficult for many other people within the groups to join in with. The sense of sadness at what had changed was more commonly compounded by a wish to forget about themselves and be forgotten about by others. In many group sessions, it was hard to stay with these themes, sometimes because group participants preferred to talk about other, less threatening issues, sometimes because others in the group were critical of this way of talking.

Trying to forget about it

Actively trying not to think about what was happening to them was often a way of coping for participants within the group. For Stan, the nights were a place of refuge where he could forget about what was happening: 'I can't wait for the night; I can go to sleep, I can forget about the dementia for a while.' As a participant in another group remarked, the problem with his memory was not what he forgot, but what he remembered.

This is natural and to be expected: some people find it easiest to be preoccupied with business, to go on with life and to shut out their awareness of what they cannot bear to contemplate. This can happen in so many ways, so instinctively within a group, that it can be hard to notice. Various strategies for living were described:

- To get by day by day, to live in the here-and-now and never think about tomorrow until it comes. Some group members explicitly stated that this was something that it was 'best not to talk about'.
- To treat dementia as if it were a battle. As one woman said, the goal is 'Never to give up, always to keep fighting on.'
- To search for a cure. Some participants seemed to be preoccupied with finding the right medication, a solution that would take their problems away.
- To laugh it off. Laughter is important in groups, and the sessions were often very funny places to be. Making a joke out of despair was, however, one way in which emotional pain could be avoided. Not everyone in the groups found it helpful to laugh all the time, but for some, laughter was always the best medicine.
- To strike a bargain. Some participants were adamant that, although they had Alzheimer's disease, this affected them in only some ways, or even not at all. One man said that it was a disease that affected only his memory; it would never affect his intellect. Another woman, who had attended a previous programme, spoke over and over again in every group she attended of how, although she had Alzheimer's, this had thankfully not affected her memory.
- To fight the old battles. One man said that he would be all right if only his wife didn't nag him so. He said that he had always felt that way, and that it was because he had switched off in the past that he could now not switch himself back on again. The emotional tensions in his marriage seemed to have been a pervasive feature of his life, with or without dementia.

When emotionally painful material is pushed away, there is inevitably a cost. To borrow a metaphor from Watzlawick et al. (1974), when you walk around the living room with your eyes closed, you're likely to bump into the furniture. Trying not to think about a situation does not mean that the problems will go away – but what does go away, over time, is your ability to deal with the problems meaningfully. The problem with not thinking about what has happened is that what is pushed away is not just the sense of anger and injustice, the vulnerability, but also the chance to think about and make sense of the present, and to plan for the future.

Trying to be forgotten

Some participants were happy to be in the group but wanted to listen and not to talk – they seemed to want to be forgotten about in the group, much as they seemed to want to be forgotten about in life. When these participants did talk, they often spoke about wanting to hide away, to be of as little bother to others as possible. Being quiet in the group seemed to be a way of being forgotten about and of hiding their disability.

For some people in the groups, allowing themselves to be forgotten was one of the few acts of caring left available to them: Molly spoke repeatedly through a session of how her husband struggled to care for both herself and their handicapped daughter. When their second daughter, who lived in Australia, came to visit, Molly told the group that she would go into a nursing home for respite care. The first thoughts of the group facilitators were to suggest that she might feel excluded and shut out. As the groups progressed, however, it became clear that Molly's sense of herself as a burden on her husband was utterly distressing to her. By staying in respite care, she could help him to enjoy his time with both his daughters without having to worry about her. Her wish to withdraw seemed to be her way of expressing her love for her husband.

INFLUENCING GROUP PROCESSES

Groups for people with dementia tend to be a combination of two different strands of work:

- In *educational* groups, the emphasis is on teaching people about their illness and encouraging them to use a variety of strategies in order to facilitate their adjustment to their impairments; such strategies may be talks from visiting speakers (e.g. McAfee et al. 1989), information on Alzheimer's disease (e.g. Haggerty 1990) and teaching memory strategies (e.g. Thrower 1998).
- In *emotionally-focused* groups, the emphasis is on helping people to share their experiences with others. These groups tend to last for about an hour and a half, and use a variety of potentially therapeutic interventions, including

anxiety management skills (e.g. Marshall 2001), focusing on relationship issues (e.g. Hawkins and Eagger 1999) and considering how to cope with the loss of independence (e.g. Barton et al. 2001).

Although some of the groups that we established as part of the Dementia Voice Group Psychotherapy Project included teaching relaxation skills, the predominant focus was on helping people to think and talk about their experiences. Just as there were some in a group who were able to talk about their feelings, so there were others who were more aware of wanting to do something. As group leaders, we tried to manage this tension between feeling and doing in many ways.

Talking about the problems people faced

When participants first came to a group, they sometimes felt a need to tell others how wonderful they thought the group was going to be, how things in their life would be fine from now on; beginning to admit to others in the group that they were not coping was often hard. As group therapists, it is important to listen hard for signs that life is not satisfactory for some people.

When participants disclose that they have worries or concerns, it is important for these voices to be heard and brought back to the group. As problems were talked about and shared, so came the hope that if other people were in the same position, this process could in some way be survived. One of our tasks as therapists was to bear the awfulness while still holding on to the possibility of hope and thereby to suggest that these things can be survived in some sense.

It is only by holding on to and making sense out of what is happening that people are able to achieve some sort of emotional mastery. In working and talking within a group, individuals began to put some shape to their fears and concerns – the 'thing' inside that they had kept hidden gradually began to be named. This process of naming and giving shape to the internal world is gradual because the 'thing' that is the person's experience of dementia is often so overwhelming that it can only be brought into awareness piece by piece. An analogy here is that of entering a bright room from a dark corridor – we can do this at first only by closing our eyes and averting our gaze. Then we can gradually begin to open our eyes but still shield them from the glare of the light by holding our fingers in front of our faces. As we become accustomed to the light, we can gradually begin to explore the interior of the room with our eyes open.

Reflective listening

The central counselling approach adopted by the facilitators within the groups was resolution therapy, a form of therapeutic intervention specifically developed for work with people with dementia (Goudie and Stokes 1989; Stokes and Goudie

1990). Based on humanistic ideas of counselling, resolution therapy offers a means by which the often-hidden emotional messages underlying the actions and language used by people with dementia are sensitively reflected back to them. This can be an effective way of helping people with dementia to make sense of what has been happening to them. A fuller description of the use of this style of working within a group setting with people with dementia can be found elsewhere (Cheston 1998; Cheston and Jones 2000).

Telling stories

One way of making sense of experiences that may be common within groups for people with dementia is telling stories about past events. Cheston (1996) has argued that telling such stories has two functions within a group: as a means of establishing a collective identity for participants as people who have shared similar experiences; and as a means of making links between the past and the present, and thereby making sense of traumatic or difficult experiences.

Within a group setting, it is important to be open to the fact that almost everything that is talked about can be interpreted as having an emotional significance. This is particularly relevant as a way of understanding the significance of the stories that are told within the group. One participant in a group that was part of the Dementia Voice Group Psychotherapy Project told a series of stories about events that had occurred to him throughout his life. A common theme within these stories was related to threat, but in telling the stories, the man spoke of different elements of threat – of wondering whether the threat was real, of understanding whether the threat could be avoided and, finally, of realizing that although the men in the stories had died, they had left something of value behind them. The exploration of threat in his stories paralleled a movement within the groups from the first session, when he had confidently told other participants that he – and they – would all regain their abilities, to the final session, when he spoke movingly of how true friendship involved telling other people the truth, no matter how painful this was.

Telling stories can therefore be a powerful and indirect way of addressing underlying fears and concerns. As one emotion is addressed, more and more layers are revealed, like peeling an onion. In listening to one emotional theme in a story, other, secondary, emotions can become apparent. These often relate to shame and embarrassment – emotions that concern the process of being in a group and having others see a more vulnerable side of oneself.

Pain enacted within the groups

People often come to a psychotherapy group frightened and uncertain. Being frightened, people with dementia may turn away from themselves; as one woman who attended our groups said, 'That's when the curtain comes down and I don't want to think any more.' Attending a group provides a chance to compare oneself with the others in the group, almost as if they were a mirror. The emotional response to looking in this mirror can vary. Sometimes it can be frightening, if one sees oneself as one may become; sometimes, it means regaining a view of oneself that has been lost – one again sees oneself as someone who is supportive, empathic and caring. At other times, it means becoming at ease with oneself, peeking between the cracks of one's fingers to learn that the face in the mirror is one that has always been there. It involves learning to tolerate oneself again.

In looking at themselves in the mirror that others bring to the group, participants may wonder whether the mirror is cracked, whether it might distort their image, whether the reflection that they see is a true one. Conflict between group members can be one way of disavowing the relevance of the reflection – and facilitators have to be able to help the group to view such conflict as an understandable part of the horror and fear that looking in a mirror can bring. As with any extreme form of emotion, it is important that facilitators help participants to feel that the emotions can be contained and managed within the group.

It is important that all the voices of participants within the group are heard. Loud and dominant voices all too often act to prevent alternative viewpoints being expressed. The voices that are excluded are sometimes those which suggest that all is not well, that life may never be the same again and that this is a fearful process. Once again, it is the facilitators' role to enable the group to understand that the apparent failure of the group may reflect the difficulties of looking truthfully in the mirror.

| *Case 1* | Since he had been diagnosed with Alzheimer's at the age of 59, Peter had lost his job, his company car and his driving licence. Peter clearly felt these losses deeply as for him they meant that he was no longer |

the breadwinner for the family, the person others looked up to and respected, the friend who drove to the match on Saturday. His grieving often took the form of tearful anger.

As the group began to meet, the sense that this was a safe place to talk developed. The loss of his driving licence was particularly painful for Peter, and he spoke movingly in one session of how he had one day taken the car keys from the shelf where they were kept and gone out to the car. He had lovingly stroked the bonnet of the car, walking all round it just to feel its touch. He had then put the keys into the lock, opened the door and once again sat in the driving seat. For the first time in years, he had put the keys into the ignition and turned the engine on. Peter cried in the group as he talked about how he wanted to drive the car away, but he knew that his family were watching him from inside the house, worried about what he would do. He eventually turned the ignition off, got out of the car and walked back into the house.

During the final session, Peter was able to say that, although he was saddened by the loss of his licence, he felt that he was now not as angry. He felt there were other things in life that were important, and he was wondering about selling his car at some point. Outside the group, Peter reflected on the impact that the group had had upon him to the research officer who was evaluating it, saying, 'I can see that it helps to talk about stuff in that group.'

CONCLUSION

The central element of group work is offering people the time and space to think about themselves in the context of other people, others both similar and dissimilar to themselves. The process of meeting others in a similar position brings both hope and threat: hope because experiencing others in a similar position means having a sense of not being on one's own; threat because change involves adapting to uncertainty. A central task for group facilitators is to manage the tensions within the group as participants deal with these two themes. In doing so, the group members alternate between approaching and avoiding the nature of their similarity.

When the groups in the Dementia Voice Group Psychotherapy Project worked well, they seemed to provide a half-way house, a safe house in which the participants were able to talk with a sense that they could explore the world because they were among friends in the true sense of friendship – people who would understand because they themselves had a similar experience.

These groups provided a setting in which people could gain a sense that they had not been forgotten, that they would be remembered, that what had happened had been important. As one group member said, 'Just because I've got a failing memory, doesn't mean that I'm a failure.'

REFERENCES

Barton, J., Piney C., Berg, M. and Parker, C. 2001: Coping with forgetfulness group. *Newsletter of the Psychologists' Special Interest Group in the Elderly* **77**: 19–25.

Cheston, R. 1996: Stories and metaphors: talking about the past in a psychotherapy group for people with dementia. *Ageing and Society* **16**: 579–602.

Cheston, R. 1998: Psychotherapeutic work with dementia sufferers. *Social Work Practice* **12**: 199–207.

Cheston, R. and Jones, K. 2000: A place to work it all out together. *Journal of Dementia Care* **8**: 22–4.

Cheston, R, Jones, K. and Gilliard, J. The impact of group psychotherapy with people with dementia. *International Journal of Geriatric Psychiatry* (under review).

Clare, L. 2001: Managing threats to self: the phenomenology of early stage Alzheimer's disease. Paper presented to the BPS Annual Conference, 30 March, Glasgow.

Feil, N. 1990: *Validation: the Feil method*. Cleveland, Ohio: Edward Feil Productions.

Feil, N. 1992: Validation therapy. *Geriatric Nursing* May/June: 129–33.

Feil, N. 1993: *The validation breakthrough: simple techniques for communicating with Alzheimer's-type dementia*. Baltimore: Health Promotions.

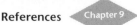

Goudie, F. and Stokes, G. 1989: Dealing with confusion. *Nursing Times* **20:** 38.

Haggerty, A. 1990: Psychotherapy for patients with Alzheimer's disease. *Advances* **7:** 55–60.

Hawkins, D. and Eagger, S. 1999: Group therapy: sharing the pain of the diagnosis. *Journal of Dementia Care* **6:** 12–14.

Kitwood, T. and Benson, S. eds. 1995: *The new culture of dementia care.* London: Hawker Publications.

McAfee, M., Ruhl, P., Bell, P. and Martichuski, D. 1989: Including persons with early stage Alzheimer's disease in support groups and strategy planning. *American Journal of Alzheimer's Disease and Related Disorders and Research* Nov/Dec: 18–22.

Marshall, A. 2001: Coping in early dementia: the findings of a new type of support group. Unpublished Phd thesis. Guildford: University of Surrey.

Stokes, G. and Goudie, F. 1990: Counselling confused elderly people. In: Stokes, G. and Goudie, F. eds. *Working with people with dementia.* Bicester: Winslow, 181–90.

Thrower, C. 1998: Support and a crucial sense of belonging. *Journal of Dementia Care* **6:** 18–20.

Watzlawick, P. Weakland, J. and Fisch, R. 1974: *Change: principles of problem formation.* New York: Norton.

Yale, R. 1995: *Developing support groups for individuals with early stage Alzheimer's disease: planning implementation and evaluation.* Baltimore: Health Professions' Press.

Positive communication with people who have dementia

Jonathan Parker

Communication is an active process but one that can easily be ignored in daily life. Although we may acknowledge its importance, especially within our personal and social lives, it is not something that most of us tend to analyse deeply most of the time. It is only when communication becomes difficult for some reason, such as when travelling abroad and not being able to speak or understand the language, or when something goes wrong with a close relationship, that our minds focus more keenly on the importance and intricacies of communicating with others.

Conceptually and theoretically, the term 'communication' is complex. Here, these complexities will be explored in relation to people with dementia, who often have specific and profound communication difficulties – both expressive and comprehensive. These difficulties are often compounded by personal, professional and social assumptions, and by expectations regarding communication, especially with respect to dementia.

This chapter considers positive ways of communicating with people who have dementia. Interpersonal communication provides the focus, but social practices and abstract communication are also discussed. There is a brief consideration of communication theory, followed by a review of research concerning communication and people who have dementia. The implications for practice are illustrated throughout by the use of case study material.

The key elements of this chapter concern the exploration of the different levels and types of communication applicable to dementia care, the articulation of positive communicative approaches for working with people who have dementia and how we can apply these in practice.

COMMUNICATION: DEFINITIONS AND PARAMETERS

Communication concerns interacting with another and involves giving, receiving, interpreting and acting upon or responding to information. There are many types of communication that are useful when working with people who have dementia (Figure 10.1).

It is speech that most frequently comes to mind when thinking about communication, but not everyone is able to communicate using speech. In addition, some verbal responses, for example grunts and 'uh-huhs', do not use recognized speech or language. This is important to consider when working with people with dementia, who may have impaired expression and articulation.

There are non-verbal ways of communicating, such as nodding, leaning towards a person and maintaining eye contact, that involve the bodies of those interacting. Identifying and developing skills in using non-verbal communication may be particularly important for working with people who have dementia given the often-continuing sensitivity to non-verbal signs and cues (Tibbs 2001). Non-verbal communication carries with it a range of cultural rules and norms that form part of the lexicon of acceptability and difference. It is vital to be sensitive to cultural diversity when working with people whose other means of communication are impaired (*see* Chapter 13).

There is a means of communicating by failing to respond. When, for example, someone does not return your messages and telephone calls, avoids being in the same room as you and ignores all your attempts at making eye contact or starting

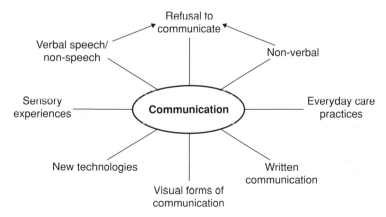

Figure 10.1 Possible communication types for working with people who have dementia

a conversation, he or she may be presenting a very clear message indeed! It is important to remember that such a null response is possible when working with a person with dementia. To attribute a lack of response solely to the dementia may be more comfortable but may fail to acknowledge a strongly 'communicated' message stating 'I don't want to talk' or 'I would rather talk to someone else.' These are not easy things to 'hear', but it is important to accept that people who have dementia are individuals, with their own personalities and ways of expressing emotion. Each person who has dementia has his or her own experience and understanding of it (Bender and Cheston 1997).

At the level of service delivery, communication also involves what we may term 'care texts' – the ways in which social and health care practices, as well as family care-giving practices, communicate information and aspects of self-worth and value. In this sense, the care environment 'speaks' or communicates a view on how dementia should be seen and how the person who has dementia should be treated. Because communication is interactive, this message is heard and responded to by those with dementia and those caring for individuals who have dementia. This 'common sense' approach not only communicates a message to people with dementia, or to their carers about dementia, but also tends to impede communication that falls outside the expected or assumed parameters. If, for example, it is considered unlikely that the person with dementia can hold a conversation, meaningful utterances might be discounted and views expressed might not be heard or acted upon, because it is taken as self-evident that the person cannot communicate. It may also result in mistaken interpretations or indeed mean that efforts to 'hear' the person are not given due attention.

Case 1   Breda moved into a nursing home 6 months ago. She was described as 'difficult', as 'prone to tantrums' and as having 'lost her ability to communicate in a meaningful way'. Care staff were at a loss when Breda began shouting 'Ribs, ribs!' She did not appear to be in pain and had no history of physical complaints, and examination by the doctor identified no medical condition causing her 'pain'. The nursing home staff then contacted Breda's daughter, who laughed and described Breda's favourite meal of 'ribs'. Breda was offered her favourite meal – her shouting lessened, and the interaction between her, the nursing home staff and her daughter increased.

Written communications are important, but written information has the capacity to exclude as well as include, and a person-centred approach is crucial for ensuring inclusive practices. Written agreements, or care plans, to make transparent services, and the expectations that people can have of the services provided, have become increasingly important. Descriptions of care agencies, residential homes and so on provide information on which informed choices can be made. For those people who have never had or have lost the written word, or find it daunting, the use of such information can, however, exclude them from making choices. Written information may give the power of choice to a third party, maybe a relative or friend, who may not always know the wishes of the person for whom the services are required. Interpersonal communication is essential in searching out the views of the person who will receive the services.

Case 2 Martha, a new social work care manager, was planning for a review of Elspeth Morris, a 93-year-old woman with dementia who lived at home supported by an intensive range of care services. When completing the section 'User's views of service', Martha asked her team leader how user involvement contributed to the review. Martha was taken aback when her team leader said. 'Simply put "EM has dementia." They'll know she can't be asked to comments on services.'

It may be that new technologies and wider abstract communicative media such as the visual arts, film, television, painting, music and aural media, and olfactory, gustatory and tactile sensations may also be developed to facilitate communication with people who have dementia.

In summary, there are many ways to communicate, including:

- Verbal – speech based, non-speech based
- Non-verbal – body language, micro skills, deliberate non-communication
- Everyday care practice – social and care-giver practice
- Written communication strategies
- Visual communication strategies
- New technology communications.

All these aspects of communication are important for those working with people who have dementia. Communication is also important for carers interacting with the person with dementia, for people who have dementia themselves and between people with dementia in care settings.

AN OVERVIEW OF COMMUNICATION THEORY

Where dementia is concerned, there has been an increasing emphasis on promoting positive and effective communication (Goldsmith 1996; Kitwood 1997; Cheston and Bender 1999). At the same time, the concerns of care staff and family care-givers often centre on communication losses and deficits. An understanding of communication theory in practice is therefore important when considering communication with people who have dementia.

Classical communication theories rely on both verbal and non-verbal expressions (Klein and White 1996). These traditional approaches to communication theory suggest (Randall and Parker 2000, p. 69) that it:

examines the processes that communication involves: the selection of a means of conveying a message (language, gesture, writing) the decoding of the message by the recipient (hearing, seeing, reading), and making a response on the basis of the interpretation (reply).

Communication theory holds as axiomatic the fact that action is taken in relation to information received. Information is interpreted, evaluated and processed. Feedback is then sent to the person initiating the communication, who can judge how that individual has processed the information. This model simplifies what happens in reality when a range of other personal and social factors may influence either the initial communication or the respondent's understanding and reply.

A cursory glance indicates that this theory of communication has clear consequences for those who have dementia. A person wishing to communicate with another individual must be understandable if the communication is to be effective. Recipients need to be able to hear, see and/or read depending on the type of communication sent. They must also be able to interpret or decode the communication. Expectations, past experiences and assumptions are also important. This is a simple description of a very complex process that may not always be possible when, for some reason, communication is impaired.

The standard medical paradigm emphasizes pathology. In dementia, pathology is assumed to cause specific and global difficulties, including impaired communication (Stuart-Hamilton 2000). The clinical picture of dementia and associated cognitive, emotional and behavioural changes presents potential challenges to communication at a number of levels, for example:

- Communication with the person who has dementia
- Communication by the person who has dementia
- Communication between people with dementia and significant others
- Communication between social and health care practitioners and people with dementia
- Communication between social and health care practitioners and family caregivers supporting and/or intimately related to people with dementia
- Communication between professionals and services or organizations working with people who have dementia
- The wider communication and dissemination of information aimed at policy change and development.

The person with dementia may begin to develop a range of expressive and comprehensive difficulties. These may be grouped under the broader categories of dysphasia affecting spoken communication, and alexia and agraphia with respect to the written word (Lishman 1987). The consequences of these difficulties are legion and individually experienced. The effects on close relationships also depend on the history of those relationships, personality factors, the expectations of the partner, significant other or carer, and his or her willingness and capacity to adapt. Gelder et al. (1989) point out that the clinical features of dementia are to some extent determined by the person's personality before dementia. This may mean that the previously social, conversational person may strive to maintain a communicative facade whereas the isolated or non-sociable person may not.

Speech quality, such as tone and volume, is particularly important to communication. Syntactical errors (getting sentences jumbled) and nominal dysphasia (forgetting the names of people or objects) are common and can be particularly distressing to carers, who may believe that forgetting their name or something important is personally directed. As the dementia progresses, the person may lose speech altogether or only make noises. Other cognitive factors, such as deficits in attention and working memory, and disruptions of memory-encoding processes, may make accurate the interpretation and recall of communication and responding more difficult.

Case 3a Peggy Moran was 86 years old and had lived in Greendales residential care home for the previous 3 years. She was a widow with two daughters, one of whom lived nearby and visited regularly each month. The second daughter lived in California but wrote frequently and had visited her mother twice since she had moved into Greendales.

Peggy had significant communication difficulties, which had become progressively worse over the 3 years. She had had very little speech on entering the home; the only words she now uttered were when she sang parts of hymns that were said, by her daughter, to be her favourites – 'There is a green hill far away' and 'Guide me, Oh thou great Jehovah' – and one or two words that she called out from time to time.

Staff found Peggy hard to communicate with, often receiving very little response. When helping her to dress or bathe, she sometimes simply complied, but at other times she shrieked or struck out at staff.

The most difficult incidents occurred at night. Peggy seemed on occasions to be afraid of the dark. She would scream, for up to 3 or 4 hours, and seemingly be inconsolable, often shouting 'Dolly.' Staff did not know how to respond and had taken to sitting with her in one of the day rooms and giving her a toy doll that one of them had brought in. Some staff worried that they were acting inappropriately by giving her the doll, whereas others assumed that since she had dementia, there was no point worrying – if something calmed her down, it should be used.

Features of communication

Information may be processed on a selective basis. It may be that the negative side of communication is seen but the good points are minimized or completely ignored. This depends to a large extent on the past experiences and learning of those communicating, as well as on local and cultural factors. It is important for care-givers and health and social care staff working with people who have dementia to be aware of the way in which they speak. They need to develop specific ways of conveying information or asking questions that accord with past and present preferred ways of communicating with the person with dementia. In the case of Peggy, staff had begun to assume that Peggy could not communicate because of her conversational problems and perceived 'challenging behaviours'. Information on Peggy was processed selectively on the basis of assumptions both about her as a person and about dementia.

There may also be information-processing problems, which can affect perception, evaluation and feedback. This is certainly possible for many people with dementia. For Peggy, staff became blocked in developing and testing alternative ways of interpreting information, her shouts, her screams and her singing.

It is important to remember that communication must be seen in context. Relevant factors concerning the situation, others involved and perceptions of past experiences lead to different forms of communication. By experimenting with others, we form patterns of communication that help to regulate and make our relationships predictable. Although Peggy's communication difficulties were acknowledged, the patterns of communication that had developed were ignored. Staff provided responses to Peggy's distress that were functional for her, although were limited to giving her a doll or sitting with her when she was upset and screaming. Staff also interpreted this behaviour/communication as Peggy being 'difficult or her dementia causing communication problems'.

Aspects of power in communication theory

We may see communication patterns developing in our day-to-day work situations, and the responses we make to individual events, and the developed 'team response' (care-text), needs to be examined in relation to communication and power.

Power is an important concept in communication theory. Interactions may be equal between people (symmetrical relationships), or fixed and unequal roles may be assigned (complementary relationships). The latter is likely between social and health care practitioners and medical practitioners because of received discourses of care (Parker 2001). Inequalities of power are perhaps more keenly experienced by family carers and especially by those who have dementia.

The assumed global relevance of social psychological models of communication that emphasize individualism is being called into question, so new theories and models that take into account cultural, regional and local contexts should be developed. Triandis (1994) highlights the fact that communication theories are mainly derived from an observation of Western cultures. There needs to be a degree of redress that acknowledges cultural diversity and works with this to find the most effective means of communication (Airhihenbuwa and Obregon 2000).

COMMUNICATING WITH PEOPLE WHO HAVE DEMENTIA: THE EVIDENCE FROM RESEARCH

The limitations of communication theory must be acknowledged. A knowledge of the rules of communication can, however, help health and social care workers in establishing constructive relationships. Much of the increase in appreciation of the needs and personhood of the person with dementia can be traced to pioneers such as Kitwood (1997) and the greater emphasis on the possibilities of psychotherapy (Cheston and Bender 1999). These moves have also emphasized communication. Indeed, Kitwood's development of dementia care mapping is predicated on the understanding that the person with dementia is communicating by his or her behaviour (Kitwood and Bredin 1992). By learning to 'read' dementia care situations, social and health care staff can identify situations of well-being/ill-being and thereby improve and enhance that care.

Research indicates that communication with people who have dementia is possible. Goldsmith's (1996) exciting study concerning 'hearing the voice' of people who have dementia challenged many of the prevailing myths that people with dementia had all lost the ability to communicate and there was little, if any, point in attempting to consult with them. Allan (2001) has extended this work and identified an array of techniques that can be successfully employed by social and health care practitioners and family carers in communicating with people with dementia.

Allan's (2001) research explored ways in which staff could consult people with dementia about their views of services in a way that recognized continuing personhood (*see also* Bamford and Bruce 2000; Barnett 2000; Parker et al. 2001). The research was collaborative, with a process that encouraged and supported staff to develop individual approaches to communication and consultation in residential and nursing settings. Allan found that 'many people with dementia, including those with significant communication difficulties, can, with the right kind of support, take an active role in communicating their feelings about services' (2001, p. 9). A difficulty for care services was highlighted in the increasing emphasis on well-defined procedures for assessing performance and making decisions that could detract from the complex, uncertain and time-consuming process involved in listening to people with dementia.

Allan (2001) emphasized the importance of finding the right words, not using jargon and working towards the right level of communication by starting more generally and modifying one's approach accordingly. The relationship with the person with dementia was central. Importantly, she indicated that communication and consultation are integral to good everyday care practice. Communication is not an independent activity to be undertaken apart from other tasks. She described three main categories of working with people with dementia:

- Working with pictures
- Communications during the completion of other activities
- Focusing on non-verbal forms of communication.

Photographs, magazine pictures and pictures for recognition purposes employed in teaching were used to establish links. These allowed people to tell their stories and were seen as promoting an enjoyable social activity, increasing communication so that experiences and perceptions of care could be discussed. Importantly, the use of pictures brought up a considerable amount of information concerning people's personal lives and preferences. Staff taking part in the project also acknowledged the importance of non-verbal communication in presenting wishes and feelings. Staff were supported and assisted to develop their knowledge of self and others by observing non-verbal responses. During help with personal care, food-tasting sessions or going for walks, people were encouraged to talk and converse without feeling 'on the spot' and possibly worrying about communication deficits.

Allan grounded her research in daily practice and stressed (Allan, 2001, p. 66) that communicating with people with dementia can be a gift of all care staff given the opportunity to develop their skills and knowledge:

> Although getting started on finding ways to communicate with people and promote their involvement can be difficult, it is important not to think of these activities as 'rocket science'. As these examples demonstrate, it is about creating opportunities for people to bring to bear these very human processes and qualities that we all value and appreciate in our relationships.

Allan acknowledged that many factors need to be taken into account and that it is not always easy to communicate with people with dementia. The individual experience of dementia and the particular mood, physical, social and temporal environments, staff factors and organizational factors all need to be taken into account.

Developing positive communication with people who had dementia had added benefits:

- Increased staff confidence
- The development of knowledge and skills
- Deepened relationships
- An awareness of the impact of services.

Allan concluded that although there are many ways of communicating with people with dementia, these need to be developed individually. They must give maximum control to the individual and should be integrated into everyday practice (*see also* Killick and Allan 2001).

WAYS AND METHODS OF COMMUNICATING: TRANSLATING RESEARCH INTO PRACTICE

Sensory, as well as cognitive, impairment may contribute to communication difficulties (Mentis and Briggs-Whittaker 1995) so language should always be clear, understandable and grounded in the context of the person. Everyday arte-facts, including photographs, pictures, ornaments and furniture, should be used to facilitate communication. Care routines need to be flexible enough to accom-modate change in wishes but should be regular to assist understanding of the environment. Positive communication with people who have dementia demands good listening and information-gathering skills, checking information and using it in a sensitive, person-centred way. This may occur in the following areas:

- Making assessments and conveying service information
- Developing and maintaining constructive and therapeutic relationships
- Contributing to environmental design to aid communication.

Developing positive communication skills is also important for family carers. Health and social care practitioners can model and teach the use of constructive, everyday approaches to aid communication. Care-givers may find the strain of constantly interpreting and perhaps misinterpreting conver-sation to be threatening and humiliating, and may consider it less challenging to withdraw from conversation altogether. It is important to assist people to continue trying to find ways of communicating as this can increase both satis-faction (Neustadt 2001) and well-being (Berkman 2000). Killick (1999) describes the stories most prominent in people's minds that express deep emotions in unconventional yet poetic ways. Listening is important, but it is not a special skill; instead it is a matter of learning empathy, self-effacement and the art of keeping silent.

Making assessments and conveying service information

Health and social care staff have a duty to convey honest, supportive information to people with dementia and their carers (Audit Commission 2000; Tibbs 2001). Payne (1997) identifies four aspects of communication with service users. These concern assessment and information-gathering tasks such as:

- Gaining information
- Giving feedback
- Giving information
- Reframing information.

These uses of communication are central to developing good practice. The *National Service Framework for Older People* (Department of Health 2001) promotes a single assessment process to ensure enhanced care practice. Practitioners will need to be able to make individual, needs-focused assessments that take into consideration cultural factors and, as far as possible, include service users. This demands good communication skills and knowledge as well as an emphasis on the relational aspects of communication.

Practitioners need to prepare a clear picture of possible and probable clinical features with a view to supporting the person with dementia and his or her carers in developing ways of managing these (Cheston and Bender 1999). Effective communication on the part of practitioners uses those interpersonal skills and methods which aid the development and maintenance of relationships. These skills and methods can be used equally effectively by family care-givers and others.

Understanding interpersonal communication and family communication patterns is very important for health and social care practitioners and must take local and cultural factors into consideration. General patterns of communication are developed over time and may represent key processes by which the relationship is conducted at that local level. The concept of relational communication suggests that listening is central to the enactment, development and maintenance of both personal and social relationships, and involves three elements – cognitive (understanding), affective (caring) and behavioural (interactive) (Halone and Pecchioni 2001). Elements of relational communication can be developed if one partner in a relationship has dementia.

People with dementia and their relatives have often built up specific listening patterns that are important to the continuance of their relationship. When these processes are disrupted, relatives and people significant to the person with dementia may need help and assistance to find and practise new ways of listening to and communicating with that person. Vittoria's (1998) research into 'communicative care' suggests that reciprocal processes of communication in care settings can help to counteract devaluation and loss of self by increasing opportunities for social interaction and emphasizing peoples' worth as individuals (*see also* Innes and Capstick 2001). The positive effects of communication depend, states Vittoria, on the quality of the relationship created between service users and staff. It is crucial to acknowledge, however, that creating positive relationships is neither easy nor static, demanding constant revision to listening and communication processes and a continuous attempt to develop innovatory and constructive ways of communicating (Beach and Kramer 1999).

Validation work developed as a specific way of working with unresolved issues and staying with people and their concerns (Feil 1992, 1993; *see also* Chapter 9). In this approach, practitioners accept that there is meaning behind the confused words and behaviour of people who have dementia and accept the struggle to resolve past conflicts. A woman seeking a 'lost child' would, for example, not necessarily be distracted from her thoughts and feelings, but the practitioner would acknowledge how she felt and explore with her what that meant for her. It might not be possible to establish what events lay behind this search, but the acceptance of that woman's emotions would convey a validation of her worth as a human being.

The strengths of validation lie in its acceptance of the diversity of experiences and in developing deep 'listening' to feelings as well as words. It has been challenged as leading to collusion with falsehoods and therefore being patronizing. However, it approaches people with dementia as being valuable, unique human beings and is one that practitioners can adopt in everyday practice by conveying empathy, genuineness and warmth. It is a method that can be developed by family care-givers and can provide a framework for understanding seemingly bizarre, confused and sometimes upsetting behaviours. It is also effective in increasing well-being (Toseland and Diehl 1997).

The use of reminiscence, life story and biographical methods has increased in recent years (Gibson 1998). Although there are differences in technique and application, these methods honour the importance of the individual's story and place in history, which is essential in developing effective communication (Broadbent 1999). Key memories of an individual's life can be triggered by photographs or personal objects, and social interaction can be increased (*see* Chapter 4). General reminiscence can take place in informal or more formal groups, whereas individual methods of life review and life story work can be used to engage and form relationships, to collect important information for care plans and reviews or to resolve past issues. These methods use everyday media and can be undertaken while completing everyday tasks. Internalizing the practice of searching for, introducing and developing possible triggers is not time-consuming, validates the individual by conveying interest, may bring forth personal information and can increase satisfaction.

Communication has both a biographical and a historical context. This means that a person's life, experiences and learning build a vast storehouse of communicative possibilities. These are in turn influenced by and impact upon the wider historical, political and social events occurring within the lifespan of that individual and the others with whom he or she interacts (Parker 2001). Recognizing the centrality of personal experiences and historical context is fundamental to person-centred dementia care.

Now let's return to the case of Peggy.

Case 3b A new member of care staff, Linda, was appointed as Peggy's key worker. She was not burdened with preconceived assumptions about Peggy's behaviour and sought to build life story information to identify the likes, wants, wishes and significant events of Peggy's life. Linda, like other staff, found that Peggy was difficult to engage but did seem to enjoy company and having her hand held. In collecting background information from Peggy's daughter, she found out that Peggy's older sister – Dolly –had died in a house fire at night when she was 7 years old. This information helped Linda and the other care staff to understand Peggy's distress. It confirmed the importance of validating the feelings and words of others and the importance of collecting accurate life history information. Having this information did not dramatically change Peggy's communication abilities, but it did assist communication between the staff and family carers, and helped them give Peggy better care when she was distressed.

Environment and communication

Changes to the environment and routine can help to improve communication and can be taught to care-givers and social and health care staff. Orange and Lubinski (1996) suggest that specific times, tasks or daily activities can be used to enhance communication. For example, establishing set mealtimes, identifying the person's stated preferences and setting up a routine for preparing for the meal and clearing away afterwards may afford the chance to discuss everyday issues in an everyday situation.

The importance of the physical environment is recognized in reality orientation (Holden and Woods 1988) and in environmental design. It is important to ensure that environments are constructed to minimize stress and confusion (Marchello et al. 1995), allowing people to navigate successfully and ground themselves in familiar and safe situations. This makes positive communication more likely. Design parameters communicate information, which has meaning for our understanding of communication with people who have dementia as much as it has for wider social life. There appears to have been some success in designing accessible living spaces to improve the lives of people with dementia (Marshall 1997; Coleman 2000).

Case 4 Alan, who had dementia, had been living on his own since his wife's death 7 years previously. He was physically fit and continued his hobby of growing clematis plants. His daughter had paid for the renovation and extension of his kitchen as a present. She was perplexed when Alan began to lose his way around, stopped going into the garden, forgot to eat or drink unless prompted and appeared increasingly sad. Alan and his daughter were visited by a community psychiatric nurse and social worker, who suggested a reorienting programme, labelling cupboards and foods, and using arrows to point to key items. At first, Alan's daughter thought that this might appear patronising, but Alan agreed to the programme. After 3 weeks, Alan had regained his confidence and re-established many routines. For Alan, known places and familiarity communicated a sense of belonging and identity.

CONCLUSION

It is fundamental to remember that positive communication is not something that is the preserve of health and social care practitioners: everyone can develop these methods. The role of the practitioner is to educate and model positive communication. To do this effectively, practitioners must adopt and immerse themselves in person-centred approaches to dementia care. This again represents one of the standards (Standard 2: Person centred care) of the *National Service Framework for Older People* (Department of Health 2001). If communication with people who have dementia it is to be positive, it is essential that a person-centred value base be promoted. Communication is interactive and intersubjective, traversing different areas and levels. This demands an appreciation of the 'other'. Positive communication is 'talks' *with* rather than *at* in all its forms and varieties.

This gives rise to a number of implications for social and health care practice, related to:

- Training issues and skills development
- Supervision issues
- The importance of practitioner research
- An emphasis on value-based and person-centred care.

With adequate attention to the above, positive communication can be enhanced and promoted. The two fundamental points to consider are that communication is possible and that it can be achieved in everyday situations: it is not beyond the reach of family carers or health and social care staff.

REFERENCES

Airhihenbuwa, C.O. and Obregon, R. 2000: A critical assessment of theories/models used in communication for HIV/AIDS, *Journal of Health Communication* 5 (suppl.): 5–16.

Allan, K. 2001: *Communication and consultation: exploring ways for staff to involve people with dementia in developing services*. Bristol: Policy Press/Joseph Rowntree Foundation.

Audit Commission 2000: *Forget me not: mental health services for older people*. London: Audit Commission.

Bamford, C. and Bruce, E. 2000: Defining the outcomes of community care: the perspectives of older people with dementia and their carers. *Ageing and Society* **20:** 543–70.

Barnett, E. 2000: *Including the person with dementia in designing and delivering care: 'I need to be me!'* London: Jessica Kingsley.

Beach, D.L. and Kramer, B.J. 1999: Communicating with Alzheimer's residents: perceptions of care providers in a residential facility. *Journal of Gerontological Social Work* **32** (3): 5–27.

Bender, M. and Cheston, R. 1997: Inhabitants of a lost kingdom: a model of the subjective experiences of dementia. *Ageing and Society* **17:** 513–32.

Berkman, L.F. 2000: Which influence cognitive function: living alone or being alone? *Lancet* **355:** 1291–3.

Broadbent, I. 1999: Using the biographical approach. *Nursing Times* **95** (39): 52–4.

Cheston, R. and Bender, M. 1999: *Understanding dementia: the man with the worried eyes*. London: Jessica Kingsley.

Coleman, R. 2000: Design for later life: beyond a problem orientation. In: Warnes, A.M., Warren, L. and Nolan, M. eds. *Care services for later life: transformations and critiques.* London: Jessica Kingsley, 219–42.

Department of Health. 2001: *National service framework for older people.* London: Stationery Office.

Feil, N. 1992: *Validation: the Feil method.* Cleveland, Ohio: Edward Feil Productions.

Feil, N. 1993: *The validation breakthrough.* Baltimore: Health Professions Press.

Gelder, M., Gath, D. and Mayou, R. 1989: *Oxford textbook of psychiatry,* 2nd edn. Oxford: Oxford University Press.

Gibson, F. 1998: *Reminiscence and recall: a guide to good practice,* 2nd edn. London: Age Concern England.

Goldsmith, M. 1996: *Hearing the voice of people with dementia.* London: Jessica Kingsley.

Halone, K.K. and Pecchioni, L.L. 2001: Relational listening: a grounded theoretical model. *Communication Reports* **14:** 59–71.

Holden, U. and Woods, R. 1988: *Reality orientation,* 2nd edn. New York: Churchill Livingstone.

Innes, A. and Capstick, A. 2001: Communication and personhood. In: Cantley, C. ed. *A handbook of dementia care.* Buckingham: Open University Press, 135–45.

Killick, J. 1999: Eliciting experiences of people with dementia. *Generations* **23:** 46–9.

Killick, J. and Allan, K. 2001: *Communication and the care of people with dementia.* Buckingham: Open University Press.

Kitwood, T. 1997: *Dementia reconsidered: the person comes first.* Buckingham: Open University Press.

Kitwood, T. and Bredin, K. 1992: Toward a theory of dementia care: personhood and well-being. *Ageing and Society* **12:** 269–87.

Klein, D. and White, J. 1996: *Family theories.* London: Sage.

Lishman, W.A. 1987: *Organic psychiatry: the psychological consequences of cerebral disorder,* 2nd edn. Oxford: Blackwell Scientific Publications.

Marchello, V. Boczko, F. and Shelkey, M. 1995: Progressive dementia: strategies to manage new problem behaviors. *Geriatrics* **50:** 40–3.

Marshall, M. 1997: Therapeutic design for people with dementia. In: Hunter, S. ed. *Dementia: challenges and new directions.* London: Jessica Kingsley, 181–93.

Mentis, M. and Briggs-Whittaker, J. 1995: Discourse topic management in senile dementia of the Alzheimer's type. *Journal of Speech and Hearing Research* **38:** 1054–66.

Neustadt, G.K. 2001: Side by side travelling the road – and sharing the load – of Alzheimer's disease. *ASHS Leader* **6:** 4–9.

Orange, J.B. and Lubinski, R.B. 1996: Conversational repair by individuals with dementia of the Alzheimer's type. *Journal of Speech and Hearing Research* **39:** 881–95.

Parker, J. 2001: Interrogating person-centred dementia care in social work and social care. *Journal of Social Work* **1:** 329–45.

Parker, J., Penhale, B., Manthorpe, J. and Bradley, G. 2001: Hearing what users say: the importance of training for high quality management in dementia care. *Managing Community Care* **9:** 29–34.

Payne, M. 1997: *Modern social work theory,* 2nd edn. Basingstoke: Macmillan.

Randall, P. and Parker, J. 2000: Communication theory. In: Davies, M. ed. *The encyclopaedia of social work.* Oxford: Blackwell, 69.

Stuart-Hamilton, I. 2000: *The psychology of ageing: an introduction*, 3rd edn. London: Jessica Kingsley.

Tibbs, M.A. 2001: *Social work and dementia: good practice and care management*. London: Jessica Kingsley.

Toseland, R.W. and Diehl, M. 1997: The impact of validation group therapy on nursing home residents with dementia. *Journal of Applied Gerontology* **16:** 31–51.

Triandis, H.C. 1994: *Culture and social behavior*. New York: McGraw-Hill.

Vittoria, A.K. 1998: Preserving selves: identity work and dementia. *Research on Aging* **20:** 91–136.

Younger people with dementia: coming out of the shadows

Maria Parsons

It is ironic, given the subsequent neglect of people younger than 65 years of age with dementia, that Alois Alzheimer's case reports of what subsequently became known as Alzheimer's disease featured the dementing condition of a woman in her early 50s. In the ensuing decades, the interest in presenile dementia or early-onset dementia has been overtaken by a concern about meeting the needs of older people, among whom dementia is increasing exponentially, with significant rises in the very elderly (Melzer et al. 1997). Studies setting out the significant social and economic consequences of dementia for the individual and society (Knapp et al. 1998), and government policy and directives for service develop-ment, have focused almost entirely on older people (Audit Commission 2000; Department of Health 2001), serving to reinforce the social construction of old age as one of senility and disability, and to marginalize younger people with dementia.

Of the 900 000 people with dementia, some 18 000 are estimated to be under 65 years old (Newens et al. 1993). A numerically much smaller, more dispersed popu-lation of people with younger-onset dementia has nevertheless been identified as a distinct group by policy-makers, service-planners and providers (Williams 1995; ADS 1996; Department of Health 1999; NHS Executive South East 2000), as having different needs that require specialist resources (Delaney and Rosevinge 1995; Williams 1995; Whalley 1997; Harvey 1998).

The drivers for change have been many. Society's awareness of dementia has increased, in part because of the development of a new culture of dementia care, which has challenged neuropathological definitions of dementia, taking the view that neurological impairment is only one element in a dementing process involving biological, psychological and socio-cultural variables that interact to shape and mediate the individual's unique experience of dementia (Kitwood and Bredin 1992). These ideas have influenced formal services by shifting care practice from a medical to social model, and by focusing attention on the lived experience of the person with dementia, at whatever age this occurs.

Other developments include national initiatives such as CANDID, providing on-line information, advice and support to people with early-onset dementia and their families (Harvey et al. 1998), and the Alzheimer's Society's Younger People and Dementia project, a catalyst for service development in local authority social services departments (Williams et al. 1996). At a regional level, many of the UK dementia services development centres have led research and service evaluation contributing to the growth of knowledge on younger people and their needs (Cox 1991; Parsons 1999; Cantley et al. 2000). Locally, 'champions' in health and social services often pioneer service development (Gutteridge 2001), sometimes in partnership with carers (Pointon 2001), and the voices of younger people have begun to be heard (Goldsmith 1996; Killick 1999). More recently, the National Service Framework for Older People (Department of Health 2001, p. 106) has required health and local councils responsible for care to 'review current arrangements, in primary care and elsewhere, for the management of dementia in younger people, and agree and implement a local protocol across primary care and specialist services'.

THE NATURE OF DEMENTIA

A cruel and arbitrary condition, dementia is characterized by the death of cells in crucial areas of the brain, causing memory impairment and over time affecting all activities dependent on cognition. Life course theory provides a framework for exploring the changes, adaptations and transitions experienced by individuals as they move through the lifespan (Hagestad and Neugarten 1985). The occurrence of dementia in younger people is especially disruptive and, given the stage of life reached, affects the clinical features of dementia, giving rise to unique experiences in younger people (Woodburn and Johnstone 1999). Researchers and those developing formal services have sought to elucidate the nature of such differences and the implications they might have for the type of help and support required by individuals and carers.

Dementia is usually defined as a syndrome, manifested in a distinct pattern of symptoms, that can be caused by more than 70 diseases, although 70–80 per cent of those affected are estimated to have Alzheimer's disease, vascular dementia or dementia with Lewy bodies (Wilcock et al. 1999). This does not, however, hold for younger people, in whom the range of dementia-causing diseases is much wider (Harvey 1998) and rare forms of dementia more common. Hence, although Alzheimer's disease is the largest single cause of dementia overall, it affects only 34 per cent of younger people, who are more likely to have mechanical, metabolic, endocrine or toxic dementias or a dementia caused by an infection (Harvey 1998).

Diagnosis is acknowledged to be more difficult and protracted in younger people (Lloyd 1993; Luscombe et al. 1998), misdiagnosis (Newens et al. 1993) or a lack of accurate diagnosis occurring (Ryan 1994) for a significant number. Because of the age of onset, approximately 20 per cent of instances of dementia in people under 65 years of age may be regarded as treatable, or the aggravating factors as remediable (Wilcock et al. 1999), but, with the exception of depression, treatment is unlikely to be successful. A higher rate of psychiatric morbidity has been reported among younger people (Newens et al. 1993; Ferran et al. 1996), who have fewer physical problems (Fossey and Baker 1995) and a higher level of physical activity (Delaney and Rosevinge 1995), making them less prone to death from physical causes, and for whom progressive dementias are therefore inevitably terminal (McWalter and Chalmers 1999).

It has been suggested that dementia may be more severe, and the deterioration more rapid, in younger people than in those who are older (Keady and Nolan 1994b). Other studies however, take the opposite view, arguing that the severity of the disease at the time of identification is a key factor in predicting survival and rate of progression (Christie and Wood 1988; Newens et al. 1993).

Alzheimer's disease has a gradual and insidious onset and a progressive course. The early symptoms resemble depression, anxiety or emotional stress, diagnosis becoming possible only when specific features manifest themselves. Alzheimer's disease appears in different forms and subsets, some of which are inheritable. Three genes have been identified in early-onset familial Alzheimer's disease (Lovestone 1998), although a relatively small number of families is affected (Pollen 1994). As in other dementias, including Huntingdon's disease, disease-causing genes that are inherited in an autosomal dominant manner will be passed relentlessly down from generation to generation from male to female and vice versa (Lovestone 1998).

Vascular dementia accounts for 18 per cent of all dementias in people aged under 65. Because of the interruption of blood supply to the brain, strokes are a common cause of cognitive impairment, which then follows a stepwise progression. People more prone to vascular dementia include those with untreated high blood pressure, the rate of which is high among some black minority groups, suggesting an increased risk of vascular dementia in such individuals (Patel et al. 1998).

Studies show that approximately 17 per cent of those under 65 are affected by dementia with Lewy bodies (Tobianksy 1994). Common features of this condition include those normally associated with psychotic illnesses, such as hallucinations, delusions and mood disturbances. Those with dementia associated with Lewy bodies are more susceptible to falls. Neuroleptics are contraindicated and should not be used (McKeith et al. 1992).

Frontotemporal dementias appear to be more commonly diagnosed among younger people, affecting some 12 per cent of all those with dementia, and may be more common in men (Ratnavelli et al. 2002). A deterioration of personality and behaviour is often accompanied by social disinhibition. Psychological symptoms include mood changes, emotional instability and a lack of concern for others. Frontal dementia is usually clinically indistinguishable from this. The most noticeable change in a younger person who has Pick's disease, a dementia with frontotemporal dominance, may be gradual disintegration of language (not just speech) over an indeterminate length of time, memory, attention, personality and behaviour all deteriorating as well (Bayer 2000).

Approximately 50 per cent of individuals with Huntingdon's disease show symptoms of dementia before they are 65 years old, the most prominent manifestations being movement and non-cognitive features. Although the chorea causes considerable disability, it is the dementia component of the illness that challenges carers and others.

It is estimated that 20–30 per cent of those affected by Parkinson's disease also have dementia, which develops in the later phases of the illness and, in combination with involuntary movements, ridigity, stiffness and tremor, results in complex health and social care needs. Supranuclear palsy is principally caused by Steele–Richardson–Olszewski disease, but the degree of dementia seen in this condition is variable, and other signs and symptoms, not unlike those of Parkinson's disease, are typical of the corticobasal degeneration.

Dementia is a prominent feature of the very rare new variant form of the prion diseases known as Creutzfeldt–Jacob disease, which is caused by a virus transmitted in infected material, in the human case, beef from infected cattle. Creutzfeldt–Jacob disease typically affects young adults, who begin to develop psychiatric and neurological symptoms. Damage to the brain, which is characteristically sponge-like at post mortem, confirms spongiform encephalopathy. In one study of the first 100 cases, the median age of onset was found to be 26 (range 12–74) years and the median duration of disease 13 months (Spencer et al. 2002).

About 8–16 per cent of people with AIDS have a type of dementia caused by the human immunodeficiency virus damaging the white matter of the brain, usually in the later stages of the disease. Dementia is also a late feature of syphilis, a sexually transmitted disease now much rarer in the UK because treatment is available that halts its progression.

Dementia sometimes results from pressure on parts of the brain as a result of tumours, subdural haematomas or normal-pressure hydrocephalus. Surgical interventions aim to remove the cause of the pressure or repair the site of the damage. More rarely in younger people, hypothyroidism or vitamin B12 deficiency may produce a dementia with disturbances of balance, walking or vision. Treatments are available for both of these, although the dementia is rarely reversible.

Almost all younger people with Down's syndrome possess an extra chromosome 21, which triggers the production of the beta-amyloid protein found in the neurofibrillary tangles associated with Alzheimer's disease. Prevalence increases from 8 per cent in people aged 35–49, to 55 per cent in the 50–59-year age group and 75 per cent in those over 60, although a sizeable group do not develop dementia, other factors probably precipitating the onset of the disease (Cooper 1999).

Alcohol abuse can result in reversible changes in motor and cognitive functioning, and is associated with neurological diseases, principally Wernicke's encephalopathy, often manifested in Korsakoff's amnesiac syndrome, a psychiatric disorder. Wernicke–Korsakoff's syndrome, as it is therefore known, is caused by severe thiamine (vitamin B1) deficiency resulting from poor nutrition. It has an acute onset and is characterized by gait difficulties, global confusion and problems with eye co-ordination. Treatment can effect recovery.

INCIDENCE AND PREVALENCE

Health and social services are required to undertake locality population needs assessments to identify potential requirements that can be used in service commissioning and planning (Department of Health 1989). Obtaining reliable epidemiological data on younger people with dementia is, however, problematic given the size and dispersed nature of the group (Newens et al. 1993; Woodburn and Johnstone 1999), the sporadic nature of many dementias among those included and the quality of the available data (McWalter and Chalmers 1999).

A longitudinal study by Harvey (1998) of younger people with dementia in two London boroughs provides a reliable information base for service-planning and provision. Over a two-and-a-half year period, the study sought to identify all cases of young-onset dementia in Hillingdon and Kensington and Chelsea, as well as the different dementias involved. This highlighted 185 cases, giving a prevalence of 67.2 cases per 100 000 at risk in the 30–64-year age group. Hence, in a population of 200 000–250 000, there might be 100–150 younger people with dementia. Extrapolated to the whole of the UK (Harvey 1998), the estimated number of cases was 16 737 (95 per cent confidence interval 13 975–19 879), of whom:

- 900 would be under the age of 40
- 2700 were expected to be under the age of 50
- 12 000 would be under 60.

The generalizability of the study remains contested as random variations have been identified in other population need assessments (Whalley et al. 1995;

McWalter and Chalmers 1999), and local prevalence figures are likely to be influenced by ease of access to information and formal services (Parsons 1999). Statutory organizations and voluntary agencies both report an increase in the number of younger people known to have dementia following the development of specialist services (Cantley and Smith 1999), and as these develop, it will be important to gather bottom-up information from case files and reassess incidence and prevalence.

THE NEEDS OF YOUNGER PEOPLE WITH DEMENTIA

Empirical research into the needs of younger people with dementia is sparse in comparison to the multitude of local studies and project reports (Furst and Sperlinger 1993; Quinn 1996; Fuhrmann 1997). Most studies include the views of statutory and voluntary agencies, and often carers, but the service-user perspective is largely neglected (Beattie et al. 2002). There are few published studies of consultation with younger people and their carers (Quinn 1996; Keady and Nolan 1999; Killick 1999), although locality projects usually include interviews with service users and carers (Parsons 1999; Reed et al. 2000). Accounts written by younger people with dementia chronicle their thoughts, feelings and experiences, providing invaluable insights into their support needs (Davis 1989; Friel-McGowin 1993).

Ostensibly, people with dementia are not consulted as it is believed that it is difficult to elicit their views. However, 'For people with dementia to be present only through the proxy voice of their carer or by having research done unto them (with or even without their consent) is no longer a tenable position' (Clarke and Keady 2001, p. 41). Researchers have begun to address a range of issues relating to the participation of people with dementia in research and recent work has included those with dementia reflecting on research (Wilkinson 2001).

Studies overwhelmingly show that many of the needs of those with young-onset dementia differ from those of older people (Cox and McLennan 1994; Williams et al. 1996; Keady and Nolan 1999). Younger people present very specific and often highly individual needs, reflecting differences in the socio-cultural and economic context of dementia within their everyday lives (Tindall and Manthorpe 1997; McLennan 1999; Downs 2000). The experience of dementia among younger people from black minority ethnic groups has not yet been identified, although services for those with dementia from minority groups are fragmentary (Patel 1998) and their needs are not identified in any systematic way (Daker-White et al. 2002).

INFORMATION: NOW AND LATER

For most individuals and their families, needs arise at different stages, and interventions may be more effective if made during key events and points of transition.

Information needs predominate during the pre-recognition stage, to the time of first contact with medical or social care professionals and then throughout the course of the illness. Information may not need to be complex. One carer described 'how she was driven to distraction by her husband's hiding and hoarding, until it was explained this may be a response to him losing so much of himself that he was trying to stop other things being lost on which she reflected: "When we understand we can make allowances"' (Pointon, in Fountain 2002, p. 13).

Information needs to be easily accessed, available in different formats and include diagnosis and prognosis, sources of help and support, and contact details. General practitioners, usually the first professionals to be contacted by concerned individuals and their families, are generally not able to offer information on dementia (Audit Commission 2000). Carers therefore report frustration until contact with the Alzheimer's Society or more specialist groups, such as the Huntington's Society or Pick's Disease Group, is made.

DIAGNOSIS AND MULTIDISCIPLINARY ASSESSMENT

It is important to diagnose the type of dementia as accurately and as early as possible in order to provide individuals and their families with comprehensive information and access to appropriate support and treatment. As younger people with dementia are an extremely heterogeneous population, and the impact on individuals and families is profound, specialist assessment is deemed essential (Department of Health 2001). Assessment needs to be accurate, comprehensive, multidisciplinary and co-ordinated (Alzheimer's Disease Society 1991, 1995; Cox 1991), but the experience of individuals and carers is very often one of 'falling through the net' (Cox 1999, p. 76).

In the absence of a clear care pathway and established protocols between primary and secondary care, younger people with dementia, their families and general practitioners access specialist assessment and diagnosis via different routes (Cox 1999; Clarke 2000). Clinical diagnosis is a core component in assessment, but research shows that this may be made by many different specialisms, including adult psychiatry and neurology (Allen and Baldwin 1995). More recently, the Royal College of Psychiatrists (1999) has published a position statement that makes the case for diagnosis to be undertaken by a consultant, based in old-age psychiatry but specializing in younger people, who would be able to draw on the department's resources and expertise related to dementia and manage clinical care more appropriately.

Assessment usually includes a detailed individual and familial history, magnetic resonance imaging scans, blood tests, electroencephalograms, neuropsychological tests, lumbar punctures and very occasionally a brain biopsy. The ideal model for multidisciplinary assessment in secondary care is thus a specialist unit or memory clinic. There has been a substantial growth in the number of the latter following the licensing of cholinesterase inhibitor drugs and the development of younger-onset services (Lindsay et al. 2002). Most have moved beyond 'labelling', offering comprehensive and expert assessment services that are highly regarded by individuals and families (McLennan 1999; Wilcock et al. 1999).

BEYOND TREATMENT

Following diagnosis, drug treatment may be offered for non-cognitive symptoms. Some younger people may be suitable for one of the three drugs – donepezil (Aricept), rivastigmine (Exelon) and galantamine (Reminyl) – licensed by the National Institute of Clinical Excellence for the symptomatic treatment of Alzheimer's disease, which are available via the National Health Service (NHS) subject to certain conditions (Department of Health 2001). These drugs influence the cholernergic neurotransmitter system, slowing down the rate of functional decline and ameliorating non-cognitive features of the illness. More research is needed on the impact of anti-dementia drugs on individuals and families (Wimo et al. 1999).

However, given the range of different types of dementia, 'psychological approaches to intervention … are likely to be needed whatever welcome pharmacological breakthroughs are around the corner' (Woods 1999a, p. 245). Younger people with dementia face a number of crises and different kinds of loss for which non-drug treatments, especially psychosocial interventions and therapeutic activities, may be useful. For optimal benefit, these must be individualized, based on careful neurological assessment and, if used to address specific problem behaviours, preceded by assessment and observation. Interventions can include cognitive management techniques such as reality orientation (Camp et al. 1996), or behavioural approaches, particularly in relation to personal care such as continence. More latterly, interest in the person's subjective world has led to the application of established therapeutic techniques such as psychotherapy (Cheston and Bender 1999), groupwork (Yale 1999), reminiscence and life review work (Gibson 1994).

EMPLOYMENT AND MEANINGFUL OCCUPATION

Younger people with dementia, especially men, are more likely to be working, and their employment will inevitably be curtailed through early retirement, redundancy or dismissal (Seddon 1999). For most adults, work provides income, self-esteem and financial and psychological security, and its loss has many implications for family members (Woods 1999b). Over 50 per cent of carers also have to give up their job or reduce their hours (Delaney and Rosenvinge 1995), although some employers are able to offer a degree of flexibility to meet changing needs (Seddon 1999). Ultimately, however, in order to remain in employment, carers need to be able to access locally based facilities, age-appropriate services and activities with flexible opening hours. Transport is a key element of such provision (Fossey and Baker 1995; Williams et al. 1996; O'Donovan, 1999).

The ending of employment also removes structure and meaningful occupation for many younger people with dementia, and, in the absence of such daily rhythm, individuals often experience a loss of self-esteem and depression (Woods 1999a, b). Those who have worked in the domestic sphere also face difficulties when their capacity for undertaking home-making tasks diminishes. There are, however, few appropriate services available to meet the need for meaningful daytime occupation for younger people, who often have a high level of stamina and fitness.

Statutory or voluntary day care is usually offered in centres, which cater primarily for older people with dementia and are very rarely appropriate. According to a number of studies, most younger people prefer individualized support that is tailored to their needs. Such a preference may include The Clive Project (2001), which provides paid carers who are matched as far as possible with younger people, with the aim of enabling them to continue with their interests, lifestyle and quality of life throughout the illness (Gutteridge 2001). Where such projects are run in rural areas, they are costly (Parsons 1999), as are other forms of intensive one-to-one support (Fox 1995).

MEETING SOCIAL NEEDS WITHOUT STIGMA

Many social activities and interests enjoyed by adults are contingent not only on employment and income, but also on social skills that become impaired by dementia. Studies show that contact with friends and colleagues, and visits outside the home, declines, giving rise to unmet social needs (Parsons 1999; Reed et al. 2000). Day centre attendance is rarely a substitute for the richness of ordinary life so, in many areas, small-scale facilities and activities have been developed such as the Alzheimer's café (Redwood 2001) projects, or simply as places to be, for example the SPECAL project (Pritchard and Dewing 1999).

FINANCIAL AND LEGAL SECURITY: SEEKING ADVICE

Many families make considerable financial sacrifices to continue caring (Stewart 1998). One carer calculated that he had forgone salaries and a pension amounting to £360 000, which were 'replaced' by a total of £7300 in state benefits over the 5 years he spent caring for his wife (ADS Suffolk, Age Concern Suffolk and Suffolk Council Social Services 1999). Families often become dependent on state benefits as carers cease employment (Harvey 1998). As cognitive health declines and the capacity to make decisions reduces, the need for financial and legal planning becomes paramount. Families need, ideally with the younger individuals themselves, to discuss and consider how to safeguard their income and assets and what options are available. Specialist guidance for people with dementia and their families is considered to be inadequate as social workers, who are often best placed to offer advice, generally lack sufficient expertise to provide information (Langan and Means 1995), and those seeking information may turn to voluntary organizations or lawyers who specialize in this area.

FAMILY LIFE

As the condition of the younger person begins to decline, the dementing process affects both the family's relationships with the outside world and the dynamics of relationships within the family system (Tindall and Manthorpe 1997). Families usually develop coping strategies, seeking to restore equilibrium and normalize their situation. Clarke (1999) emphasizes the need for community-based professionals, such as community psychiatric nurses, care managers and direct carers, to respect these by developing support strategies and commission services that complement the ways in which families manage to carry on with their daily lives.

Studies demonstrate the importance of continuity in professional support offered to carers. Community psychiatric nurses (Adams 1999), Dementia Relief Trust nurses (Jarvis et al. 1992) and workers from voluntary agencies are most likely to fulfil this role, although Fountain (2002) argues the case to involve social workers. Such a relationship can engender a gradual sharing of information and advice through the peaks and troughs of illness (McLennan 1999) and is the core of family-centred work. This enables professionals to access the knowledge base of the family, promoting positive relationships to enhance the well-being of the person with dementia (Clarke 1999).

The support needs of primary carers of younger people with dementia, usually spouses, are reported to be high (Freyne et al. 1999), although the nature of the stressors changes. At the outset, the emotional impact of diagnosis and the provision of psychological support for a physically fit relative who may be depressed, have mood swings or become agitated often results in anxiety problems (Harvey 1998) and a deterioration in mental health (Quinn 1994). Towards the end of the illness, carers are more involved in meeting physical care needs and require practical assistance and training in lifting (Pointon 2001).

There are sometimes highly complex issues to address surrounding the genetic implications of the illness for those individuals and families in which inheritable diseases are causing dementia. Genetic testing and counselling programmes for early-onset familial Alzheimer's disease and frontotemporal dementia report beneficial results (Steinbart et al. 2001), and are increasingly being offered at specialist clinics and hospitals in the UK and Europe. In the absence of a cure, a number of families with younger-onset dementia often do not seek genetic testing, especially as the results have already been used to discriminate against some people with dementia (Lovestone 1999). Bio-ethical and legal debates in the field continue as more genes are identified, and the announcement of preimplantation diagnosis for a form of Alzheimer's disease caused by a gene mutation presents perhaps the starkest indication of future challenges (Verlinsky et al. 2002).

The effects of the dementing process impact on most spheres of personal and sexual relationships between spouses (Parsons 1999), but there is a paucity of research in this area (Cox and McLennan 1994; Cox 1999), and little is known about dementia among people who are lesbian or gay (Ward 2000). The quality of the relationship before the onset of illness is, however, an important indicator of how well a couple cope with additional stress (Harvey 1998). Studies of hetero-sexual older people indicate that a high level of non-cognitive symptoms and high expressed emotion in the carer are both correlates of a poorer outcome for the relationship (Fearon et al 1998). The gender of the partner affected by dementia appears to influence the continuity and quality of sexual relationships, men without dementia reporting a higher rate of sexual satisfaction than women whose husbands are affected.

The effect of dementia in a parent on younger children cannot be overestimated (Robertson 1996). Although children are likely to be beyond primary school age, their parent's dementia may come at a time when the pressures of schooling and adolescence coincide with caring responsibilities in which there is a role reversal (Quinn 1996). Children's behaviour often changes, attention-seeking, alterations in school performance, sleeping difficulties and hypochondria having all been reported (Robertson 1996). Children and young people who live in families with a parent with dementia need to discuss their experiences away from their day-to-day situation and to hear clear explanations (Gilliard 1999). Explanatory booklets written for children can have a useful role (Hann 1998).

FINAL TRANSITIONS

There is often a significant deterioration in the condition of the younger person or an increase in the psychological and behavioural symptoms of dementia; this, coupled with carer stress, may lead families to consider increasing the amount of support or finding an alternative to informal care. Studies show a paucity of age-appropriate respite or residential care, little specialist provision being available to meet the often-complex needs of people with dementia caused by different diseases in each locality (Cox 1999).

Younger people are frequently admitted to nursing homes for older people or, following protracted negotiations with funding agencies, to specialist units that may be a long distance from home (Cox 1991). One specialist housing project offers a pioneering model of support to a small group of younger people with dementia who are supported by a high ratio of staff to residents (Cantley and Smith 1999), but this a rare form of provision. A model of care that offers a flexible range of provision, matching the needs of individuals and carers with day, respite and residential care, is seen as ideal (Cox 1999). Most younger people wish to die at home, support to do this varying from area to area. Specialist terminal care facilities or hospices for people with cognitive degenerative diseases have yet to be developed in the UK.

SERVICE DEVELOPMENT: NEXT STEPS

Although younger people with dementia are not a homogenous group, most studies make the case for distinctive care or specialist service provision (Alzheimer's Disease Society 1991; Quinn 1996; Robertson 1996; Keady and Nolan 1999). Research indicates that the most effective models of care are age appropriate and flexible, responding to the cognitive and physical changes in a non-institutionalized setting, alongside person-centred service provision that needs to include high-quality residential care (Sperling and Furst 1994; Williams et al. 1996; Fuhrmann 1997). This service model is, however, some way from being achieved, for the following reasons.

First, there is a dearth of specialist services, and specialist provision is anomalous (ADS 1995). Many areas have significant service gaps, as illustrated by findings from a national survey which showed that 87 per cent of health authorities possessed no specific services for younger people (Newens et al. 1995), even though most perceived a need to have them. Only 12 of the 304 NHS trusts surveyed had established specialist services (Barber 1997), a more recent regional survey reporting only two specialist services in the south west of England (Daker-White et al. 2002). In the six health authorities surveyed by Williams et al. (1995), existing services for younger people with dementia were limited and the care given deemed inadequate.

Second, services have clearly developed in an incremental fashion using no standard model of care (Ferran et al. 1996; Keady and Nolan 1999; Woods 1999a) across health and social services, the voluntary sector and often independent agencies. Existing specialist services, particularly those offering day or residential care, or community support, tend to be underdeveloped, operate almost autonomously (especially if they are located in voluntary organizations) and do not liaise with other services, either directly or adequately (Williams et al. 1996). Many services are delivered through singleton development workers or very small teams (Dementia Plus 2002). This fragmentation contributes to the lack of a co ordinated integrated pathway that hinders service development, yet partnership between the voluntary and statutory sector is crucial if a model of integrated, multidisciplinary and collaborative working is to be achieved (Cox 1991, Quinn 1996; Williams et al. 1996; Cox and Keady 1999; Keady and Nolan 1999).

The threshold of 65 years of age reflects the current division between the organization of acute and elderly care, and may serve as a barrier to providing effective services and care (Cox 1991; Cox and McLennan 1994). Most of the generic services available are designed and set within an older person's perspective, which is generally seen as being inappropriate (Furst and Sperlinger 1993; Barber 1997; Roarty 1998b; Woods 1999a), but no comparative studies exist to test whether providing services for people on the basis of need rather than age is a more satisfactory arrangement. A choice does, however, need to be offered.

Finally, policies advocating early intervention and prevention have not yet been comprehensively applied, and most services for people with dementia appear to be reactive, generally attempting to support people with severe conditions (Keady and Nolan 1999). These findings echo those emerging from research into local authority eligibility criteria, which showed that service allocation was geared to people with dementia who had a very high dependency level (Blackman and Parsons 1999). Bureaucracy can nevertheless be ameliorated, as proved by a recommendation included in good practice guidelines for social services staff supporting people with CJD, produced by the Association of Directors of Social Services, which describes how senior managers should cut through 'red tape' if necessary: 'Consider if a fast track approach is required on occasions. E.g. if there is a request for an orange badge and need is obvious, why go through a long and bureaucratic delay?' (ADS 1998, p. 4).

The way forward lies in specialist commissioning and planning. A development framework for strategic and operational planning has been provided by the Health Advisory Service report (Williams et al. 1996) and was successfully used by a multiagency project group that drew up a Specialist Services Commissioning Strategy for Younger People with Dementia in Oxfordshire (Clive Project 2001). More recent policy directives recommend regional approaches (Department of Health 2001).

At the macro level, a major decision for commissioners and planners has been where to locate services for younger people with dementia, especially as, more generally, 'services for people with dementia have always hovered uneasily between services for mental health and those for older people' (Cox 1999, p. 295). Adult mental health, with the care programme approach, floating support and assertive outreach, appears to offer a useful approach to a serious and enduring mental illness. Expertise in dementia and a social model of care tends, however, to be rooted in community health and social care services.

Service development needs to be underpinned by training and staff development, including the acquisition of specialist knowledge and person-centred skills, which are fundamental to good practice. Training is also needed to support inter-agency working and multidisciplinary collaboration (Chapman 1999). In some areas, younger-onset dementia multiagency teams are resources for other services (ADS 1995, 1996). Training programmes for supporting carers through the provision of information on coping strategies, and managing challenging behaviour, have been shown to be effective (Brodaty et al. 1997).

CONCLUSION

For younger people with dementia and their families, the experience of dementia is profound, and shifts in the philosophy, policy and practice of dementia care have at last rendered many of them visible. Epidemiological and population needs studies have identified diffuse groups among whom there are many causes of dementia, giving rise to complex and formidable needs.

The description of 'living in the labyrinth' penned by one younger person with dementia would, however, act as a metaphor for the support services currently available and the access to them: many formal services are ill prepared to meet the different needs of younger people, and specialist services are poorly developed in many areas. Many specialist services have grown incrementally across the statutory, voluntary and latterly independent sectors, but many are small scale and poorly staffed, and funding is variable. Mainstream services are geared towards meeting the needs of older people. The absence of integrated care pathways, single assessment and a single point of entry to this constellation of different services has resulted in anomalies, individuals and families experiencing the sensation of 'falling through the net'.

Policy directives are, however, in place, and strategic specialist service-commissioning and planning should provide a clear structure, welding together disparate parts into a co-ordinated whole of valued services that focus on the younger person with dementia and the support carers.

REFERENCES

Adams, T. 1999: Developing partnership in the work of community psychiatric nurses with older people with dementia. In: Cox, S. and Keady, J. eds. *Younger people with dementia: planning practice and development.* London: Jessica Kingsley, 292–304.

Allen, H. and Baldwin, B. 1995: The referral, investigation and diagnosis of pre-senile dementia: two services compared. *International Journal of Geriatric Psychiatry* **10**: 185–90.

Alzheimer's Disease Society. 1991: *Declaration of rights for younger people with dementia and their carers.* London: ADS.

Alzheimer's Disease Society. 1995: *Services for younger people with dementia.* London: ADS.

Alzheimer's Disease Society. 1996: *Younger people with dementia: a review and strategy.* London: ADS.

Alzheimer's Disease Society, Age Concern Suffolk and Suffolk Council Social Services. 1999: *Too young! A report on younger people with dementia in Suffolk.* Suffolk: Ipswich ADS.

Alzheimer's Disease Society, CJD Support Network/Association of Directors of Social Services. 1988: *Good practice guidelines for social services professionals.* London: ADS.

Audit Commission. 2000: *Forget me not. Services for older people with mental health problems.* London: Audit Commission.

Barber, R. 1997: A survey of services for younger people with dementia. *International Journal of Geriatric Psychiatry* **12**: 951–4.

Bayer, T. 2000: Rarer causes of dementia. *Signpost* **4:** 4–7.

Beattie, A., Daker-White, G., Gilliard, J. and Means, R. 2002: Younger people in dementia care: a review of service needs, service provision and models of good practice. *Aging and Mental Health* **6:** 205–12.

Blackman, T. and Parsons, M. 1999: *Social care services for adults in Staffordshire: a study of decision making.* Oxford: Oxford Brookes University.

Brodaty, H., Gresham, M. and Luscombe, G. 1997: The Prince Henry Hospital dementia caregivers training programme. *International Journal of Geriatric Psychiatry* **12:** 183–92.

Camp, C., Foss, J.W., O'Hanlon, A.M. and Stevens, A.B. 1996: Memory interventions for persons with dementia. *Applied Cognitive Psychology* **10:** 193–210.

Cantley, C. and Smith, M. 1999: *An independent supported living house for people with early onset dementia: evaluation of a dementia care initiative project.* Newcastle: Dementia North, University of Northumbria.

Cantley, C., Fox, P. and Barber, B. 2000: *Better services for younger people with dementia? Findings from a regional survey of service planning and development.* Northumbria: NHS Northern and Yorkshire Regional Office, Dementia North.

Chapman, A. 1999: Training and younger people with dementia: a shared learning perspective. In: Cox, S. and Keady, J. eds. *Younger people with dementia: planning, practice and development.* London: Jessica Kingsley, 282–91.

Cheston, R. and Bender, M. 1999: *Understanding dementia. The man with worried eyes.* London: Jessica Kingsley.

Christie, A.B. and Wood, E.R.M. 1988: Age, clinical features and prognosis. *International Journal of Geriatric Psychiatry* **8:** 553–9.

Clarke, C. 2000: Professional practice with people with dementia and their carers: help or hindrance. In: Adams, T., Clarke, C.L. and Cantley, C. eds. *Dementia care: developing partnerships in practice.* London: Baillière Tindall.

Clarke, C. and Keady, J. 2001: Getting down to brass tacks. A discussion of data collection with people with dementia. In: Wilkinson, H. ed. *The perspectives of people with dementia: research methods and motivation.* London: Jessica Kingsley.

Clive Project. 2001: *Developing Oxfordshire's services for younger people with dementia.* Commissioning strategy report. Oxford: Clive Project.

Cooper, S. 1999: Learning disabilities and dementia. In: Cox, S. and Keady, J. *Younger people with dementia: planning practice and development.* London: Jessica Kingsley, 292–304.

Cox, S. 1991: *Pre-senile dementia: an issues paper for service planners and providers.* Stirling: Dementia Services Development Centre.

Cox, S. 1999: Opportunities and threats: multi-agency perspectives and person-centred planning. In: Cox, S. and Keady, J. eds. *Younger people with dementia: planning, practice and development.* London: Jessica Kingsley, 69–88.

Cox, S. and Keady, J. 1999: Changing the mind-set: developing an agenda for change. In: Cox, S. and Keady, J. eds. *Younger people with dementia: planning practice and development.* London: Jessica Kingsley, 292–304.

Cox, S. and McLennan, J.M. 1994: *A guide to early onset dementia.* Stirling: Dementia Services Development Centre.

Daker-White, G., Beattie, A., Means, R. and Gilliard, J. 2002: *Serving the needs of marginalised*

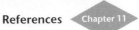

groups in dementia care: younger people and minority ethnic groups. Bristol: University of the West of England.

Davis, R. 1989: *My journey into Alzheimer's disease.* Amersham: Scripture Press.

Delaney, N. and Rosevinge, H. 1995: Pre-senile dementia: sufferers, carers and services. *International Journal of Geriatric Psychiatry* **10:** 597–601.

Dementia Plus. 2002: *Early onset dementia in Worcestershire 1999/2000. A report for Worcestershire Health Authority.* Wolverhampton: University of Wolverhampton, West Midlands LEDC for Older People, Centre for Health Practice: Research and Development.

Department of Health. 1989: *Caring for people. Community care in the next decade and beyond.* London: HMSO, Cm 849.

Department of Health. 1999: *National service framework for mental health: modern standards and service models.* London: DoH.

Department of Health. 2001: *National service framework for older people.* London: Stationery Office.

Downs, M. 2000: The socio-economic context of dementia: an idea whose time has come? *Ageing and Society* **20:** 369–75.

Ferran, J., Wilson, K., Doran, M., Ghadiali, E., Johnson, F., Cooper, P. and McCracken, C. 1996: The early onset dementias: a study of clinical characteristics and service use. *International Journal of Geriatric Psychiatry* **11:** 863–9.

Fearon, M., Donaldson, C., Burns, A. and Tarrier, N. 1998: Intimacy as a determinant of expressed emotion in carers of people with Alzheimer's disease. *Psychological Medicine* **28:** 1085–90.

Fossey, J. and Baker, M. 1995: Different needs demand tailored services. *Journal of Dementia Care* Nov/Dec: 22–3.

Fountain, R. 2002: Should social services departments employ specialist young onset dementia social workers? Unpublished MSc dissertation, University of Oxford.

Fox, J. 1995: *Supported employment and early onset dementia: a pilot study.* Maidstone: Kent Care, Kent County Council Social Services.

Freyne, A., Kidd, N., Coen, R. and Lawlor, B.A. 1999: Burden in carers of dementia patients: higher levels in carers of younger sufferers. *International Journal of Geriatric Psychiatry* **14:** 784–8.

Friel-McGowin, D. 1993: *Living in the labyrinth: a personal journey through the maze of Alzheimer's.* Cambridge: Mainsail Press.

Fuhrmann, R. 1997: *Early onset dementia in the Brighton, Hove and Lewes area: prevalence and service needs.* Brighton: University of Sussex.

Furst, M. and Sperlinger, D. 1993: *'Hour to hour, day to day': a survey of the service experiences of carers of people with pre-senile dementia in the London borough of Sutton.* Sutton: St Helier NHS Trust.

Gibson, F. 1994: What can reminiscence contribute to people with dementia? In: Bornat, J. ed. *Reminiscence reviewed: evaluations, achievements, perspectives.* Buckingham: Open University Press, 46–60.

Gilliard, J. 1999: Young carers: individual circumstances and practice consideration in dementia caregiving. In: Cox, S. and Keady, J. eds. *Younger people with dementia: planning, practice and development.* London: Jessica Kingsley, 196–202.

Goldsmith, M. 1996: *Hearing the voice of people with dementia: opportunities and obstacles.* London: Jessica Kingsley.

Gutteridge, T. 2001: Meeting a special need for confidence and independence. *Journal of Dementia Care* **8:** 20–4.

Hagestad, G.O. and Neugarten, B.L. 1985: Age and the life course. In: Binstocl, R.H. and Shanas, E. eds. *Handbook of aging and the social sciences.* New York: Van Nostrand Reinhold, 35–61.

Hann, L.1998: *The milk's in the oven: a booklet explaining dementia for children.* London: Mental Health Foundation.

Harvey, J. 1998: *Younger onset dementia: epidemiology, clinical symptoms, family burden, support and outcome.* London: NHS Executive North Thames.

Harvey, R., Roques, P., Fox, N. and Rossor, M. 1998: CANDID – counselling and diagnosis in dementia: a national telemedicine service supporting the care of younger patients with dementia. *International Journal of Geriatric Psychiatry* **13:** 391–88.

Jarvis, J., Jason, J. and Butterworth, M. 1992: *The Admiral Nurse Project: a service for carers of people with dementing illness: a critical appraisal of the service from the carers' point of view.* London: Dementia Relief Trust.

Keady, J. and Nolan, M. 1994: Younger-onset dementia: developing a longitudinal model as a basis for a research agenda and as a guide to interventions with sufferers and carers. *Journal of Advanced Nursing* **19:** 659–69.

Keady, J. and Nolan, M. 1999: Family caregiving and younger people with dementia: dynamics, experiences and service expectations. In: Cox, S. and Keady, J. eds. *Younger people with dementia: planning, practice and development.* London: Jessica Kingsley, 203–22.

Killick, J. 1999: 'Dark head amongst the grey': experiencing the worlds of younger persons with dementia. In: Cox, S. and Keady, J. eds. *Younger people with dementia: planning, practice and development.* London: Jessica Kingsley, 153–72.

Kitwood, T. and Bredin, K. 1992: Towards a theory of dementia care: personhood and well-being. *Ageing and Society* **12:** 269–87.

Knapp, M., Wilkinson, D. and Wrigglesworth, R. 1998: The economic consequences of Alzheimer's disease in the context of new drug developments. *International Journal of Geriatric Psychiatry* **13:** 531–43.

Langan, J. and Means, R. 1995: *Personal finances, elderly people with dementia and the new community care.* London:Anchor Housing Association.

Lindsay, J., Marudkar, M., van Diepen, E. and Wilcock, G. 2002: The second Leicester survey of memory clinics in the British Isles. *International Journal of Geriatric Psychiatry* **17:** 41–7.

Lloyd, M.P. 1993: *Early onset dementia in the Maidstone area: identifying needs of sufferers and carers.* Maidstone: Maidstone Health Authority, Mid Kent Social Services.

Lovestone, S. 1998: *Early diagnosis and treatment of Alzheimer's disease.* London: Martin Dunitz.

Lovestone, S. 1999: *Genes and everything.* Seminar paper given as part of Oxford Dementia Centre Research Seminar series, 1998–1990, Oxford.

Luscombe, G., Brodaty, H. and Freeth, S. 1998: Younger people with dementia: diagnostic issues, effects on carers and use of services. *International Journal of Geriatric Psychiatry* **13:** 323–30.

McKeith, I.G., Fairbairn, A. and Perry, R. 1992: Neuroleptic sensitivity in patients with senile dementia of the Lewy body type. *British Medical Journal* **314:** 266–70.

McLennan, J. 1999: Assessment and service responses for younger people. In: Cox, S. and Keady, J. eds. *Younger people with dementia: planning, practice and development.* London: Jessica Kingsley, 17–36.

McWalter, G. and Chalmers, J. 1999: Needs assessment: individual and strategic care planning. In: Cox, S. and Keady, J. eds. *Younger people with dementia: planning, practice and development.* London: Jessica Kingsley, 52–68.

McWalter, G., Toner, H., Corser, A., Eastwood, J., Marshall, M. and Turvey, T. 1994: Needs and needs assessment: their components and definitions with reference to dementia. *Health and Social Care* **2:** 213–19.

Melzer, D., Ely, M. and Brayne, C. 1997: Cognitive impairment in elderly people: a population based estimate of the future in England, Scotland and Wales. *British Medical Journal* **315:** 462–483.

Newens, A., Forster, D. and Kay, D. 1995: Referral patterns and diagnosis in pre-senile Alzheimer's disease: implications for general practice. *British Journal of General Practice* **44:** 405–7.

Newens, A., Forster, D., Kay, D., Kirkup, W., Bates, D. and Edwardson, J. 1993: Clinically diagnosed pre-senile dementia of the Alzheimer type in the Northern health region: ascertainment, prevalence, incidence and survival. *Psychological Medicine* **23:** 631–44.

NHS Executive South East Regional Specialised Commissioning Group. 2000: *Annual Report 1999/2000.* London: NHS Executive.

O'Donovan, S. 1999: The service needs of younger people with dementia. *Signpost* **4:** 6.

Parsons, M. 1999: *The Clive Project: an evaluation report.* Oxford: Oxford Dementia Centre, Oxford Brookes University.

Parsons, M. 2001: Living at home. In: Cantley, C. ed. *A handbook of dementia care.* Buckingham: Open University Press.

Patel, N., Mirza, N.R., Lindblad, P., Amstrup. K. and Samaoli, O. 1998: *Dementia and ethnic minority older people: managing care in the UK, Denmark and France.* Lyme Regis: Russell House.

Pointon, B. 2001: Whose service is it? A pressing need for change. *Journal of Dementia Care* **9:** 23–5.

Pollen. 1994: *Hannah's heirs. The quest for the genetic origins of Alzheimer's disease.* Oxford: Oxford University Press.

Pritchard, E. and Dewing, J. 1999: *An evaluation of SPECAL (Specialised Early Care for Alzheimer's): a multimethod evaluation of the SPECAL services for people with dementia.* Oxford: Royal College of Nursing Institute.

Quinn, C. 1996: *The care must be there: improving services for people with young onset dementia and their families.* London: Dementia Relief Trust.

Ratnavelli, E., Brayne, C., Dawson, K. and Hodges, J.R. 2002: The prevalence of frontotemporal dementia. *Neurology* **58:** 1615–21.

Redwood, K. 2001: All in the same boat. *Journal of Dementia Care* **9:** 9.

Reed, J., Cantley, C. Stanley, D., Clarke, C., Banwell, L. and Capel, S. 2000: *An evaluation of the Lewis project: a service for people with early onset dementia.* Newcastle: Centre for Care of Older People, University of Northumbria at Newcastle.

Roarty, E. 1998: *Lothian early onset support service: annual report 1997–1998.* Edinburgh: Alzheimer Scotland.

Robertson, S. 1996: *Younger people with dementia: the impact on their children.* Stirling: Dementia Services Development Centre.

Royal College of Psychiatrists. 1999: *Services for younger people with Alzheimer's disease and other dementias.* London: Royal College of Psychiatrists.

Ryan, D.H. 1994: Misdiagnosis in dementia: comparisons for diagnostic error rate and range of hospital investigation according to medical speciality. *International Journal of Geriatric Psychiatry* **9:** 141–7.

Seddon, D. 1999: Negotiating caregiving and employment. In: Cox, S. and Keady, J. eds. *Younger people with dementia: planning, practice and development.* London: Jessica Kingsley, 173–95.

Spencer, M.D., Knight, R.S.G. and Will, R.G. 2002: First hundred cases of new variant Creutzfeld Jakob disease: retrospective case notes review of early psychiatric and neurological features. *British Medical Journal* **324:** 1479–82.

Sperlinger, D. and Furst, M. 1994: The service experiences of people with pre-senile dementia: a study of carers in one London Borough. *International Journal of Geriatric Psychiatry* **9:** 47–50.

Steinbart, E.J., Smith, C.O., Poorkaj, P. and Bird, T.D. 2001: Impact of DNA testing for early-onset familial Alzheimer disease and frontotemporal dementia. *Archives of Neurology* **58:** 1828–31.

Stewart, A. 1998: Alzheimer's disease: a review of current economic perspectives. *Ageing and Society* **18:** 586–600.

Tindall, L. and Manthorpe, J. 1997: Early onset dementia: a case of ill-timing? *Journal of Mental Health* **6:** 237–49.

Tobiansky, R. 1994: Diffuse Lewy body disease. *Journal of Dementia Care* **2:** 26–7.

Verlinsky, Y., Rechitsky, S., Verlinksy, O., Masciangelo, C., Lederer, K. and Kuliev, A. 2002: Preimplantation diagnosis for early-onset Alzheimer disease caused by V7171 mutation. *Journal of the American Medical Association* **287:** 1038–40.

Ward, R. 2000: Waiting to be heard: dementia and the gay community. *Journal of Dementia Care* **8:** 24–5.

Whalley, L. 1997: Early onset dementia. In: Hunter, S. ed. *Dementia challenges and new directions.* London: Jessica Kingsley, 71–7.

Whalley, L.J., Thomas, B.M., McGonigal, G., McQuade, C.A., Swingler, R. and Black, R. 1995: Epidemiology of presenile Alzheimer's disease in Scotland (1974–88) I. Non-random geographical variation. *British Journal of Psychiatry* **167:** 728–31.

Wilcock, G.K., Bucks, R.S. and Rockwood, K. eds. 1999: *Diagnosis and management of dementia. A manual for memory disorders teams.* Oxford: Oxford University Press.

Wilkinson, H. ed. 2001: *The perspectives of people with dementia: research methods and motivation.* London: Jessica Kingsley.

Williams, D. 1995: Services for younger sufferers of Alzheimer's disease. *British Journal of Psychiatry* **166:** 699–700.

Williams, R., Barrett, K., Muth, Z., Barker, W., Bingley, W. and Brooke, N. 1996: *Mental health services: heading for better care: commissioning and providing mental health services for people with Huntingdon's disease, acquired brain injury and early onset dementia.* London: HMSO.

Wimo, A., Winblad, B. and Grafstrom, M. 1999: The social consequences for families with Alzheimer's disease patients: potential impact of new drug treatment. *International Journal of Geriatric Psychiatry* **14:** 338–47.

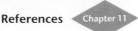

Woodburn, K. 1999: Epidemiological issues and younger people with dementia. In: Cox, S. and Keady, J. eds. *Younger people with dementia: planning, practice and development.* London: Jessica Kingsley, 37–51.

Woodburn, K. and Johnstone, E. 1999: Ascertainment of a population of people with early-onset dementia in Lothian, Scotland. *International Journal of Geriatric Psychiatry* **14:** 362–7.

Woods, B. 1999a: Younger people with dementia: psychosocial interventions. In: Cox, S. and Keady, J. eds. *Younger people with dementia: planning, practice and development.* London: Jessica Kingsley, 245–60.

Woods, B. 1999b: Promoting well-being and independence for people with dementia. *International Journal of Geriatric Psychiatry* **14:** 97–109.

Yale, R. 1999: Support groups for people with early stage Alzheimer's Disease. In: Cox, S. and Keady, J. eds. *Younger people with dementia: planning, practice and development.* London: Jessica Kingsley, 261–81.

Practice systems

Helping families cope with dementia

Chapter

12

Helping families cope with dementia

Alison Marriott

> Imagine you are trying to plan a holiday. You don't know how to get to where you want to go or what to pack. You don't know what your journey will be like or whether you will like the place where you are heading . . .

This is how one woman described the experience of facing the task of caring for her husband after his diagnosis of Alzheimer's disease had been confirmed. She was unsure how his illness might progress, what it would require of her or how to prepare herself for it. She did not know who to ask for advice or whether she really *wanted* to know what to expect. Her experience reflects the many uncertainties involved in caring for and supporting a family member who has a diagnosis of dementia, and the effects upon family members may be immense. This chapter will present an overview of:

- The effects of caring for a family member with dementia
- Care-giver assessment
- The mediating factors in care-giving that make a difference to the experience of being a family care-giver
- Models of care-giving
- Intervention approaches that can be used when working together with families.

THE EFFECTS OF CARING

There are approximately 5.7 million informal carers in the UK, many of whom are providing care to a member of their family (Office of Population Censuses and

Surveys 1997). Of these, 855 000 carers provide care for over 50 hours a week, which would cost an estimated £34 billion a year to fund if using statutory services. Most people with dementia live in the community, and approximately two thirds have a main identifiable carer (Wenger 1994). Coping with a family member with a diagnosis of dementia is one of the significant roles that family care-givers adopt, and there is considerable evidence to suggest that this is one of the most difficult caring roles. Caring for a family member with Alzheimer's disease appears to be associated with higher levels of psychological morbidity and stress than does caring for older people with enduring physical health problems (Gonzalez-Salvador et al. 1999), and there appears to be a range of psychological and physical effects associated with this role.

PSYCHOLOGICAL EFFECTS

Supporting a family member with dementia may have a direct effect upon the psychological well-being of the carer. Depression is very common, and carers often report anxiety symptoms and high levels of stress, which are often directly associated with the demands of caring for someone with dementia. Estimates of psychological distress vary depending upon the methodology of the study quantifying them, the measuring instrument used and the type of sample, but depressive symptoms have been reported in about half of carers (Clair et al. 1995). In a review of studies using psychiatric diagnostic criteria (DSM-III-R; American Psychiatric Association 1987), Russo et al. (1995) reported major depression in 6–10 per cent of care-givers and generalized anxiety in 6 per cent.

Carers commonly worry about difficulties arising from the person's illness, such as what might happen if they went out and left the person with dementia unattended, or how they can cope with challenging behaviours associated with the dementia. Carers have to cope with continual adjustment to the changing demands of the illness and its unpredictable symptom course. In addition, they may worry about becoming too ill to continue caring, or have concerns about the future if the person with dementia outlives them. One 82-year-old man who had cared for his wife during her gradually progressive dementia described how one source of comfort arising from her death from an unrelated illness was that he no longer had to worry about what would happen to her if she outlived him and had to be cared for by someone else.

Many carers coping with a family member with dementia find their role unexpected and unwelcome. They may resent the demands of caring or feel sad that it prevents them fulfilling life experiences that they had hoped to enjoy at that particular time in their lives. When the resources that carers perceive themselves to have are outweighed by the requirements for care demanded of them, they are more likely to experience stress and to perceive the role of care-giver as burdensome. When the burden of care becomes too much, their ability to provide quality care is likely to decline, and there is an increased chance that the person with dementia will move into institutional or residential care. Psychological morbidity in care-givers is often a major determinant of nursing home placement for people with dementia (Gilleard et al. 1984).

Although the psychological impact of care-giving upon family care-givers is therefore a very important factor for services to address, in the interests of both the carer and the person with dementia, it is also important to recognize that many family care-givers do experience satisfaction associated with the care-giving role. A study by McKee et al. (1997) found that many carers reported coping well with their role. The Carer Satisfaction Scale is a measure that outlines a number of positive effects associated with care-giving, including having an opportunity to repay past kindness, being closer to the person and trying to maintain the individual's dignity and self-esteem. Taking account of any satisfactions related to caring will be important to a comprehensive assessment when working with carers, particularly when drawing up strengths/needs lists, as described later in this chapter. This can help to consider constructively the strengths that are brought to the care-giving role.

Apart from the psychological impact of care-giving, the task of supporting a family member with dementia may have other consequences, including a negative impact on the physical health of the carer (Schulz and Williamson 1997). Many carers of older people may themselves be experiencing the increased number of physical problems often associated with ageing but may, because of the demands of caring, be less able to take time out to attend to their own physical health care needs. There may also be a reduction in the time that carers spend in social activities and interests, particularly if they cannot leave the person with dementia alone or find it difficult to continue to engage in activities that they would, prior to the illness, have enjoyed sharing with the person with dementia.

It may be difficult for carers to continue in full-time employment, and many carers, particularly women, give up paid employment (Yee and Schulz 2000), with the accompanying financial implications and potential dependence upon welfare benefits. This may have a marked effect upon families caring for someone with a young-onset dementia as the carer may be a spouse caring for someone of working age who can no longer work, and may also find the demands of caring incompatible with their own continuing employment.

CARE-GIVER ASSESSMENT

When considering the effects of care-giving, the use of a formal and standardized assessment will supplement the process. There are a number of measures, drawn from the wider psychological literature, that are available to assess specific aspects of psychological state, as well as more specific care-giver measures. The General Health Questionnaire (Goldberg 1978) has often been used in carer research to consider the psychological morbidity of carers and as a general measure of care-giver distress, as have other measures of psychological state such as the Beck Depression Inventory (Beck 1988). More specific measures to assess care-givers have been developed covering a range of domains, including carer burden, strain and methods of coping. Examples here include the Zarit Burden Inventory (Zarit et al. 1980) and the Screen for Caregiver Burden (Vitaliano et al. 1991), which conceptualizes the care-giver burden in terms of its subjective and objective aspects.

The Ways of Coping Inventory of Folkman and Lazarus (1980) has been widely used to consider carers' coping styles, and the Dementia Caregiver Checklist is a comprehensive checklist derived from carers' own descriptions of caring for someone with dementia that describes 44 common care-giving experiences. The carer is asked to indicate the problems that have occurred and to rate how stressful they are and how able the carer feels to cope with them. In practice, this is a useful way of considering, together with family members, many aspects of care-giving and to pinpoint those areas which the carer is finding particularly difficult. It can therefore be used to identify areas for intervention with the carer. This measure was used to assess carers and to develop specific problem areas for intervention in the carer intervention study for carers of people with Alzheimer's disease described in Marriott et al. (2000).

Gathering information about the family care-giver, supplemented by assessment measures, is an important precursor to providing appropriate means of help and support. Assessment will, however, also require an awareness of the mediating factors in care-giving since these may affect the way in which the family care-giver is able to offer care.

MEDIATING FACTORS IN CARE-GIVING

Although different carers will share similar experiences of family care-giving, a care-giver's experience will be mediated by a complex set of interacting contexts, which make each situation unique. The nature of the experience will be determined by factors associated with:

- The person with dementia
- The carer
- The relationship between the carer and the care recipient
- The context in which care takes place.

The person with dementia

The cognitive changes associated with dementia clearly have implications for family members. The resulting changes in functioning mean that carers usually become involved in supporting the person with activities of daily living, personal care tasks and other tasks that rely on an intact memory and language functions, as well as on visuospatial abilities. The type of dementia diagnosed also appears to have some impact upon a carer's experiences. The generally more gradual progression of Alzheimer's disease may have a different effect upon care-givers from that of the more stepwise progression of a vascular dementia or the fluctuating course found in Lewy body dementia. Vetter et al. (1999) compared the care-givers of people with a diagnosis of Alzheimer's disease with those caring from individuals with cerebrovascular dementia and found that the latter diagnosis imposed a greater burden in the earlier stages of the illness, whereas the Alzheimer's disease care-givers experienced more burden in the later stages.

There is relatively little research, however, comparing the differential effects of care-giving according to the type of dementia, and it is therefore currently not clear whether the same mediating factors and carer interventions are applicable across different diagnostic profiles. There is, however, a developing consensus that the *non-cognitive* effects of dementia, rather than the cognitive effects *per se*, appear to be particularly significant with respect to carers' psychological well-being (Clyburn et al. 2000).

Non-cognitive features and care-giving

Non-cognitive features are the symptoms such as depression, hallucinations and behavioural changes associated with the dementia. Donaldson et al. (1997) found that depression, sleep disruption and wandering were especially stressful for carers. Behavioural changes such as wandering can be difficult for carers to manage in themselves, but they can also have secondary effects, such as increasing the carer's anxiety about the person's safety if he or she should wander out; there may thus be an increased pressure upon the carer to supervise the person more closely. This may in turn have an effect upon the behaviour of the person with dementia.

| **Case 1** | Mrs Jones, who had Alzheimer's disease, became more agitated and disorientated as the result of a urinary tract infection and frequently walked around the house. Her husband became concerned that she |

might wander out of the house and began to supervise her more closely. Mrs Jones became more agitated as a result of her reduced personal space and tried to walk away from her husband, including attempting to go out of the house to get away. His anxieties about the potential risk of wandering were confirmed by this, and he continued to try to supervise her even more closely, leading to an incident in which Mrs Jones tried to push her husband out of the way.

This is an example of how a physical health change led to a behavioural change in the person with dementia, which in turn led to difficulties for the carer in coping with the change and then to an exacerbation of the situation. The carer's appraisal of the person's agitation as a risk factor for wandering is also very important to the interactions that developed, and a further consideration of the role of cognitive factors will follow.

The carer

Although the term 'carer' has been used liberally throughout this chapter, there may be risks in applying this label to people who are supporting a family member with dementia. Labels such as this tend to encourage automatic beliefs and assumptions about what 'carers' are like and what 'carers' may need or may benefit from. These assumptions may be based on our knowledge of some of the themes described as commonly shared experiences of care-giving but may not take full account of individual differences. A comprehensive assessment will help to reduce any tendency, which the application of a label may have, to dehumanize the person to whom it applies and make him or her appear 'other' from ourselves or without unique characteristics. Kitwood (1997) has written eloquently about person-centred care for an individual with dementia and proposed an equation incorporating this:

$$D \text{ (Dementia)} = P + B + H + NI + SP$$

which suggests that personality (P), biography (B), physical health (H), neurological impairment (NI) and social psychology (SP) are *all* important to understanding the needs of the person with dementia. However, just as all individuals with dementia will possess their own unique 'equation', family care-givers will also have their unique 'care-giver equations'.

The care-giver equation is likely to be made up of many factors, including 'givens' about the carer, such as the carer's gender, cultural group, type of relationship to the care recipient and longstanding personality features. It will, however, also be influenced by factors, which vary according to the situation facing the carer, such as carers' levels of information and knowledge about the situation they are facing, their appraisal of the situation, the coping strategies that they may bring to and acquire as a result of care-giving, and their previous and current levels of psychological distress. If all care-giver equations were the same, every family carer would experience the challenge of care-giving in the same way and intervention would be more straightforward. The challenge in assisting care-givers is to try to understand and formulate the important dimensions in each carer's situation and to work with the carer on intervention approaches that best address his or her particular equation.

Many of the factors that have been found to be significant in determining carers' experiences are based upon group statistical findings relating to a large number of carers, and there will clearly be individual differences, which need to be considered. However, the features identified in this type of research, such as those outlined below, give a helpful indication of the potential effects of particular carer characteristics, which can direct our thinking when working with individual carers.

Approximately two thirds of family care-givers for those with dementia are spouses, women representing 73 per cent of all carers (Tebb and Jivanjee 2000). Women may be more likely than men to experience the negative effects of care-giving. This may be because of a number of factors, including different coping styles, different competing family responsibilities and demands for time, women's persistence with caring over a longer period, more participation in 'hands-on' and time-consuming tasks by women, a greater likelihood that females will report distress and a greater chance that male carers will share care with other family members (*see* Yee and Schulz 2000 for a review). There is some evidence to suggest that gender differences reduce as the time spent caring rises, women maintaining a similar level of distress, but men's distress increasing over time (Yee and Schulz 2000). Previous experience of mental health problems has been associated with an increased vulnerability of carers (Russo et al. 1995), and the carers' personality features may be important in terms of their coping style (Hooker et al. 1994).

The carer's cultural group and ethnicity may also be important to the experience and appraisal of caring (*see* Chapter 13). Knight et al. (2000) found that black carers reported a lower level of burden than, but a similar level of anxiety and depression to, white carers. Aranda and Knight (1997) have considered stress outcomes for different cultural groups in some detail. Some of the other mediating factors associated with the carer, such as coping strategies, appraisal and stress have been incorporated into various models of care-giving, which are outlined in more detail below.

The carer–care recipient relationship

Although factors related to the person with dementia and the carer mediate the experience of care-giving, the nature of the relationship between the carer and the care recipient is important. Interpersonal relationships between people with dementia and their carers have been found to be characterized by more hostility and less affection than relationships between carers and people with other mental health problems (Orford et al. 1987). Many carers report difficulties arising from a change in relationship with the person, which is often associated with the 'loss' of the person as previously known, this being caused by the cognitive and personality changes associated with dementia. Carers who are spouses have been found to exhibit more distress than non-spouse carers (Brodaty and Hadzi-Pavlovic 1990), which may be partly the result of the alteration in a longstanding relationship and intimacy.

The carer's perception of the interpersonal relationship with the care recipient also seems to be an important mediator of distress as negative perceptions of the pre-morbid relationship have been linked to increased distress (Gilleard et al. 1984), and carers who maintain positive feelings towards the person with dementia report a lower level of strain associated with caring (Morris et al. 1988).

The care context

When working with family care-givers, it is important to consider the support system within which care is taking place. This includes factors such as social support available to the carer and also formal support systems. Evidence relating to the value of various forms of social and formal support is presently equivocal, but there does not appear to be a clear and direct link between an increased quantity of support and improved carer well-being. The carer's perception of the quality of the relief offered is important (Coen et al. 1997) and providing more in terms of formal support may not always help the situation unless the support clearly targets difficulties identified by the carer. Bruce and Paterson (2000) found that a significant proportion of carers reported that difficulties with health care agencies contributed to their stress.

Care-giver models

Models of care-giving have attempted to integrate some of these factors that mediate the experience of care-giving. Models such as Pearlin et al.'s (1990) stress process model provide a theoretical basis for trying to understand the complex interactions involved in care-giving, as well as a framework to generate testable ideas for research. They can also generate ideas for formulating and intervening with carers. Lazarus and Folkman's (1984) influential stress appraisal and coping model proposes that stress occurs when there is a shortfall between the demands of the situation and the carer's ability to cope with these demands. The carer's coping style is considered, often facilitated by the use of the Ways of Coping Checklist (Folkman and Lazarus 1980). Coping has been characterized as either 'problem focused' (i.e. focusing on stress by acting on the situation) or 'emotion focused' (i.e. internally reappraising the stressful situation), and research has identified that problem-focused coping is generally a more effective strategy for carers to adopt than emotion-focused coping.

It may, however, not always be possible to apply problem-focused coping strategies to some of the characteristics found in dementia, and flexibility in coping style may be important. McKee et al.'s (1997) paper assessed coping strategies in 228 carers, half of whom were caring for someone with dementia. They found that the carers appeared to have a dominant 'first-line' method of coping, which they used until it was no longer effective, when other, more context-specific coping strategies began to be utilized. The flexibility and ability to adapt in this way may well have an impact upon the capacity to cope with caring, and this type of research has interesting implications for care-giver intervention directed at developing effective strategies to help carers cope. Other models considering care-giving include Wilson's model of family care-giving (Webb and Morries 1994), the ecological model of care-giver isolation (Tebb and Jivanjee 2000) and the existential model (Farran 1997).

INTERVENTION APPROACHES

A range of intervention approaches has been developed and applied to the care of people with dementia. Donaldson et al. (1998) suggest three broad ways in which strategies may be effective:

1. Altering the symptoms of the illness (using medication and behavioural management approaches)
2. Reducing the carer's exposure to these symptoms (by respite care and carer support services)
3. Changing the care-giver's responses to the illness (by means of individual or family therapy for carers).

There have been a number of recent reviews of the area, including Zarit and Leitsch's (2001) appraisal of important factors to consider when developing and evaluating community-based programmes, Pusey and Richard's (2001) review of psychosocial interventions for the carers of people with dementia, which suggested that individualized problem-solving and behaviour management approaches were effective, and Cooke et al.'s (2001) review of psychosocial and psycho-educational approaches, which pointed to the effectiveness of social and cognitive interventions, such as problem-solving and social support. The reviews acknowledge the methodological problems of most of the studies, such as small sample sizes, inadequate controls, short follow-up periods and a lack of specificity related to the components of the treatments used. Charlesworth (2001) has also discussed factors that may strengthen the validity of systematic reviews of intervention in the area.

In order to demonstrate some of the clinical applications of intervention strategies with carers, the remainder of this chapter will focus on the intervention that we undertook in Manchester with the carers of people with Alzheimer's disease. This evaluated the effects of cognitive behavioural family intervention in a randomized controlled trial incorporating a range of approaches for carers, including the provision of information on dementia, stress management and carer-coping strategies (Marriott et al. 2000). It included strategies that addressed the three areas proposed by Donaldson et al. (1998) above as techniques were directed at behavioural management and improving carer support within an individualized therapeutic approach for carers. This intervention approach, comprising 14, once-fortnightly sessions, had a positive effect upon stress and depression in family care-givers as well as significant results in terms of the behavioural disturbance and activities of daily living of people with dementia. The treatment used in this study was based on a written protocol that clearly outlines the approach used in each treatment session (Table 12.1), some aspects of which are outlined in more detail with illustrative case examples below.

Table 12.1 Structure of cognitive-behavioural therapy intervention for the carers of people with dementia

Session number	Intervention
1–3	Education/information-giving
4	Stress assessment
5–9	Stress management
10	Coping skills: introduction and assessment
11, 12	Coping skills: patient behaviour management
13, 14	Coping skills: coping with feelings of loss

Education/information-giving

Sessions 1–3 involved a thorough assessment of the carer's current understanding of dementia using the Knowledge about Dementia Interview. These initial sessions aimed to improve the carer's knowledge using an integrative approach, based on the work of Tarrier and Barrowclough (1986) with schizophrenia. This approach recognizes that carers' and professionals' understandings of dementia are likely to differ and proposes that, rather than beginning with professionals outlining their understanding of dementia for the carer, it is more effective to try to understand the *carer's* model of the illness and then to try to provide an accessible alternative to inaccurate beliefs about the illness, which may in turn affect the carer's strategies for care. Carers were given written information booklets outlining dementia, coping with caring and advice about services, but the therapy sessions were based around individualized case examples for each carer.

Case 2   In this particular case, the carer believed that her husband's memory problems were caused by Alzheimer's disease but that his poor hygiene was really due to laziness. This belief was affecting the carer's approach to her husband as she was able to be supportive and understanding towards his memory problems but was less tolerant of his poor hygiene, which she perceived to be 'deliberate' rather than attributable to the illness. This led to an insistence by the carer that her husband attend to his hygiene, followed by his inability to do so and subsequent rows. Broadening the carer's knowledge base, supplemented by written materials describing how dementia can affect motivation and self-care skills, enabled her to perceive and manage this situation differently.

| Case 3 | In this case, the carer believed that his wife's dementia had begun when they moved house, and he felt he had caused her illness by insisting on the move. This belief was affecting the carer's mood as |

he felt responsible for both the house move and his wife's memory problems. Providing information on the biological basis of dementia, and the ways in which disorientation can be helped by placing furniture and possessions in familiar places and trying to re-establish a routine after the move, helped this carer to take positive steps towards establishing a new routine and feeling less responsible for the problem. During discussion, this man was also able to recall examples of how his wife's memory changes had been affecting her abilities before the move, which challenged his initial belief that her problems had been entirely precipitated by his decision to move house.

The education/information-giving sessions were an important precursor to the later cognitive aspects of the intervention as they helped in understanding the carer's knowledge and beliefs about the illness and how these might affect their caring strategies. There is variable research evidence on the impact upon carers of discrete educational programmes. Coen et al. (1999) found that a dementia carer education programme had no significant impact on quality of life, burden or well-being. Graham et al. (1997) reported that more knowledgeable carers had a lower level of depression but a higher rate of anxiety. Although carer education programmes appear on the whole to improve carers' knowledge of dementia, there is equivocal evidence about whether they help to reduce carers' burden or stress. Our study demonstrated that there were considerable individual differences in how information-giving affected carers' emotional state, and, when working with carers, it is always important to consider what the likely impact of information will be. It would seem most appropriate to provide information in an accessible form, based on an understanding of the carers' current level of knowledge and their particular concerns, and to provide follow-up support and the opportunity for them to ask further questions.

Stress management

Sessions 4–9 addressed the area of carer stress, covering the behavioural, physical, cognitive and affective aspects of stress. A range of techniques for stress management, including progressive muscle relaxation and tension-scanning, was introduced, and carers were taught to review their psychological responses to the stress of caring by using practical examples from their own experiences and by challenging their existing cognitions:

- What evidence do you have for that thought?
- Is there another way of looking at the situation?
- Are your judgements based on what you felt rather than what you did?

- What if that happens; would it be so bad?
- Are you expecting too much of yourself?
- Are you thinking in black-and-white, all-or-nothing terms?
- Are you overestimating how responsible you are for the way things turn out?
- Are you overestimating how much control you have over things?

Behavioural responses to stress were addressed by encouraging carers not to use avoidant, self-sacrificing or isolating approaches and by encouraging them to consider their own needs and to develop effective social supports and resources. Goal-setting was used to help carers define each step involved in, for example:

- Discussing their problems with another person
- Asking a family member for help
- Asking a friend who has stopped visiting to visit again
- Increasing pleasurable activities in their daily routine.

Carers often feel overwhelmed or think that it will not be possible to take these steps, when it is initially suggested that they may be helpful. They may feel that they do not have time to spend on themselves and may believe that they should always put the needs of the care recipient before their own. It is therefore important, with the carer, to work through the process of identifying the possible consequences of this for the carer's own well-being, to consider in a practical, step-by-step way how carers may take time out from caring, and to support and encourage them to consider their own needs if this approach is to be effective.

Coping skills training

The final sessions of the intervention addressed coping skills to help carers develop a range of effective strategies for dealing with difficult care-giving situations. The Dementia Caregiver Checklist was used to produce examples for each carer of problem areas, a strengths/needs list being produced with each carer (Box 12.1).

In the behavioural management part of the coping skills training, the carer was introduced to an 'antecedents, behaviour, consequences' (ABC) approach to behavioural analysis, and specific behaviours identified by the carer were targeted using this approach. Problem-focused and emotion-focused ways of coping were also considered, specific examples were targeted with the carer in which:

- The situation was more amenable to practical intervention as the stress was arising from the nature of the behaviour (e.g., the person with dementia waking several times a night or being incontinent).

- The carer's expectations of or reactions to the person were the main determinants of carer stress (the carer, e.g., misinterpreting a behaviour as intentional or being embarrassed by person's behaviour).
- The situation was amenable to both practical intervention and an alteration in carer response.

Box 12.1 Example of a strengths/needs list

Needs the carer may have:

- Specific symptoms the carer is finding it difficult to address
- Stress related to changes in role that the carer is experiencing
- Difficulties the carer is having in distinguishing behaviour caused by the dementia from behaviour caused by other factors

Strengths the carer may have:

- Effective life skills, such as good time management
- A good relationship with the person
- Social support
- A willingness to ask for help when it is needed
- Willingness to take time away from the person with dementia

---

The final aspect of the coping skills intervention focused on the feelings of loss that many carers of people with dementia experience. This provided an opportunity to talk through feelings of loss and how they affected the carer in order to try to reframe some aspects of loss as changes requiring adjustment and adaptation, emphasizing the person's retained skills and (using the Carer Satisfaction Scale) some of the satisfactions of caring where appropriate.

This intervention approach was effective compared with that of people receiving treatment as usual from standard old age psychiatry services and was maintained over the follow-up period after treatment had ended. It introduced a wide range of approaches for carers, drawing on what is known about carer experiences of loss, stress and depression, and tried to provide carers with ways of coping with the non-cognitive aspects of dementia, which are known to be highly related to carer stress and burden. It is currently not clear whether it is more effective to introduce specific intervention approaches for carers facing specific challenges associated with their role as these arise, or to introduce a wide range of approaches to carers, as in the above study, which the carer may be able to utilize as the illness progresses and the carer faces changing challenges. If the experiences of caring for someone with dementia are like the journey described by the carer in the opening paragraph of this chapter, the greater the carer's flexibility in terms of their information base, stress management techniques and coping strategies, the better equipped they may be to sustain their difficult role.

REFERENCES

American Psychiatric Association. 1987: *Diagnostic and statistical manual of mental disorders*, 3rd edn revd. Washington DC: APA.

Aranda, M.P. and Knight, B.G. 1997: The influence of ethnicity and culture on the caregiver stress and coping process: a sociocultural review and analysis. *Gerontologist* **37:** 342–54.

Beck, A. 1988: *Beck depression inventory*. New York: Psychological Corporation.

Brodaty, H. and Hadzi-Pavlovic, D. 1990: Psychosocial effects on carers of living with persons with dementia. *Australian and New Zealand Journal of Psychiatry* **24:** 351–61.

Bruce, D.G. and Paterson, A. 2000: Barriers to community support for the dementia carer: a qualitative study. *International Journal of Geriatric Psychiatry* **15:** 451–7.

Charlesworth, G. 2001: Reviewing psychosocial interventions for family carers of people with dementia. *Aging and Mental Health* **5:** 104–6.

Clair, J.M., Fitzpatrick, K.M. and Gory, M.E. 1995: The impact of psychosocial resources on caregiver burden and depression. *Sociological Perspectives* **38:** 195–215.

Clyburn, L.D., Stones, M.J., Hadjistavropoulos, T. and Tuokko, H. 2000: Predicting caregiver burden and depression in Alzheimer's disease. *Journal of Gerontology: Social Sciences* **55B:** 2–13.

Coen, R.F., O'Boyle, C.A., Coakley, D. and Lawlor, B.A. 1999: Dementia carer education and patient behaviour disturbance. *International Journal of Geriatric Psychiatry* **14:** 302–6.

Cooke, D.D., McNally, L., Mulligan, K.T., Harrison, M.J.G. and Newman, S.P. 2001: Psychosocial interventions for caregivers of people with dementia: a systematic review. *Aging and Mental Health* (2): 120–35.

Donaldson, C., Tarrier, N. and Burns, A. 1997: The impact of the symptoms of dementia on caregivers. *British Journal of Psychiatry* **170:** 62–8.

Donaldson, C., Tarrier, N. and Burns, A. 1998: Determinants of carer stress in Alzheimer's disease. *International Journal of Geriatric Psychiatry* **13:** 248–56.

Farran, C.J. 1997: Theoretical perspectives concerning positive aspects of caring for elderly persons with dementia: stress/adaptation and existentialism. *Gerontologist* **37:** 250–6.

Folkman, S and Lazarus, R.S. 1980: An analysis of coping in a middle-aged community sample. *Journal of Health and Social Behaviour* **21:** 219–39.

Gilleard, C.J., Belford, H., Gilleard, E., Whittick, J.E. and McKee, K. 1984: Emotional distress amongst the supporters of the elderly mentally infirm. *British Journal of Psychiatry* **145:** 172–7.

Goldberg, D.P. 1978: *Manual for the General Health Questionnaire*. Windsor: NFER Nelson.

Gonzales-Salvador, M.T., Arango, C., Lyketsos, C.G. and Barba, A.C. 1999: The stress and psychological morbidity of the Alzheimer patient caregiver. *International Journal of Geriatric Psychiatry* **14:** 701–10.

Graham, C., Ballard, C. and Sham, P. 1997: Carers' knowledge of dementia, their coping strategies and morbidity. *International Journal of Geriatric Psychiatry* **12:** 931–6.

Hooker, K., Frazie, L.D. and Monahan, D.J. 1994: Personality and coping among caregivers of spouses with dementia. *Gerontologist* **34:** 386–92.

Kitwood, T. 1997: *Dementia reconsidered: the person comes first*. Buckingham: Open University Press.

Knight, B.G., Silverstein, M., McCallum, T.J. and Fox, L.S. 2000: A sociocultural stress and coping model for mental health outcomes among African American caregivers in Southern California. *Journal of Gerontology: Psychological Sciences* **55B:** 142–50.

Lazarus, R.S. and Folkman, S. 1984: *Stress, appraisal and coping*. New York: Springer Publishing.

McKee, K.J., Whiitick, J.E., Ballinger, B.B. et al. 1997: Coping in family supporters of elderly people with dementia. *British Journal of Clinical Psychology* **36:** 323–40.

Marriott, A., Donaldson, C., Tarrier, N. and Burns, A. 2000: Effectiveness of cognitive-behavioural family intervention in reducing the burden of care in carers of patients with Alzheimer's disease. *British Journal of Psychiatry* **176:** 557–62.

Morris, R.G., Morris, L.W. and Britton, P.G. 1988: Factors affecting the emotional well-being of the caregivers of dementia sufferers. *British Journal of Psychiatry* **153:** 147–56.

Office of Population Censuses and Surveys. 1997: *The General Household Survey 1995*. London: HMSO.

Orford, J., O'Reilly, P. and Goonatilleke, A. 1987: Expressed emotion and perceived family interaction in the key relatives of elderly patients with dementia. *Psychological Medicine* **17:** 963–70.

Pearlin, L.I., Mullan, J.T., Semple, S.J. and Skeff, M.M. 1990: Caregiving and the stress process: an overview of concepts and their measures. *Gerontologist* **30:** 583–94.

Pusey, H. and Richards, D. 2001: A systematic review of the effectiveness of psychosocial interventions for carers of people with dementia. *Aging and Mental Health* **5:** 107–19.

Russo, J., Vitaliano, P.P., Brewer, D.D., Katon, W. and Becker, J. 1995: Psychiatric disorders in spouse caregivers of care recipients with Alzheimer's disease and matched controls: a diathesis-stress model of psychopathology. *Journal of Abnormal Psychology* **104:** 197–204.

Schulz, R. and Williamson, G.M. 1997: A two-year longitudinal study of depression among Alzheimer's caregivers. *Psychology and Aging* **3:** 139–46.

Tarrier, N. and Barrowclough, C. 1986: Providing information to relatives about schizophrenia: some comments. *British Journal of Psychiatry* **149:** 458–63.

Tebb, S. and Jivanjee, P. 2000: Caregiver isolation: an ecological model. *Journal of Gerontological Social Work* **34:** 51–72.

Vetter, P.H., Krauss, S., Steiner, O. et al. 1999: Vascular dementia versus dementia of Alzheimer's type: do they have differential effects on caregiver burden? *Journal of Gerontology: Social Sciences* **54B:** 93–8.

Vitaliano, P.P., Russo, J., Young, H., Becker, J. and Maiuro, R.D. 1991: The screen for caregiver burden. *Gerontologist* **31:** 76–83.

Webb, L. and Morries, N. 1994: Wilson's model of family caregiving. *Nursing Standard* **8:** 27–30.

Wenger, G. 1994: Dementia sufferers living at home. *International Journal of Geriatric Psychiatry* 9721–33.

Yee, J.L. and Schulz, R. 2000: Gender differences in psychiatric morbidity among family caregivers: a review and analysis. *Gerontologist* **40:** 147–64.

Zarit, S.H. and Leitsch, S.A. 2001: Developing and evaluating community based intervention programmes for Alzheimer's patients and their caregivers. *Aging and Mental Health* **5:** 84–98.

Zarit, S.H., Reever, K.E. and Bach-Peterson, J. 1980: Relatives of the impaired elderly: correlates of feelings of burden. *Gerontologist* **20:** 649–55.

Developing ethnically sensitive and appropriate dementia care practice

Anthea Innes

In this chapter, I focus on ethnically sensitive practice. 'Ethnicity' is a socially constructed term, the relationship between ethnicity and dementia being a neglected area of research, both generally and particularly in the UK. We are now beginning to appreciate that services that are ethnically sensitive may not be ethnically appropriate. Moreover, racism is a disagreeable feature of service provision and must be addressed at the interpersonal, organizational and institutional levels.

Dementia is a key and growing issue for all minority ethnic groups in the UK. The experiences of dementia in minority ethnic groups have generally not been well documented in the UK, although the prevalence of dementia among the members of such communities would be expected to increase as they age (Ahmad and Walker 1997). Few research studies in the UK have ethnicity as a central aspect of the experience of dementia and dementia care, much of the literature stemming from work in North America.

This chapter begins by considering definitions of ethnicity, followed by an exploration of the literature related to dementia and ethnicity. Two hypothetical case studies, drawing on issues raised in previous research work in Bradford

(Innes et al. 2001a, b), provide examples of families from minority ethnic communities and their experience of service provision. The chapter ends by suggesting implications for the development of ethnically and culturally sensitive and appropriate dementia care provision.

WHAT IS ETHNICITY?

Ethnicity is a concept that is distinct from but related to the concept of 'race'. Both terms are socially constructed, but there are important differences in the ideology underlying their use.

'Race' is a term that brings to bear negative stereotypical beliefs and prejudices towards individuals and groups, most commonly as a result of physical attributes such as skin colour and facial features. 'Race' is often used to describe an attribute of a racialized group (Miles 1993), that is, a group that is perceived negatively as a result of physical features and other perceived attributes. Such beliefs provide a 'rationale' for racist views and behaviours.

The term 'ethnicity' is perhaps preferable as it acknowledges that everyone, and not just those groups easily identifiable as 'different' as a consequence of physical attributes, has an ethnic identity. Ethnicity can thus be defined (Blakemore and Boneham 1994) as an identification with:

- A distinctive culture (e.g. norms, beliefs, social systems, diet and dress)
- A language
- A community system, often linked to religious beliefs
- A sense of shared heritage and historical origin.

It is, however, often difficult to disentangle the terms 'race' and 'ethnicity' as they can be used synonymously and are often employed to describe physical characteristics rather than an identification with cultural practices, norms and beliefs.

MULTIPLE JEOPARDY

'Triple jeopardy' is the term used to describe the disadvantaged position of older people from minority ethnic groups, who are 'at risk because they are old, because of the physical conditions and hostility under which they have to live, *and* because services are not accessible to them' (Norman 1985, p. 1). People with dementia may be at an even greater disadvantage given the stigma attached to dementia within society as a whole (Kitwood 1997) and particularly within minority ethnic communities (Yeo and Gallagher-Thompson 1996). This has led to the suggestion that people with dementia from minority ethnic groups are open to quadruple jeopardy (Bowes and Wilkinson 2002).

It is easy to develop the notion of multiple jeopardies if gender, class, sexual orientation and physical disability are added to the equation. It can thus be argued that people with dementia from minority ethnic groups, along with others with dementia who are disadvantaged according to characteristics such as gender and class, are likely to experience greater disadvantage and more unsatisfactory service provision than people with dementia from the white majority population. Intersecting identities thus contribute to the experience of dementia, ethnicity being but one component of this experience.

What do we know about dementia in minority ethnic groups?

The inappropriateness of services for minority ethnic groups has been discussed in the literature (Gunaratnam 1991; Ahmad and Walker 1997; Mays 1998). Numerous authors argue that culturally sensitive services are required that respond to the specific needs of minority populations (Ahmed and Webb-Johnson 1995; Boneham et al. 1997; Dilworth-Anderson and Gibson 1999; Lau and Zane 2000). The added stigma of mental health problems (Yeo 1996; Rait and Burns 1997; Shah 1998) may also contribute to a lack of awareness and/or use of the services currently available (Alvidrez 1999; Kosloski *et al.* 1999).

Minority ethnic groups' experiences of dementia have not been well documented in the UK (Manthorpe 1994). It has been suggested that dementia tends to be 'hidden' within minority ethnic communities (Brownlie 1991; Anderson and Brownlie 1997). This was also indicated in a literature review on the topic of dementia and minority ethnic groups (Patel et al. 1998) exploring material from the UK, Denmark and France. This review pointed to a lack of culturally sensitive service provision and noted that, although dementia within minority communities tends to be hidden, this does not mean that it is absent.

In addition, white minority ethnic groups are often excluded from culturally sensitive service provision because they are 'invisible'; indeed, the only major review of minority ethnic communities and dementia in the UK (Patel et al. 1998) does not refer to any white minority group. In the UK, white minority ethnic groups, such as Polish and Ukranian communities, are, as a result of, migration patterns more likely to have reached old age than are those from Asian, Chinese and African Caribbean communities (Scott 2000; Ziarksi 2000) and thus stand in need of culturally appropriate service provision now. If dementia is hidden within these communities, the uptake of available dementia services may be low here (Bowes and MacDonald 2000).

Research has demonstrated that South Asian carers experience difficulty when caring for family members (who do not have dementia) and therefore need help from outside the family; this is despite the common belief that people from South Asian communities 'look out for their own' (Atkin and Rollings 1993). The stress and strain of caring generally (Ungerson 1987), and caring for a person with dementia specifically, has been well documented (Gilleard 1984; Morris et al. 1991; Clarke and Keady 1996; Nolan et al. 1996). The supposition that belonging to a particular ethnic group will eliminate the need for support services is open to debate. Indeed, research from the US clearly demonstrates a need for cultural sensitivity in service provision for a range of minority ethnic groups, for example black elderly (Daniels-Lewis and Chavis-Ausberry 1996; Dilworth-Anderson and Gibson 1999), American Indians (Cross 1996; Josea-Kramer 1996) and Hispanics (Gallagher-Thompson et al. 1996).

Dementia within the Chinese community has been underresearched despite there being a UK population of around 160 000 Chinese people (Office of Population Censuses and Surveys 1993). As a result of migration patterns, the Polish community also has a large proportion of elders (Ziarski 2000). As Polish and Chinese communities have a larger number of elders than the other ageing minority ethnic populations, it is these communities, and such others as those of Italian and Jewish origin, who are likely to be experiencing the impact of dementia now but who have a low level of awareness of dementia and a low knowledge and uptake of services.

Work in the USA suggests that a diagnosis of dementia in Chinese families can, because of the stigmatizing view of mental illness within Chinese culture (Lee 1982; Phillips 1993), trigger strong negative responses and a desire to keep the dementia hidden within the family (Elliott et al. 1996). A study in London in the late 1980s found that 90 per cent of Chinese older people interviewed had received no help from social workers, meals-on-wheels or community nurses despite there being an observed need for these (Chiu 1989). More recently, Yu (2000) found that use of social services among Chinese older people was low and that 97 per cent of those interviewed had difficulty using services. There have been calls for service providers to be aware of cultural beliefs and preferences when providing care in a multi-ethnic society, staff training being emphasized as a means of attaining culturally sensitive service delivery (Henley and Scott 1999). The extent to which this is happening in practice is open to question.

Recent government initiatives such as the *National Care Standards for Scotland* (Scottish Executive 2001) highlight the need for culturally appropriate services for all older people from minority ethnic communities, as does the *National Service Framework for Older People* (Department of Health 2001). This recognition comes at a time when there is little baseline knowledge or understanding of the incidence of dementia in, or the needs of people with dementia and their families from, minority ethnic groups (Scott 2000). There is thus a need for further research in this area.

What does 'ethnically sensitive' or 'ethnically appropriate' care provision entail?

'Ethnically sensitive' can imply the need for an awareness of other cultures, leading to a 'checklist approach' (Smaje and Field 1997) often being adopted in the development of existing services for people from minority ethnic groups. Providing services for those from minority ethnic groups with dementia and their families is much more than understanding religion and language, as has been suggested (Tibbs 1998), although this may be a common starting point. Knowledge of dietary and religious preferences and the availability of translated information and interpreters are to be welcomed, as these may enhance minority ethnic elders' experience of services, but it does not follow that an ethnically or culturally appropriate service is available (Innes et al. 2001b). Culture may encompass religion and language, but there are several other components of central importance. These include individuals' personal beliefs and values, family dynamics and practices, and relationships within the wider community.

A model for cultural competence (Purnell 1998) provides a framework for considering social and cultural factors that may influence the experience of dementia of, and service provision for, any one individual. Such an approach recognizes the personhood of the individual with dementia (Kitwood 1997). In addition, multiple identities or oppressions can be taken into account, for example the impact of people's gender, their family relationships, their social status and the support available within the community (Andersen and Collins 1995). The multifaceted nature of the care experience becomes apparent when not just the ethnic group of the person with dementia is considered.

Case 1   Aliya, aged 22, cared at home for her grandfather, Iqbal, who was 86 and had dementia, with some assistance from her sister-in-law and uncle. Although the family network was strong, there were certain elements of care that she and her family found difficult, for example washing and dressing her grandfather when he wet or soiled himself. The reason Aliya gave for this was 'In our religion we're not supposed to look there!'

But when the family approached their general practitioner, he was unsympathetic to the demands that caring was placing on the family, stating, 'Well, there's enough of you to all do your share.' When problems of personal care were raised, the general practitioner advised 'Put him in a nursing home then.' This was not perceived as a viable option for the family, Aliya stating: 'In our community we are meant to look after our elders; people would think we'd abandoned him, he'd think we'd abandoned him.'

Private home care assistants were brought in to help with personal care, but Iqbal bit them when they attempted to assist him, which resulted in the agency refusing to provide further care. The cost of care from other local agencies led Aliya to find out about the financial help available to her. Social services proved useful, helping to fill out the benefit forms. The problems of caring continued, however, with no suggestion from the service providers about the possibility of breaks for the family and for Iqbal through day or respite care, although Aliya had requested that Iqbal be considered for such services.

This case suggests that the general practitioner lacks knowledge or understanding of the religious and cultural beliefs of Iqbal and his family. Similarly, the agency providing the care assistants did not explore the option of male carers to assist with personal care. Furthermore, the affordable help was withdrawn from the family. Neither the general practitioner nor social services provided sufficient information or a full assessment of Iqbal and his care situation. Although financial help might have been forthcoming, practical help and respite for both Iqbal and his family were neither suggested nor explored. The belief of the general practitioner that 'there are enough of you' reflects and perpetuates the perception that Asian families will 'look out for their own' (Atkin and Rollings 1993).

Case 2   Mr Salapa, 88 years of age, cares for his wife, who is 84, at home. Mrs Salapa, who has dementia, becomes extremely anxious when her husband is not around. She no longer understands or speaks English, reverting to her original language, Polish. Because of this and her anxiety, Mr Salapa has decided that day care is inappropriate. A home help comes in to assist with household tasks, giving Mr Salapa the opportunity to shop locally for food. Mrs Salapa has become accustomed to the home help, and they communicate a little non-verbally. Mr and Mrs Salapa sometimes both go to their church, but transport poses a difficulty as Mrs Salapa has mobility problems. They do, however, attend the local Polish community centre once a week, the community centre providing transport, and Polish-speaking staff and volunteers enabling Mrs Salapa to participate in conversation and events. The local priest and church members occasionally visit, but Mr and Mrs Salapa are considered to be a low priority as neither are 'seriously ill' or ill enough to be in hospital. Mr and Mrs Salapa live a quiet and fairly isolated life but are happy that they have one another.

At first sight, the above case study suggests no immediate problems. Mr and Mrs Salapa have one another for company, and the limited input from the home help enables Mr Salapa to go out alone once a week. In addition, they go out as a couple to the Polish community centre. Mrs Salapa, however, only gets to church if transport can be arranged, despite both Mr and Mrs Salapa having a long history of active involvement in church activities. Other than the Polish community centre, no services are staffed by Polish-speaking workers, so Mrs Salapa would find it difficult to use mainstream services staffed by English-speakers. Therefore, although some services are not taken up, this does not mean that there are no service needs. White minorities may be at a double disadvantage: they are invisible as they appear to have assimilated within the majority white population. This is further compounded by their dementia being managed and hidden within the family, suggesting a lack need for services. This is, of course, not necessarily the case.

EXAMPLES OF ETHNICALLY APPROPRIATE SERVICE PROVISION

The Polish community centre mentioned above clearly meets a community need in the provision of services to Polish-speaking members that would otherwise be unavailable. This is an example of a community-led initiative driven, staffed and used by members of the Polish community. Other services have similarly evolved from community-led concerns, resulting in the members of such communities campaigning for services or staffing initiatives to be used by members of the local population.

In Edinburgh, for example, a sheltered housing complex for older Chinese people has been developed (Munday 1996) in response to the unsuitability of sheltered housing designed primarily with the white majority population in mind. Similarly, the Edinburgh Chinese Elderly Support Association has developed a meals-on-wheels service that provides traditional Chinese food by contracting out the service to a local Chinese restaurant. Although these services are not specifically for people with dementia, they are geared towards older people, and a number of people with a probable dementia use them.

In Scotland, there is one Polish community worker with the organization Alzheimer Scotland Action on Dementia who has had the challenge of beginning to work with Polish elders and providing information (also translated into Polish) on dementia to a population previously neglected by mainstream service providers. This is not to say that lunch clubs and day care services have not been developed for older Polish people generally – indeed they have (Scott 2000) – but services specifically for older people with dementia from a minority ethnic group have been overlooked.

Information on dementia has been translated into a number of minority languages by the Alzheimer's Society of England and Wales. Such leaflets are to be welcomed, but the effectiveness of both Alzheimer Scotland Action on Dementia and Alzheimer's Society leaflets has yet to be fully evaluated in terms of the impact that these have for people with dementia and their families.

MANAGEMENT/SERVICE DEVELOPMENT ISSUES

The above discussion suggests a number of management and/or service development issues:

- Identifying 'hidden' minority ethnic groups
- Providing information
- Recruiting and retaining staff who speak community languages
- Staff development
- Developing individualized, culturally appropriate services.

The identification of hidden minority ethnic groups who may be experiencing dementia, yet who may be missing out on mainstream services, is worth exploring given the likelihood of a large number of people with dementia in such minority populations. White minority groups are more likely to be overlooked as they may appear to have assimilated within the white majority population. Migration

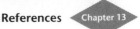
patterns (e.g., identifying areas to which Polish people moved to at the end of the Second World War) may provide one means of identifying localities with a potentially high level of older people from minority groups.

Providing information on dementia to minority ethnic communities has begun in the work of the Alzheimer's Society and Alzheimer Scotland Action on Dementia. Producing information on the services available and developing consultation on those required are further areas of development. For this to be successful, schemes such as those employing outreach workers with an understanding of the cultural taboos surrounding mental health and disability are recommended, such workers being able to work from the inside of minority groups to identify modes of service delivery that are acceptable.

Culturally appropriate services cannot be developed without the willingness of service providers to become culturally competent, which includes the flexibility to address wider issues of culture, ethnicity and racism. For example, developing and understanding role tensions such as the gender and age status of an individual, which may bring rewards, combined with the loss of status accompanying perceptions of dementia equating to madness, may lead to difficulties for the individual, family and community in meeting the care and cultural needs of an individual with dementia.

Not only do service providers need to be aware of differences in cultures, but systems and procedures also need to be in place to contribute to service users' satisfaction. Educating staff on cultural differences has been advocated as a way forward to ensure cultural competence and tackle interpersonal racism and prejudice. If resources are not made available and alternative modes of service delivery are not developed, staff may find it difficult, if not impossible, to provide a service that meets the aspirations and needs of its users, that is, services that are non-discriminatory, open and equitable for all ethnic groups.

REFERENCES

Ahmad, W.I.U. and Walker, R. 1997: Asian older people: housing, health and access to services. *Ageing and Society* **17:** 141–65.

Ahmed, T. and Webb-Johnson, A. 1995: Voluntary group. In: Fernando, S. ed. *Mental health in a multi-ethnic society: a multi-disciplinary handbook.* London: Routledge, 73–86.

Alvidrez, J. 1999: Ethnic variations in mental health attitudes and service use among low income African American, Latina, and European American young women. *Community Mental Health Journal* **35:** 515–30.

Andersen, M. and Collins, P. 1995: *Race, class and gender.* Belmont: Wadsworth.

Anderson, I. and Brownlie, J. 1997: A neglected problem: minority ethnic elders with dementia. In: Bowes, A.M. and Sim, D.F. eds. *Perspectives on welfare: the experience of minority ethnic groups in Scotland.* Aldershot: Ashgate.

Atkin, K. and Rollings, J. 1993: *Community care in a multi-racial Britain: a critical review of the literature.* London: HMSO.

Blakemore, K. and Boneham, M. 1994: *Age, race and ethnicity: a comparative approach.* Buckingham: Open University Press.

Boneham, M.A., Williams, K.E., Copeland, J.R.M. et al. 1997: Elderly people from ethnic minorities in Liverpool, mental illness, unmet needs and barriers to service use. *Health and Social Care in the Community* **5**: 173–80.

Bowes, A. and MacDonald, C. 2000: *Support for majority and minority ethnic groups at home – older people's perspectives.* Social Work Research Findings no. 36. Edinburgh: Scottish Executive, Central Research Unit.

Bowes, A. and Wilkinson, H. 2002: South Asian people with dementia: research issues. In: Wilkinson, H. ed. *The perspectives of people with dementia.* London: Jessica Kingsley, 223–41.

Brownlie, J. 1991: *A hidden problem? Dementia among minority ethnic groups.* Stirling: University of Stirling, Dementia Services Development Centre.

Chiu, S. 1989: Chinese elderly people: no longer a treasure at home, *Social Work Today* 10 Aug: 15–17.

Clarke, C.L. and Keady, J. 1996: Researching dementia care and family care giving: extending ethical responsibilities. *Health Care in Later Life* **1**: 87–95.

Cross, A. 1996: Working with American Indian elders in the city. In: Yeo, G. and Gallagher-Thompson, D. eds. *Ethnicity and the dementias.* London: Taylor & Francis, 183–6.

Daniels-Lewis, I. and Chavis-Ausberry, M.S. 1996: African American families: management of demented elders. In: Yeo, G. and Gallagher-Thompson, D. eds. *Ethnicity and the dementias.* London: Taylor & Francis, 225–34.

Department of Health. 2001: *National service framework for older people.* London: Department of Health.

Dilworth-Anderson, P. and Gibson, E.B. 1999: Ethnic minority perspectives on dementia, family care giving, and interventions. *Generations, Journal of the American Society on Aging* **XX111**: 40–5.

Elliott, K.S., Minno, M.D., Lam, D. and Mei Tu, A. 1996: Working with Chinese families in the context of dementia. In: Yeo, G. and Gallagher-Thompson, D. eds. *Ethnicity and the dementias.* London: Taylor & Francis, 89–107.

Gallagher-Thompson, D., Talamantes, M., Ramirez, R. and Valverde, I. 1996: Service delivery issues and recommendations for working with Mexican American family caregivers. In: Yeo, G. and Gallagher-Thompson, D. eds. *Ethnicity and the dementias.* London: Taylor & Francis, 137–49.

Gilleard, C.J. 1984: *Living with dementia.* London: Croom Helm.

Gunaratnam, Y. 1991: Breaking the silence: Asian carers in Britain. In: Bornat, J., Johnson, J., Pereira, C., Pilgrim, D. and Williams, F. eds. *Community care: a reader.* Basingstoke: Macmillan, 114–23.

Henley, A. and Scott, J. 1999: *Culture, religion and patient care in a multi-ethnic society.* London: Age Concern England.

Innes, A., Ashraf, F., Ismail, L. and MacKenzie, J. 2001a: Supporting family carers of people with dementia from minority ethnic groups. *Generations Review* **11**: 19–20.

Innes, A., Ashraf, F., Ismail, L. and MacKenzie, J. 2001b: The importance of cultural competence in dementia care. *Journal of Dementia Care* **9**: 2–3.

Josea-Kramer, B. 1996: Dementia and American Indian populations. In: Yeo, G. and Gallagher-Thompson, D. eds. *Ethnicity and the dementias.* London: Taylor & Francis, 175–80.

Kitwood, T. 1997: *Dementia reconsidered: the person comes first*. Buckingham: Open University Press.

Kosloksi, K., Montgomery, R.J.V.M. and Karner, T.S. 1999: Differences in the perceived need for assistive services by culturally diverse caregivers of persons with dementia. *Journal of Applied Gerontology* **18:** 239–56.

Lau, A. and Zane, N. 2000: Examining the effects of ethnic specific services: an analysis of cost-utilization and treatment outcome for Asian American Clients. *Journal of Community Psychology* **28:** 63–77.

Lee, E. 1982: A social systems approach to assessment and treatment for Chinese American families. In: McGoldrick, M., Giordano, J., Pearce, J.K. and Giordano, J. eds. *Ethnicity and family therapy*. New York: Guilford Press, 527–51.

Manthorpe, J. 1994: Reading around: dementia and ethnicity. *Journal of Dementia Care* **2:** 22–4.

Mays, N. 1998: Elderly South Asians in Britain: a survey of relevant literature and themes for future research. *Ageing and Society* **18:** 71–97.

Miles, R. 1993: *Racism after race relations*. London: Routledge.

Morris, R.G., Woods, R.T., Davies, K.S. and Morris, L.W. 1991: Gender differences in carers of dementia sufferers. *British Journal of Psychiatry* **158:** 69–74.

Munday, E. 1996: An evaluation of the process of housing need assessment for minority ethnic elders: a case study of 'Cathay Court' sheltered housing scheme for Chinese elders. Unpublished project. Diploma in housing studies, Edinburgh College of Art.

Nolan, M., Grant, G. and Keady, J. 1996: *Understanding family care*. Buckingham: Open University Press.

Norman, A. 1985: *Triple jeopardy: growing old in a second homeland*. London: Centre for Policy on Ageing.

Office of Population Censuses and Surveys. 1993: *1991 census: ethnic group and country of birth – Great Britain*. London: OPCS.

Patel, N., Mirza, N.R., Linbald, P., Armstrup, K. and Samaoli, O. 1998: *Dementia and minority ethnic older people: managing care in the UK, Denmark and France*. London: Russell House.

Phillips, M.R. 1993: Strategies used by Chinese families coping with schizophrenia. In: Davis, D. and Harrell, S. eds. *Chinese families in the post-Mao era*. Berkley: University of California Press, 277–306.

Purnell, L.D. 1998: Purnell's model for cultural competence. In: Purnell, L.D. and Paulanka, B.J. eds. *Transcultural health care: a culturally competent approach*. Philadelphia: F.A. Davis, 7–53.

Rait, G. and Burns, A. 1997: Appreciating background and culture: the South Asian elderly and mental health. *International Journal of Geriatric Psychiatry* **12:** 973–7.

Scott, H. 2000: Scotland. In: Huismann, A., Raven, V. and Geiger, A. eds. *Neurogenerative diseases among migrants in EU states: prevalence, care situation and recommendations*. Bielefeld: Verlag Hans Jacob, 201–33.

Scottish Executive. 2001: *National care standards for Scotland*. Edinburgh: Scottish Executive.

Shah, A. 1998: The psychiatric needs of ethnic minority elders in the UK. *Age and Ageing* **27:** 267–9.

Smaje, C. and Field, D. 1997: Absent minorities? Ethnicity and the use of palliative care services. In: Field, D., Hockey, J. and Small, N. eds. *Death, gender and ethnicity*. London: Routledge.

Tibbs, M. 1998: Special needs of minority ethnic groups. In: Benson, S. ed. *The care assistant's guide to working with people with dementia*. London: Hawker, 18–24.

Ungerson, C. 1987: *Policy is personal: sex, gender and informal care*. London: Tavistock.

Yeo, G. 1996: Background. In: Yeo, G. and Gallagher-Thompson, D. eds. *Ethnicity and the dementias*. London: Taylor & Francis, 3–7.

Yeo, G. and Gallagher-Thompson, D. eds. 1996: *Ethnicity and the dementias*. London: Taylor & Francis, 3–8.

Yu Wai Kam. 2000: *Chinese older people: a need for social inclusion in two communities*. Bristol: Policy Press.

Ziarksi, T. 2000: *The Polish community in Scotland*. Hove: Caldra House.

Supporting and supervising in dementia care

Mark Holman

Supporting people who have dementia and their carers presents personal and work-related challenges. This chapter discusses the nature of these challenges and describes how support and supervision are provided to help people to cope with, and overcome, the difficulties that they encounter when working with people who have dementia and their carers.

WHAT IS CLINICAL SUPERVISION?

Clinical supervision arose within psychotherapy, the influence of its psychotherapeutic roots being evident in current thinking on the nature of supervision. Supervisory ideas and practice spread into other areas of counselling and also social work, where Mattison (1975), for example, brought psychotherapeutic thinking to bear on casework supervision. The development of clinical supervision within nursing has, however, been slower in the UK than in the USA. The Department of Health's report *A Vision for the Future* (1993) recommended its use throughout nursing, but this remains patchy, and it has been taken up with marked enthusiasm only within mental health nursing. As clinical supervision has been adopted in an ever-widening arena, discussion continues about its definition and purpose. Bond and Holland (1998, p. 12) discuss some of these issues and suggest a series of characteristics important in any discussion of supervision. Key elements relating to the purpose of supervision comprise:

- The review of practice is central to supervision, and through it practitioners are given time to reflect upon their practice and their contribution toward shaping the relationships in which their practice takes place.

Inherent in this idea are two related beliefs, that supervision

- provides a mechanism for ensuring the quality of the service provided to patients, clients or service users, and
- plays an important part in the supervisees' continuing professional development and should take place throughout their career.

Allied to these views on the purpose of supervision are beliefs about how supervision should be structured within organizations:

- Organizations should provide a framework within which supervisory relationships may be developed. Without a commitment to, and a statement of the importance of supervision there is a risk that individual supervisory arrangements may run out of steam or get subsumed within competing organizational needs.
- Clinical supervision is separate and distinct from an organization's management structures.

CLINICAL SUPERVISION IS DISTINCT FROM MANAGERIAL SUPERVISION

Many professions, particularly in mental health and child care, have been exposed to widespread public criticism in the face of profound failures to protect members of the public. This has led to calls for a greater monitoring of their work. This increased scrutiny has in turn led to a blurring of the distinction between clinical and managerial supervision. Kearney (1998, p. 169), discussing the introduction of private sector management techniques into the public services, describes the traditional view of supervision that has prevailed in the private sector:

> supervision has been traditionally invariably understood to mean overseeing, looking at what is going on; an observation, rather than a conversation; 'walking the job' is often an important aspect of being a manager.

There is, however, a widespread suspicion of this view of supervision, particularly within nursing, where many people have worked in a negative and unsupportive environment. Bond and Holland (1998), although recognizing that managerial supervision has a place, claim that its purpose contrasts with that of clinical supervision. They argue that whereas managerial supervision has as its focus the needs of the organization and the role of that individual within the organization, clinical supervision focuses on the needs and development of individual practitioners.

SUPERVISION IN OLDER PEOPLE'S SERVICES

In addition to the demands of supporting a wide range of people, practitioners working with dementia may also experience specific problems.

Any meeting between health and social care practitioners and service users creates a tension between the degree to which the helper brings a 'professional' self and an 'ordinary' self to bear on the relationship. Menzies (1970) studied the reaction of nursing staff to the pain and suffering to which they were exposed when working with patients. She noticed that their work produced a high level of anxiety and described the adoption of professional detachment as a way in which nurses dealt with this anxiety. Menzies claimed that this was only partially successful because 'The social defences prevent the individual from realising to the full her capacity for concern, compassion and sympathy, and for action based on those feelings' (1970, p. 36).

Barker et al. (1999) also describe this split between health and social care practitioners' ordinary and professional selves. They claim that workers at the 'care face' make greater use of their ordinary selves in their dealings with service users and that this leads them to do more ordinary things for people. They illustrate this point with the example of a community psychiatric nurse working with a person with dementia who describes feeling obliged to ensure that one of his patients has fuel and basic foodstuffs as part of his contact with the person, and who says that he would take them shopping for these things if he felt it necessary.

Brandon (1987) explores the tension between the helper's professional and ordinary selves, stating that 'We can only offer ourselves, neither more nor less, to others – we have in fact nothing else to give.' For many of us working with people who have dementia, this ordinariness is central to the work that we do, and there is a possibility that this closeness will affect, in both positive and negative ways, the relationships we develop with service users. Kitwood (1997) discusses the importance of the relationships made with people with dementia, calling for 'positive person work' that addresses their emotional needs. He stresses that the first requirement of practitioners is that they are psychologically available in the relationships they form, and he believes that clinical supervision is vital if health and social care practitioners are to work effectively.

Working with people with dementia will at some point lead to practitioners encountering their own and other people's ageist attitudes. Ageism is a feature of many Western societies, and two ideas have been advanced to explain such views. First, Hughes (1995) argues that ageist thinking may originate partly from economic and political structures that force retirement on older people, who are then seen to be economically and socially redundant. Worse still, older people are, because of their economic inactivity, increasingly seen as a drain upon the resources of the young. Hughes also suggests that older people remind others of the possibility of their own physical deterioration and raise the often unwelcome, uncomfortable and distressing recognition that they will some day die. Second, Slater (1995) argues that one possible consequence of ageism is that it allows younger people to deny their own ageing and death. Such issues may be central to many of the contacts that practitioners have with older people.

Working with older people who have dementia brings particular stresses to the relationship between the worker and the service user. We all carry fears of madness, and, at times of particular life stress, it is common to hear people say that they are 'going mad' or 'losing their mind'. These fears are described by Kitwood (1997), who suggests that they are eclipsed by the fear of the complete loss of one's sense of self that appears to accompany the other losses of dementia. He claims that contact with someone who has dementia may trigger our fears of insanity and dependence, and that these fears are difficult to address because we do not know what old age has in store for each of us.

Packer (1999) describes a study she undertook with a group of staff working with people who had dementia, which confirmed these notions about the fear that arises from working with this condition. She found that ageist views within society were reflected in the attitudes of staff, who saw ageing in terms of chronic disease, physical decline and frailty. She also observed that care practitioners struggled with the demands of caring for people with dementia, particularly when trying to engage them in activities or understand what had led to angry outbursts on their part. Packer suggests that supervision is a particularly suitable vehicle for helping practitioners to cope with the frustrations and anxieties that such work imposes.

CARE SETTINGS FOR OLDER PEOPLE

Work with people with dementia takes place in a variety of settings with differing supervision and support arrangements. Supervisory structures are being developed in the UK's National Health Service, particularly under the umbrella of clinical governance, but their implementation remains patchy. In addition, as we have noted, there is a continuing tension between the need to provide managerial and clinical supervision. In contrast, the supervisory system within social services is better developed, supervision usually being provided by a worker's line manager. Supervisory structures remain, however, sketchy for the majority of those working with people who have dementia.

Home care workers and care assistants, in particular, receive very little support and supervision, yet they spend long periods of time with vulnerable people and undertake physically and emotionally demanding work. Taylor (2001), in a survey of home care workers, found that three quarters of the sample supported older people with dementia. Three quarters of the respondents felt that their work was becoming more stressful, while a quarter reported feeling that they were unsupported in their work.

Similar findings led Davies (1998) to group together a series of jobs that she defined as carework. She proposed that there are a series of defining characteristics to such jobs: they are mainly carried out by women; they do not have a sustained training structure; and they are associated with low status and low regard. Davies suggested that many of these features arose partly from an ignorance of the skills involved in this work, which was exacerbated by practitioners finding them difficult to articulate. The British Psychological Society (1994) claims, however, that the relationship between domiciliary workers and service users is central to the effective delivery of care, and it recognizes that this has both training and supervisory implications.

MODELS OF SUPERVISION

Effective support and supervision address the emotional needs of staff and the development of their skills. In addition, it provides a means for safeguarding vulnerable service users (*see* Chapter 15). Several models of supervision are outlined in the literature. Those described by Stoltenberg and Delworth (1987), Inskipp and Proctor (1988), and Hawkins and Shohet (1989) illustrate the variety of approaches that are available.

A developmental model

The developmental model devised by Stoltenberg and Delworth (1987) evolved from the supervision of counsellors and therapists. These authors suggest that the skills and techniques used by health and social care practitioners develop over time and that the supervision they receive should match their level of development. They argue that there are three stages of development – levels one, two and three, which are similar to those of novice, journeyman and expert – that health and social care practitioners may pass through.

Level one

At this level, practitioners are struggling to put theory into practice. In their work, they focus on the use of skills and techniques, and try to match their efforts against a map of the intervention they are using. This preoccupation may leave them anxious and unaware of the perspective of their service users. Health and social care practitioners at this level depend on their supervisors for guidance on case management and also look to them for encouragement that their work is satisfactory. Stoltenberg and Delworth (1987, p. 69) claim that some people remain stuck at this level, 'where they use techniques in a mechanical way, never grasp the real essence of the client, and are unaware of their own complex reactions'.

Level two

Practitioners have now gained both experience and confidence in their abilities. At this level, they are able to consider the needs of service users and adapt their skills accordingly. Their increased awareness may lead them to over-identify with a person's problems or emotional state, leading to their becoming less effective. Supervision at this level is focused less on technique and more on offering a supportive environment in which supervisees may reflect on their actions as they become increasingly independent in planning care.

Case 1 Doreen is a 72-year-old woman who lives alone in a rented bungalow. She has Alzheimer-type dementia and is unable to look after herself very well. She receives a home care package that includes four visits a day by care workers who help with personal care and getting her meals. Celia, one of the care workers, has been involved in supporting Doreen for about 6 months. Doreen has told Celia that she is afraid she might be taken into a home and would rather be dead than have this happen.

Celia notices that Doreen has become increasingly confused at night and needs more and more help to prepare for bed. She has also become anxious when left alone, and Celia has had to spend longer than her alloted time with Doreen during her evening visits. This has led to her rushing other visits and getting home late. Celia's husband has now said that she is putting Doreen before her own family and wants her to stop visiting her. Celia telephones her work supervisor to tell her that she is thinking about giving up work; when pressed, Celia tells her that she seems to worry too much about the people she visits.

Celia is at level two in terms of the developmental model. She is able to see that Doreen's abilities have declined and has adapted the help that she provides to meet Doreen's increased needs. Celia has, however, also identified with Doreen's fears of losing her independence, which has led to Celia spending some of her own time trying to compensate for Doreen's failing ability. This has had an impact on her personal life and left Celia feeling unable to cope. Celia's supervisor needs to help her to recognize her skills and develop ways of managing the emotional demands that her work places on her.

Level three

Stoltenberg and Delworth describe two stages within level three. Individuals at the first stage will have integrated their training into their personality and successfully developed their own style of working. They will try to attend to people's immediate needs yet place those needs in the wider context of the person's life. Although supervision at this level may appear to be more of a peer relationship, supervisors need to be able to retain the ability to challenge their supervisees and help them to build a realistic assessment of their strengths and weaknesses so that they can continue to develop. Stoltenberg and Delworth suggest that individuals at the second stage of level three are now well aware of their limitations and use this knowledge to seek supervision for specific cases or difficulties.

Stoltenberg and Delworth's model provides a useful way of assessing the most appropriate strategies for supervisors to adopt in their work with supervisees at different levels of development. A focus on the processes taking place in a relationship may not be helpful to the supervisee who is struggling to develop his or her knowledge and skills, whereas the provision of knowledge and information may be unhelpful to those who are more concerned with the relationships they have with service users. Stoltenberg and Delworth stress that the journey from novice to expert practitioner may not proceed sequentially through each stage and that individuals may move between levels as they develop additional skills.

The next sections outline further models of supervision, useful for those on both the 'receiving' and the 'giving' ends.

A functional model

Inskipp and Proctor (1988) outline a model that describes supervision as meeting one of three possible functions, which they describe as normative, formative and restorative. Normative tasks relate to ensuring that supervisees meet professional and organizational norms, and focus on competence and accountability. Formative tasks relate to helping a supervisee to develop understanding and skills, whereas restorative tasks offer support to practitioners who often have to struggle to manage the emotional demands that their work places upon them. These emotional demands are described in the following case study.

Case 2

Joanne is an 18-year-old woman who has just started working for a home care agency. She has been asked to visit Edith, a 92-year-old woman who has severe arthritis and memory problems, to help her regular care staff to bathe her. Joanne's work has so far mostly involved her in meal preparation, and when she sees Edith naked, she is unprepared for the sight that greets her, wrinkling her face in disgust. Edith catches this look and says to her, 'I hate my body.' This leaves Joanne ashamed that she has upset Edith, and she subsequently talks to her supervisor about the situation.

A process model

Hawkins and Shohet (1989) have developed a process model of supervision that is based within the tradition of psychotherapy. The main focus of this model is the supervisory relationship and the interpersonal forces at work within it. Supervision is based upon two interlocking systems relating to the supervisee and the service user, and the supervisee and his or her supervisor.

Case 3   David, a community psychiatric nurse, is working with Edward, who cares for his wife Sally. She has dementia and relies on Edward to help her with all aspects of her daily life. Edward is devoted to Sally and keen to continue caring for her, but he finds the demands of caring increasingly difficult. The two of them have always done things together, and Edward continues to take Sally with him when he goes shopping. This has become increasingly difficult because Sally has started to wander off when he is trying to pay for things. Edward asks David for help and says that he would like someone to go shopping with them so that he does not have to be so alert to the things that Sally is doing. David focuses on the practical difficulty that Edward describes and says that he can arrange for Sally to attend day care so that Edward can shop without distraction. Edward appears angry with David's suggestion; he tells him that he does not want Sally to go to day care and complains that no-one listens to him when he asks for help.

David describes this conversation during his supervision with Jane. She asks David to consider whether or not his solution matched Edward's request, but David tells her that his solution was perfectly adequate given the pressure that he is under at work. Jane suggests that David seems annoyed with her just as Edward had been annoyed with David. David then tells Jane that he feels she has not heard him say how much pressure he feels he is under, and together he and Jane reflect that his feeling mirrors the day-to-day pressure that Edward is feeling.

This allows David to reconsider Edward's response to his offer of day care. He recognizes that, because of his wish that he and Sally stay together, this does not reduce the pressure that Edward feels, and it therefore leaves Edward feeling dissatisfied. Having become aware of the parallels between his meeting with Edward and his supervision, David is able to consider ways in which he can pay closer attention to Edward's feelings so that they may explore other ways of helping him continually to support Sally.

Hawkins and Shohet suggest that their model separates supervision into two main categories focused on one of two factors:

- The supervisee's work – this being accomplished by the supervisee and supervisor reflecting together on written or oral accounts of the supervisee's work
- The relationship the supervisee has with the service user – this being accomplished by considering how those relationships are reflected in the relationship between supervisee and supervisor.

In Case 3, David and Jane focus initially on the content of David's therapeutic work, which corresponds to first-category interventions in Hawkins and Shohet's model. Jane's initial response retains this focus when she asks David to think more deeply about Edward and Sally's relationship. Jane senses, however, that David is annoyed by this suggestion so she shifts the focus of their conversation to a consideration of the way in which David's relationship with Edward is mirrored in his relationship with her. By doing this, Jane moves the focus of the supervision into the second category of interventions described by Hawkins and Shohet.

HOW IS SUPERVISION ORGANIZED?

Just as there are different models of supervision, so supervision may be delivered in various ways. Individual supervision may be provided through a hierarchical relationship, with a more experienced worker meeting the supervisory needs of someone who is less experienced. Hierarchical frameworks may be used within organizations for a number of reasons. A degree of quality assurance may be provided by the overview that supervisors gain of the work that is being undertaken by their supervisees, fulfilling the normative function of Proctor's model. Effective supervisory systems may also be used as part of a staff development framework.

Such hierarchical systems have, however, some disadvantages. Issues of trust between supervisor and supervisee may inhibit the effective use of supervision, supervisees often choosing not to bring their problems or weaknesses, fearing that if they do so, they will suffer outside the supervisory relationship. There are also logistical problems in ensuring that sufficient senior members of staff are available to act as supervisors. This problem is likely to be particularly acute in older people's services that employ a high number of support workers.

Individual supervision may also be provided by a peer, and there are some advantages in setting up peer supervision networks. First, the fears associated with a hierarchical structure may not apply, and supervisees may feel a greater confidence in someone who shares the same work-related experiences. Second, the pool of potential supervisors from which the organization may draw is likely to be much larger, and organizing supervision sessions may be easier. One disadvantage of peer supervision arrangements may, however, be that no-one has the final responsibility to act on poor practice or ensure that supervision actually takes place. Whereas individual supervisees may avoid supervision sessions, they may equally be prevented from attending by managers struggling to cope with work pressures. Equally, peers may lack the expertise necessary to provide each other with effective supervision: they may, for example, avoid confrontation or be unable to offer appropriate support.

Supervision may also be provided in groups, either with a group of trainees or junior practitioners receiving supervision from a group leader, or through a group of peers meeting to share problems and provide each other with mutual support. Supervision groups offer some advantages over individual supervisory structures. They provide the opportunity for members to hear a variety of differing views on problems and also to learn from the differing strategies that other members might adopt. Supervision groups are also economical in terms of both time and resources, and may offer organizations an effective alternative to implementing individual supervision. The numbers involved in a supervision group can, however, also lead to their possessing some drawbacks as there may not be enough time to address all the group members' problems, and it is easy for individuals to 'hide'. Similarly, all groups develop a life of their own, and the group dynamics may distract members from carrying out the task of supervision.

Whatever structure is adopted, supervision contracts form an important element in ensuring successful supervision. Contracts have value for both supervisees and supervisors in specifying the frequency of meetings, what will be discussed, what will be recorded and the limits of confidentiality. Contracts may also be of value to organizations in demonstrating their commitment to supervision, and, through specifying the frequency of supervisory sessions, they provide an easily auditable structure for evaluating whether or not supervision actually takes place. For a clear description of the issues considered in drawing up supervision contracts, readers are directed to Bond and Holland (1998).

TRAINING FOR SUPERVISORS AND SUPERVISEES

When asked to take part in supervisory systems, health and social care practitioners will often respond that they already provide and receive supervision. Indeed, much informal support and guidance is shared between colleagues, and Milne (1999), discussing the value of such informal support, suggests that it helps to manage stress and improve effectiveness in the workplace. Participation in structured supervision requires, however, a shift in thinking and behaviour on the part of both supervisees and supervisors. A failure adequately to prepare both parties to take part in formal supervision can lead to problems for both (*see* Brown and Ash 2001).

Supervisees need the opportunity to consider what supervision is, and most will wish to debate how it differs from management systems for monitoring their work. Proctor's model, described above, is a useful way of introducing the tasks and purpose of supervision: a description of its normative function in protecting service users from abuse may, for example, parallel a discussion on the limits of confidentiality in the supervisory relationship. Alongside this, supervisees need the opportunity to consider what they wish to gain from supervision if they are not to find the experience frustrating and sterile. Milne and Gracie (2001) emphasize the importance of the supervisee's role.

For their part, supervisors also need preparation for their role. Supervisors need to be equally clear about what supervision is and what part they play in ensuring that their supervisees are practising ethically and safely. Like their supervisees, they should have the opportunity to consider the distinctions between supervision and managerial monitoring, and these issues raise the potential of contracting as a means of safeguarding both supervisor and supervisee. Supervisors also need to be aware of the distinction between counselling and supervision. Feltham and Dryden (1994) provide a useful overview of the skills that supervisors need to deploy.

CONCLUSION

There is an increasing emphasis on supervision within organizations and the wider systems that regulate people who work with those who have dementia. The Department of Health's report *Making a Difference* (1999) suggests that clinical governance plans within the health service should ensure that nurses are able to participate in clinical supervision. Professional organizations also increasingly champion supervision, the British Association of Counselling (1993) stipulating that practitioners must receive regular supervision as a requirement of membership. There may well come a time when evidence of the receipt of supervision becomes a requirement for registration with professional bodies such as the General Social Care Council.

Implementing supervision in services for people with dementia presents a number of challenges. The increased emphasis on joint or integrated working between the health and social services may promote reviews of organizational supervisory mechanisms and lead to conflict between team managers and members who are used to differing philosophies and styles of supervision. Meaningful supervision for most support workers regrettably remains some way off. Wafer (1998) discusses strategies that care practitioners may use to help to manage the stress inherent in their work, and the fact that he does not mention supervision at all is indicative of the size of the task.

There are clear benefits of supervision for people working with those who have dementia, as well as for the organizations within which they work. Hawkins and Shohet (1989, p. 42) note the support it offers:

> The British miners in the 1920's fought for what was termed 'pit-head time' – the right to wash off the grime of the work in the boss's time, rather than take it home with them. Supervision is the equivalent for those that work at the coal face of disease, distress and fragmentation.

Graham (1998, p. 144), writing about the relationship between teacher and learner within education, borrows ideas from psychotherapy. He suggests that a 'good enough' teacher is essentially 'on the side of' the child but does not always side with him or her. This analogy also provides a useful way of describing the experience of good supervisory relationships that offer individuals support and challenge to carry on what is often difficult and demanding work.

REFERENCES

Barker, P., Jackson, S. and Stevenson, C. 1999: What are psychiatric nurses needed for? Developing a theory of essential nursing practice. *Journal of Psychiatric and Mental Health Nursing* **6:** 273–82.

Bond, M. and Holland, S. 1998: *Skills of clinical supervision for nurses*. Buckingham: Open University Press.

Brandon, D. 1987: *The trick of being ordinary: notes for volunteers and students*. London: MIND.

British Association of Counselling. 1993: *Code of ethics and practice for counsellors*. Rugby: BAC.

British Psychological Society. 1994: *Psychological well-being for users of dementia services*. Division of Clinical Psychology briefing paper no. 2. Leicester: BPS.

Brown, J.F. and Ash, B. 2001: Two heads with different tales: a look at the supervision process. *Clinical Psychology* **2:** 11–13.

Davies, C. 1998: Caregiving, carework and professional care. In: Brechin, A., Walmsley, J., Katz, J. et al. eds. *Care matters: concepts, practice and research in health and social care*. London: Sage, 131.

Department of Health. 1993: *A vision for the future. Report of the Chief Nursing Officer*. London: DoH.

Department of Health. 1999: *Making a difference: strengthening the nursing, midwifery and health visiting contribution to health and healthcare*. London: DoH.

Feltham, C. and Dryden, W. 1994: *Developing counsellor supervision*. London: Sage.

Graham, R. 1998: *Taking each other seriously: experiences in learning and teaching*. Durham: Fieldhouse Press/University of Durham School of Education.

Hawkins, P. and Shohet, R. 1989: *Supervision in the helping professions*. Milton Keynes: Open University Press.

Hughes, B. 1995: *Older people and community care: critical theory and practice*. Buckingham: Open University Press.

Inskipp, F. and Proctor, B. 1988: *Skills for supervising and being supervised*. St Leonards-on-Sea: Alexia Publications.

Kearney, P. 1998: Observing management: the contribution of observation to management in the personal social services. In: Le Riche, P. and Tanner, K. eds. *Observation and its application to social work: rather like breathing*. London: Jessica Kingsley, 169.

Kitwood, T. 1997: *Dementia reconsidered: the person comes first*. Buckingham: Open University Press.

Mattison, J. 1975: *The reflection process in casework supervision*. London: Institute of Marital Studies.

Menzies, I. 1970: *The functioning of social systems as a defense against anxiety: a report on a study of the nursing service of a general hospital*. London: Tavistock Institute of Human Relations.

Milne, D. 1999: *Social therapy: a guide to social support interventions for mental health practitioners*. Chichester: John Wiley & Sons.

Milne, D. and Gracie, J. 2001: The role of the supervisee: 20 ways to facilitate clinical supervision. *Clinical Psychology* **5:** 13–15.

Packer, T. 1999: Attitudes toward dementia care: education and morale in heath-care teams. In: Adams, T. and Clarke, C. eds. *Dementia care: developing partnerships in practice*. London: Baillière Tindall, 329–30.

Slater, R. 1995: *The psychology of growing old: looking forward*. Buckingham: Open University Press.

Stoltenberg, C. and Delworth, U. 1987: *Supervising counsellors and therapists: a developmental approach*. San Francisco: Jossey-Bass.

Taylor, M. 2001: *Homecare: the forgotten service. Report on UNISON's survey of home care workers in the UK*. London: UNISON.

Wafer, M. 1998: Stress in your life and your work. In: Benson, S. ed. *The care assistant's guide to working with people with dementia*. London: Hawker Publications, 166–7.

Chapter 15

Elder abuse and people with dementia

Bridget Penhale

There has, in recent decades, been increasing concern within Western society generally on issues relating to violence and abuse. Following a focus in the UK on child abuse in the 1970s and domestic violence in the 1980s, concern arose in the 1990s about the abuse and neglect of older people. The initial focus of interest was on the domestic or home setting. More recently, however, much needed attention has shifted to situations involving institutional settings (Stanley et al. 1999).

Elder abuse is not a new phenomenon (Stearns 1986), but it has only really been since 1988 that the problem has begun to be properly considered in the UK. Although the phenomenon was initially recognized by English doctors in the mid-1970s, it was not until the late 1980s that the issue was really addressed in the UK. In the USA, however, the problem was identified from the mid-1970s onwards and has been researched since then to try to clarify the issues and provide solutions. Other countries similarly explored the problem during the late 1980s and 90s, although some are only now beginning to consider the issues.

A steady amount of research and material on elder abuse has been accumulating, but we are still at the early stages of identification and the development of responses. It was not, for example, until 1993 that the UK government gave any clear sign that this was a problem in need of attention (Department of Health 1993), although there has since been a consistent approach from successive governments (Department of Health 2000). Abuse in institutions is an area that has been even less researched. Although there has been a lengthy tradition in the UK of scandals in institutional care, these tend to have been investigated and treated as separate inquiries into standards of care rather than as being concerned with abuse.

Elder abuse and neglect are undoubtedly complex and sensitive areas, as is also the case with child abuse and domestic violence against younger women. In addition, there have been difficulties in establishing a sound theoretical base. This is due partly to the lack of agreement concerning definitions and partly to problems in researching and responding to the topic (Ogg and Munn-Giddings 1993; Penhale 1999).

A TABOO TOPIC

Elder abuse is the most recent form of interpersonal violence to have been recognized as a problem in need of attention. It is also, however, an area that has been hidden from public concern and has been regarded as a 'taboo'. Much of the abuse that happens takes place behind closed doors and is not open to public scrutiny (Bennett et al. 1997). Making what happens in private a matter for public concern is not easy, in part because of ageism and ambivalence towards the care of older people. In addition, this is not a pleasant area to focus on, especially as it challenges some of the myths and deeply held beliefs about ageing.

It has not been easy to address this taboo and such beliefs, nor to encourage people to discuss situations, let alone to disclose them. The sexual abuse of older women is, for example, an area that has proved extremely difficult to consider, largely because many people have a problem in terms of conceptualizing older people as sexual beings.

THE IMPORTANCE OF 'NAMING'

Within the context of the hidden nature of the problem, the silencing that has occurred is understandable. Abusive situations that occur in private are not spoken about, and often not even recognized. Abusive situations that occur within institutions may, arguably, be less hidden, but they are equally likely to go unnamed. It is important therefore that, within the process of breaking the taboo, abuse is named. Furthermore, the situation should not be objectified but needs to be personalized in order that individuals' experiences can be addressed.

The power of language is important here. Aitken and Griffin (1996) and Whittaker (1996) have identified a lack of focus on gender in elder abuse through the changes in terminology seen from 1984 to 1994, from 'granny-bashing' to elder abuse (Bennett and Kingston 1993), which masks the gender specificity of abuse. This term also makes no reference to the location in which the abuse takes place. There are a number of different types of setting in which abuse and/or neglect may occur. In addition to the abuse of people in their own homes, or in a relative's home, abuse can occur in a range of institutions, including residential care homes, day care and hospitals. Abusive or neglectful situations may occur in any of these, and practitioners need to be aware of this when working in or visiting such locations.

It is also necessary to consider what is being named and who is involved in the naming so that situations are, if at all possible, recognized and dealt with by the individuals who are involved. The meanings ascribed to situations by individuals, the construction of their understandings about situations and the processes involved are also necessary components of this, although research into this type of area is comparatively rare. The fact that elder abuse was first identified by professionals should be noted here. Unlike the situation regarding violence towards young women, older people are notable by their absence from any discussion or debate concerning abuse and abusive situations unless cast in the role of 'victim', 'abuser' or concerned witness.

DIFFERING FORMS OF ABUSE

Although there is an absence of agreed or standard definitions of abuse (McCreadie 1996), most people agree on the different types of abuse. These are physical abuse, sexual abuse, neglect, financial abuse (referring also to exploitation and misappropriation of an individual's property and possessions), psychological abuse and emotional abuse. To these may be added such categories as enforced isolation and the deprivation of factors necessary for daily living (warmth, food and other items, such as teeth). Abuse within institutions encompasses, in addition to individual acts of abuse, situations that arise because of the regime or system that is operating in the unit. Abusive situations may also exist between a resident and a member of staff, initiated by the older person as protagonist, so there may be dual directionality of abuse or unidirectional abuse from a resident towards a staff member (McCreadie 1996).

As well as different types of abuse and different settings, there may be a range of different participants involved in situations. A change of setting (from home to institution perhaps) does not necessarily mean that pre-existing abuse will completely cease. It may mean that a different type of abuse then occurs or that the nature of the abuse is transformed. In addition, differing responses and interventions to relieve or prevent the differing forms of abuse may be necessary, depending on the type of abuse that is happening as well as the setting in which it is occurring. To adequately protect an older person who has been subjected to financial abuse, for example, it may be necessary to improve the security system in his or her home. Mistreatment that occurs as a result of carer stress may, however, require an approach that is more grounded in strategies involving support and assistance.

CAUSES OF ELDER ABUSE

It appears unlikely that any one factor causes abuse; there is instead more likely to be an interaction between a number of different factors. Abuse occurs for a multitude of reasons. Among the possible factors identified in the development of abuse are:

- A history of longstanding poor relationships within the family (Fulmer and O'Malley 1987; Homer and Gilleard 1990)
- The dependency of the abuser on the victim for finance (Hwalek et al. 1986), accommodation and transport (Pillemer 1986) or emotional support
- A history of mental health problems or a substance misuse problem in the abuser (Pillemer and Wolf 1986)
- A pre-existing pattern of family violence (the intergenerational transmission of violence) (Pillemer and Suitor 1988)
- The social isolation of the victim and the abuser (Pillemer and Wolf 1986).

In addition, several risk factors have been identified. These include such aspects as the presence of other stressors within the family system (e.g., unemployment, finance and overcrowding), the inability of a carer to look after the older person and inadequate support systems.

The development of conceptual frameworks related to the possible causes of family violence has so far covered a number of distinct theories drawn from the disciplines of psychology, sociology and feminism. Common themes that appear in all forms of family violence, despite differing degrees, include gender relations, power, stress, isolation and diminished resources (emotional or physical) with which to counter such difficulties.

The applicability of such areas to elder abuse and neglect has, however, not yet been fully established. More work is needed before we can be certain of the causes of different forms of family violence. Following this outline of some general aspects of elder abuse, we will now look specifically at elder abuse in relation to dementia.

DEMENTIA AND ELDER ABUSE

The first area to consider is older people with dementia. Early research on abuse suggested that the dependence of the victim was a key risk factor so we need to consider whether people with dementia and associated mental health problems are more likely than others to be the victims of elder abuse. Given the previous comments made about the general lack of research into elder abuse, it is no surprise to find that there has been limited research in this area (Manthorpe 1995) and as yet no definite answers.

There are, in the recent literature, a number of examples of elder abuse that include dementia as a component factor (Homer and Gilleard 1990; Department of Health 1992; Grafstrom et al. 1992). Few studies have, however, specifically examined the prevalence of abuse of individuals with dementia by their care-givers, although the small number that have generally identify a high rate of abuse. Two UK articles have suggested that the rate of abuse among older people with dementia is higher than would be expected looking at the overall population of people aged over 65 years (Wilson 1994; Cooney and Howard 1995).

The first study considered the level of elder abuse among older people using a psychogeriatric service and living in the community. It took the form of a survey of the perceptions of the different professional staff of the service. The research considered not just dementia but various mental health conditions, although limited information was given concerning the diagnoses of either cognitive impairments or mental health conditions. The cases were those already known to the staff involved and reported by them in the study. The findings are thus of limited relevance in this context, albeit suggestive that the rate of elder abuse is higher for clients of this type of service than for other older people (Wilson 1994).

The second article reviewed existing knowledge (at that point) concerning elder abuse and dementia (Cooney and Howard 1995). One of the studies described had been undertaken by an American group who sent out questionnaires to carers who had contacted a free dementia helpline (Coyne et al. 1993). Of the one third of carers who responded, a third (33.1%) stated that they had been physically abused by the relative with dementia, whereas 12% indicated that they had physically abused the person they cared for. This included a number of different acts such as biting, kicking and hitting.

The researchers proposed a strong association between the high physical and psychological demands often experienced by the care-givers of individuals with dementia and physical abuse. Those carers who reported abusive behaviour had been caring for longer overall and were in addition caring for longer periods during the day than those carers who did not report abuse. Within this study, there also seemed to be a relationship between those care-givers who had been abusive and those who had themselves been the subject of abuse. Slightly over one quarter of those carers who reported being abused (26%) stated that they had been abusive to their relative. In contrast, only 4.8% who had not been abused reported that they had acted abusively (Coyne et al. 1993). It is possible that aggressive or violent behaviour by the 'patient' might provoke a similar response on the part of the carer, the abuse being in effect mutual and bidirectional in certain situations.

This finding relates to earlier UK research (Levin et al. 1989) that, although not specifically considering elder abuse, looked at the situation of families caring for 'confused older people'. One of the key findings was the high risk to carers of both verbal and physical abuse by the recipient of care (Levin et al. 1989). This was echoed in a later Australian study, which asked a group of female carers of people with dementia about physical and verbal abuse and sexual violence perpetrated by the care recipient (Cahill and Shapiro 1993).

Similarly, a later American study by Pillemer and Suitor, concerning the care-givers of people with Alzheimer's disease, reported that those carers who were caring for relatives who were on occasion violent were themselves fearful of becoming violent and sometimes had aggressive feelings. Although this fear did not differ significantly between groups of married and unmarried care-givers, spouses were much more likely than other care-givers to report being both violent themselves in response to violence by the care recipient and acting on their aggressive feelings (Pillemer and Suitor 1992).

Within this study, violence also appeared to be related to disruptive behaviour on the part of the care recipient and to the care-giver and the care-receiver living together (co-residence). Care-giver distress related to people with dementia appears to be greatest when the two parties live together, perhaps because the proximity makes any stressors, tensions and conflicts more difficult to avoid (Long 1981; George and Gwyther 1986). In addition, both a higher level of stress and more frequent, perhaps unavoidable, contact seemed, in the Pillemer and Suitor study, to contribute to the positive relationship between co-residence and care-giver fear of becoming violent.

There have been a number of other studies investigating the possible links between dementia and elder abuse, some of which are relevant here. Australian research by Kurrle et al. (1992) determined that, within the sample of abused individuals, 46 per cent of those abused had a significant dementing illness, whereas approximately 65 per cent had major disabilities. A further Australian study reported on 54 cases of abuse and 100 people with dementia who had not been abused, all of the whom were the clients of a particular rehabilitation and aged care service (Sadler et al. 1995). This appeared to confirm the existence of a strong linkage between dementia and elder abuse.

When dementia was present with other pre-disposing factors, such as substance abuse or psychiatric illness on the part of the carer, or pre-existing family conflict, there was a significant risk of abuse. The mere presence of dementia, even with the existence of disturbed and aggressive behaviour on the part of the person with dementia, did not appear to result in a higher risk of either psychological or physical abuse for the person with dementia. Carers did, however, appear to be at risk of physical and/or psychological abuse (Sadler et al. 1995).

Pritchard's study of older women and men in three areas of the UK indicated that almost one third of individuals who had experienced abuse had problems relating to dementia and memory loss. A smaller number (just under 10 per cent) had other identified mental health problems (Pritchard 2000, 2001).

Homer and Gilleard, in their UK study of a population receiving regular respite care from a geriatric service, found that 45 per cent of carers reported that they had abused their relative, 14 per cent of this group admitting to physical abuse (Homer and Gilleard 1990). Of the older people receiving the service, around two fifths had been diagnosed with dementia. This study found no particular association between a diagnosis of dementia or the degree of impairment and abuse. This appears to be consistent with other research findings from the field of elder abuse indicating that the characteristics of the abusers are more relevant than those of the 'victim' (Pillemer and Wolf 1986).

The study found that violence (or a threat of violence) on the part of the person with dementia seemed to lead to a violent response by the care-giver (Homer and Gilleard 1990). The authors suggested that it was disturbed and disruptive behaviour by the care recipient, rather than simply the presence of a cognitive impairment such as dementia, that was likely to result in abuse by the care-giver.

The finding that those carers who reported being physically abusive to the person they cared for were more likely to report abuse (of themselves) by that person was duplicated in the American (Coyne et al. 1993) and Australian (Sadler et al. 1995) studies already mentioned. This suggests a degree of consistency despite cultural variability and the differing populations studied. One interpretation is that the presence of abusive or aggressive behaviour by the impaired person is a risk factor for the development and perpetuation of abusive situations. Further research would help to determine whether this finding holds for other cultures (e.g., developing countries or the Far East) and whether there are any other significant variables that need to be taken into account.

A further UK study, using an anonymous questionnaire, asked the carers of people with dementia about the possible occurrence of physical and verbal abuse and neglect of those they were caring for (Cooney and Mortimer 1995). Although there was a relatively low overall response rate (33.5 per cent), 55 per cent of those who replied admitted to at least one type of abuse, verbal abuse being the most common. Verbal abuse appeared to be linked to the degree of social isolation of the carer and to an existing poor relationship; it also appeared to be a risk factor for physical abuse. Those carers who had been caring for longer appeared to be most at most risk of abusing the person cared for. Other variables, such as satisfaction with services provided and the amount of both informal and formal support, did not appear to be related to abuse (Cooney and Mortimer 1995).

There seemed to be some evidence supporting reciprocity of abuse. Carers who admitted to either physical or verbal abuse were also more likely to report concurrent problematic abusive behaviour on the part of the care recipient. Caution should be exercised in relation to this latter finding as the response rate was low and the sample therefore small. In addition, the reports by carers were not substantiated in any objective sense. Such 'patient' variables as degrees of physical dependency or behaviour and mood disorder did not appear to be of significance as no difference was found between individuals who had been abused and those who had not. This suggests some discrepancy between carers' perceptions and the actual behaviour of the individual, a limitation of which the researchers were aware (Cooney and Mortimer 1995).

DEMENTIA CARE

There is a wealth of information, collated over the past two decades, concerning the stressful effects of care-giving, particularly in relation to dementia. Schulz et al. (1995) have provided a useful review of the psychiatric and physical effects of care-giving in situations of dementia, albeit not specifically concerning elder abuse. What is not, however, clear is the exact nature of the relationship between care-giving and stress, let alone that between stress, care-giving and abuse. Notwithstanding perceptions that much elder abuse is caused by the stress of caring, it is clear that there are many cared-for older people who are not abused even when the care-giving experience is stressful. We clearly need to develop an explanation that focuses on the differences between abusive and non-abusive situations.

Coupled with this, there needs to be a disaggregation of the apparent linkage between caring, stress and abuse. Practitioners may over-readily identify with those who abuse and consider such individuals as victims in their own right (*see also* Phillipson and Biggs 1995). Although this might, as an all-inclusive response by the caring professions, be an appropriate response to some situations, it is less than helpful. If the aetiology of abuse examines the nature of power within the dynamic of abusive relationships, such a simplistic approach is much less likely. Abusive situations might then be dealt with more effectively, although nonetheless sensitively.

Second, there has been a tendency to equate stress with a high level of physical dependency. This has resulted in a failure properly to examine the possible importance of factors such as psychological and emotional dependency (Nolan 1993). This also links to two further facts: that not all care-givers within situations of high physical dependence report a high level of stress (Nolan 1993), and that not all people who are very dependent physically are abused or neglected, as would be expected if there were a straightforward causal relationship.

Third, research by Steinmetz suggests that it is the care-giver's perception of the situation as stressful, rather than actual level of stress itself, that appears to correlate with the existence of an abusive situation (Steinmetz 1990). If situations that do not objectively appear likely to produce a high level of stress are perceived by the care-giver as stressful, a high level of stress is likely to be experienced. Abusive situations may then develop or continue. Although stress may indeed contribute to the development and continuation of abuse, it appears insufficient, in isolation, to provide a satisfactory explanation of the majority of situations of elder abuse and neglect.

Early research in elder abuse set out to determine the 'typical characteristics' of victims of abuse, resulting in some unfortunate stereotypes (Lau and Kosberg 1979; Penhale 1992). Subsequent research has focused on establishing the profiles of those who abuse. Although similar suggestions may be made concerning stereotypes, such research has been valuable because it has produced useful information about the psychopathology of a reasonable proportion of those individuals who abuse. Furthermore, it has indicated that there are likely to be a number of individuals who take on a caring role but are wholly unsuited to such a task – who are practically, psychologically, emotionally or physically unsuited to caring. People undoubtedly take on such roles for a variety of reasons, some willingly, others not.

For those with existing or previous mental health or emotional problems, or personality or relationship difficulties, the tasks associated with caring may prove too exacting. A deterioration in their own health or that of the person cared for, or additional factors complicating the situation, may lead to the development (or continuation) of an abusive relationship. A reduction in the overall availability and amount of welfare provision to assist these situations will obviously not help in the resolution of such problems.

As seen earlier, it is possible that difficult, provocative, even aggressive behaviour from the care-recipient may contribute to the development or continuation of abusive reactions on the part of the care-giver. Similar mechanisms could be present whether the care-recipient has a severe mental illness or a severe learning disability, or is significantly cognitively impaired as a result of dementia. In addition, given the possibility of aggressive or violent behaviour, it is clearly possible that a mutually abusive relationship may exist or develop within such situations. The findings of Sadler et al. (1995) suggest that other predisposing factors, such as a history of family conflict, or psychopathology on the part of the abuser, may be more likely to be of central importance in the development of abuse. Such discrepancies in the findings of different studies in part amplify some of the complexities of the field. They also indicate that no one factor provides an adequate explanation but that in many situations a number of interrelated factors can exist at the same time.

MANAGEMENT OF ABUSIVE SITUATIONS

Several non-governmental organizations have been involved in trying to raise awareness of abuse. In addition to the principal charity, Action on Elder Abuse, established in 1993, the organization Counsel and Care has been actively concerned with issues of abuse, restraint and risk-taking (see, e.g., Counsel and Care 1997, 2001, 1993). The Alzheimer's Society has also produced position statements on abuse and possible approaches to abuse prevention, such as improved service provision for carers and better systems of supervision and monitoring for care workers (Alzheimer's Society 1998).

In the UK, statutory organizations have begun to develop interventions for abusive situations, many focusing on the provision of practical support and assistance (Department of Health 1993). Respite care provision, alternative accommodation on a temporary or permanent basis, counselling for individuals or the family as a whole, or even legal remedies to resolve situations may be developed and used. The separation of individuals is generally considered to be a last resort (Department of Health 1992); when it does occur, it often entails the older person entering some form of institutional care (Bennett et al. 1997). The development of appropriate strategies should include a range of interventions with those who abuse, such as treatment for substance abuse and techniques to enhance anger management (Penhale 1993).

The assessment process should be holistic and needs led, in line with the processes of assessment and care management (Department of Health 1993). If necessary, it may also need to be abuse focused (Bennett et al. 1997). Assessment protocols to determine the extent of risk within situations are useful in this context; a number of these are now available, although have mainly been developed in America (Quinn and Tomita 1986; Breckman and Adelman 1988).

Assessment processes may vary between practitioners but should encompass a multidisciplinary approach (Department of Health 2000). As with child protection systems, skilled and qualified practitioners should undertake the most complex and difficult work. Within the assessment, there should be a full consideration of the abusive situation, including antecedents, consequences and possible future patterns. The individual's methods of dealing with the situation, including any ineffective coping strategies, also need to be taken into account. In addition, the views, beliefs and attitudes of key players in the situation on the nature and probable outcomes of the situation should be determined. A separate assessment for the abuser may be required as part of this phase. A consideration of whether it is possible to effect lasting change within the particular setting is also necessary.

Safety-planning for those individuals who require protection is an essential next step. A full assessment of the risks and level of danger involved and what might constitute adequate management of the risk(s) to the individual and others involved should also be incorporated into the process. Appropriate levels of risk management, including regular monitoring and a reassessment or review of risk, must be maintained once the degree of risk has been identified.

A focus on the needs of the individual for protection within the assessment process and subsequent care-planning stage should emphasize individual empowerment. The focus must be on the individuals, the abusive situation (or allegation) and the contributory factors and circumstances, training increasingly concentrating on such areas to assist with the development of assessment and intervention skills. Many areas are, for example, developing multiagency training initiatives, which move beyond raising awareness and include the development of those skills necessary in this type of work.

Intervention strategies can be directed at the whole family or focused on individual members (abusing or abused), and any action taken should depend on the views, wishes and needs of the individuals. If necessary, this should include a consideration of the needs of those who are cognitively impaired, the degree of impairment and their decision-making capacity.

In order to target interventions appropriately, it is necessary to try to identify the primary or main cause of the abuse. If, for example, the abuse is caused by the stress of care-giving, the provision of domiciliary services may be appropriate in order to support, alleviate and monitor the situation. If, however, the abuse results from some psychopathology of the abuser, treatment of the abuser, for example for a substance misuse problem, is more appropriate. This would be in addition to protecting the older person. The willingness of individuals to engage in interventions is important here. A successful negotiation of the boundary between the private and public worlds can be of significance in determining the outcome of interventions. Outcomes are much more likely to be successful if an individual is willing to undertake treatment for a problem.

Policies and procedures for practitioners are an essential first step in responding to the problem. In the year 2000, the government issued a guidance document, *No Secrets* (Department of Health 2000), which mandated social service departments to take the lead in co-ordinating the response to adult abuse at local level. Each social services department has to link with appropriate local agencies in order to develop multiagency policies, procedures and guidelines.

Procedures do not generally contain details of which intervention strategies to use in any given situation, the aim usually being to clarify the expectations and responsibilities of staff in the initial stages of receiving a referral and assessing or investigating a situation. The subsequent process concerning the outcome of the assessment and formulation of the care plan may also be itemized. Details of procedures concerning strategy meetings, case conferences, 'at-risk registers' and reviews are also likely to be found, together with statements concerning equal opportunities, and support for staff. Guidance documents may be developed to accompany the procedures. These aim to explain certain areas for staff, for example identifying different types of abuse and degrees of severity. Additional information and assistance for those using the procedure are also provided. Every social services department has to have in place local policies and procedures in relation to adult abuse and should be working to these with other agencies.

There are several further developments that will undoubtedly have an effect on this area. These include the establishment of the Commission for Social Care Inspection, which is charged with protective functions, relating especially to institutional settings. In addition, the implementation of relevant sections of the Care Standards Act 2000, particularly those concerning the employment of individuals who may pose a threat to the safety of children or vulnerable adults, is likely to have an increasing effect.

ISSUES RAISED

Three main areas arise with respect to protecting people with dementia from abuse. First, it can be difficult to recognize or identify situations of abuse, especially if individuals are isolated or have significant communication difficulties. Practitioners may have low or unclear expectations and may not be certain about what constitutes abuse or neglect, or what could be done about a situation. This may mean that situations are either not detected or not acted on quickly enough.

Second, in developing a response to such situations, issues of autonomy and self-determination often play a large part. If individuals lack mental capacity, some form of protection may be required. Issues of consent by individuals to particular forms of intervention are likely to be important here, and it may help to enlist the assistance of mental health professionals such as psychiatrists skilled in assessing capacity in relation to such issues. Third, the use of legal interventions, such the Theft Act 1936, in this sphere can be a sensitive and rather complex matter, perhaps because of issues of capacity and consent. It is necessary to consider carefully the extent of any harm that has resulted from the situation of abuse or neglect. In relation to an individual who lacks decision-making capacity, issues of autonomy and who takes a key role in decision-making are likely to be central.

The final point relates more generally to interventions and responses in situations of abuse. There are, increasingly, resource constraints and hard choices to be made relating to service provision and what is likely to be effective in certain situations. It is important to be realistic about the intervention used, and for this to be used with the agreement (if not full participation) of service users, their families and their carers. There may be a need to distinguish between practical and emotional forms of assistance, and if choices have to be made between different types of intervention, it may not be possible to tailor responses exactly to need. This may be particularly apparent if there are a number of individuals who have been involved in the abusive or neglectful situation, in which the provision of appropriate remedies for all concerned may not actually be possible.

CONCLUSION

As seen within this chapter, there is no evidence that dementia necessarily results in elder abuse, but it is clearly an important factor in the development and perpetuation of a number of abusive situations. As is the case with other aspects of elder abuse and neglect, research in this area is limited. A number of studies rely on reports by carers, or professionals, and discuss limited types of abuse or somewhat non-specific mental health difficulties. There are others that are not methodologically sound. As a body, such studies can hardly be considered to be conclusive. They do, however, present findings that need to be followed up by additional research in an attempt to establish their validity.

Although the exact nature of the links between dementia and abuse and the degree of importance of dementia are unclear, it appears that people with dementia who become aggressive or violent may be at increased risk of abuse, possibly within the context of an abusive relationship. The risk of abuse for individuals with dementia appears to be particularly high in the presence of other predisposing factors. A history of problematic relationship(s), substance misuse or psychiatric illness on the part of the carer, and increased vulnerability of the individual, seem to be important here. The evidence that those individuals who abuse are more likely to have substance abuse or mental health problems, including personality disorders, is currently somewhat more convincing.

We do not yet know enough about elder abuse and neglect. More needs to be done to improve the recognition of such situations and some of the causes, and further research will surely assist here. For practitioners dealing with such situations, professional and personal standards need to be acknowledged, explored and developed. Work needs to continue to establish effective systems of public accountability, including the development of clear lines of support for individuals and clear expectations of what is required. In developing care plans with the individual and other parties, practitioners need to consider the nature and extent of any cognitive impairment. In addition, they must bear in mind aspects relating to any planning for safety or protection. This will also include determining the benefits and costs, financial and otherwise, of particular interventions to ameliorate situations.

Interventions need to be appropriate and, as far as possible, sensitively tailored to meet the needs of the individuals involved. Practitioners must work to local policies and procedures, and ensure that they keep abreast of recent developments in the field. Education and training must be provided in order to increase awareness and knowledge of the problem. This will then form the framework within which appropriate responses can be developed. To act as the springboard for this, we need more research to improve our knowledge and understanding of abuse, neglect and, crucially, the extent of the linkage of these to dementia. Much work in this area is needed in order to address this most pervasive of problems. The evident commitment to achieving this is not questioned, but energy is now needed to translate this commitment into action.

REFERENCES

Aitken, L. and Griffin, G. 1996: *Gender and elder abuse*. London: Sage.

Alzheimer's Society. 1998: *Mistreatment of people with dementia and their carers*. London: Alzheimer's Society.

Bennett, G.C. and Kingston, P.A. 1993: *Elder abuse: theories, concepts and interventions*. London: Chapman & Hall.

Bennett, G.C., Kingston, P.A. and Penhale, B. 1997: *The dimensions of elder abuse: perspectives for practitioners*. Basingstoke: Macmillan.

Breckman, R.S. and Adelman, R.D. 1988: *Strategies for helping victims of elder mistreatment*. Newbury Park, California: Sage.

Cahill, S. and Shapiro, M. 1993: 'I think he might have hit me once': aggression towards caregivers in dementia. *Australian Journal on Ageing* **12:** 10–15.

Cooney, C. and Howard, R. 1995: Abuse of patients with dementia by their carers: out of sight but not out of mind. *International Journal of Geriatric Psychiatry* **10:** 735–41.

Cooney, C. and Mortimer, A. 1995: Elder abuse and dementia. *International Journal of Social Psychiatry* **41:** 276–83.

Counsel and Care. 1993: *The right to take risks*. London: Counsel and Care.

Counsel and Care. 1997: *In harm's way*. London: Counsel and Care.

Counsel and Care. 2001: *Residents taking risks*. London: Counsel and Care.

Coyne, A., Reichman, W.E. and Berbig, L. 1993: The relationship between dementia and elder abuse. *American Journal of Psychiatry* **150:** 643–6.

Department of Health. 1992: *Confronting elder abuse*. London: DoH.

Department of Health. 1993: *No longer afraid: The safeguard of older people in the domestic setting*. London: HMSO.

Department of Health. 2000: *No secrets: the protection of vulnerable adults – guidance on the development and implementation of multi-agency policies and procedures*. London: HMSO.

Fulmer, T. and O'Malley, T. 1987: Inadequate care of the elderly: a health care perspective on abuse and neglect. New York: Springer.

George, L.K. and Gwyther, L.P. 1986: Caregiver well-being: a multi-dimensional examination of family caregivers of demented adults. *Gerontologist* **26:** 253–9.

Grafstrom, M., Norberg, A. and Wimblad, B. 1992: Abuse is in the eye of the beholder. Reports by family members about abuse of demented persons in home care. A total population-based study. *Scandinavian Journal of Social Medicine* **21:** 247–55.

Homer, A. and Gilleard, C. 1990: Abuse of elderly people by their carers. *British Medical Journal* **301:** 1359–62.

Hwalek, M., Sengstock, M. and Lawrence, R. 1986: Assessing the probability of abuse of the elderly. *Journal of Applied Gerontology* **5:** 153–73.

Kurrle, S.E., Sadler, P.M. and Cameron, I.D. 1992: Patterns of elder abuse. *Medical Journal of Australia* **157:** 673–6.

Lau, E.E. and Kosberg, J.I. 1979: Abuse of the elderly by informal care providers. *Aging* **299:** 10–15.

Levin, E., Sinclair, I. and Gorbach, P. 1989: *Families, services and confusion in old age*. Aldershot: Avebury.

Long, C. 1981: Geriatric abuse. *Issues in Mental Health Nursing* **3:** 123–35.

McCreadie, C. 1996: *Elder abuse: an update on research*. London: HMSO.

Manthorpe, J. 1995: Elder abuse and dementia. *Journal of Dementia Care* Nov/Dec: 27–9.

Nolan, M. 1993: Carer-dependent relationships and the prevention of elder abuse. In: Decalmer, P. and Glendenning, F. eds. *The mistreatment of older people*. London: Sage: 148–58.

Ogg, J. and Munn-Giddings, C. 1993: Researching elder abuse. *Ageing and Society* **13:** 389–414.

Penhale, B. 1992: Elder abuse: an overview. *Elders* **1:** 36–48.

Penhale, B. 1993: The abuse of elderly people: considerations for practice. *British Journal of Social Work* **23:** 95–112.

Penhale, B. 1999: Research on elder abuse: lessons for practice. In: Slater, P. and Eastman, M. eds. *Elder abuse: critical issues in policy and practice*. London: Age Concern, 1–23.

Phillipson, C. and Biggs, S. 1995: Elder abuse: a critical overview. In: Kingston, P.A. and Penhale, B. eds. *Family violence and the caring professions*. Basingstoke: Macmillan, 181–203.

Pillemer, K.A. 1986: Risk factors in elder abuse: results from a case-control study. In: Pillemer, K.A. and Wolf, R.S. eds. *Elder abuse: conflict in the family*. Dover, Massachusetts: Auburn House, 239–63.

Pillemer, K.A. and Suitor, J. 1988: Elder abuse. In: Van Hasselt, V, Morrison, R, Belack, A. and Hensen, M. eds. *Handbook of family violence*. New York: Plenum Press, 247–70.

Pillemer, K.A. and Suitor, J. 1992: Violence and violent feelings: what causes them among family caregivers? *Journal of Gerontology* **47:** S165–S172.

Pillemer, K.A. and Wolf, R.S. eds. 1986: *Elder abuse: conflict in the family*. Dover, Massachusetts: Auburn House.

Pritchard, J. 2000: *The needs of older women: services for victims of elder abuse and other abuse*. Bristol: Policy Press.

Pritchard, J. 2001: *Male victims of elder abuse: their experiences and needs*. London: Jessica Kingsley.

Quinn, M. and Tomita, S. 1986: *Elder abuse and neglect: causes, diagnoses and intervention strategies*. New York: Springer.

Sadler, P., Kurrle, S. and Cameron, I. 1995: Dementia and elder abuse. *Australian Journal on Ageing* **14:** 36–40.

Schulz, R, O'Brien, A.T, Bookwala, J. and Fleissner, K. 1995: Psychiatric and physical morbidity effects of dementia caregiving: prevalence, correlates and causes. *Gerontologist* **35:** 771–91.

Stanley, N.; Manthorpe, J. and Penhale, B. eds. 1999: *Institutional abuse: perspectives across the lifecourse*. London: Routledge.

Stearns, P. 1986: Old age family conflict: the perspective of the past. In: Pillemer, K.A. and Wolf, R.S. eds. *Elder abuse: conflict in the family*. Dover: Auburn House, 3–24.

Steinmetz, S.K. 1990: Elder abuse: myth and reality. In: Brubaker, T.H. ed. *Family relationships in later life*, 2nd edn. Newbury Park, California: Sage, 193–211.

Whittaker, T. 1996: Elder abuse. In: Fawcett, B., Featherstone, B., Hearn, J. and Toft, C. eds. *Violence and gender relations: theories and interventions*. London: Sage, 147–60.

Wilson, G. 1994: Abuse of elderly men and women among clients of a community psychogeriatric service. *British Journal of Social Work* **24:** 681–700.

Chapter 16

Maintaining quality in dementia care practice

Dawn Brooker

This chapter focuses on the impact of quality of care as experienced by the most vulnerable group of people with dementia, those living in long-term care. Improving service quality at a macro-organizational level requires a clear understanding of what matters to people with dementia at a micro, day-to-day level. This chapter explores the latter rather than the former. For a more general discussion of quality assurance for people with dementia at an organizational level, the reader is directed to Cox (2001).

The quality of care for people with dementia in long-term care is often appalling (Marshall 2001; MacDonald and Dening 2002), but this is rarely discussed other than by those who are directly affected. Complaints about the quality of care are, for complex and multifactorial reasons, rarely made. Those who are receiving services are generally too damaged and demoralized to complain, and their relatives are too browbeaten and scared to do so. Those who are fit and well usually find the spectre of dementia too distressing and would rather focus their energy elsewhere. And those responsible for funding services and working within a cash-restricted budget usually dare not look too closely for fear of the cost of putting the situation right.

Scandals occasionally hit the media, but they usually focus on issues of physical abuse or malnourishment, episodes that are dreadful but not commonplace. Instead, most poor-quality care and neglect is psychological rather than physical. It includes incomplete assessments, no-one contacting you when they promised to, feeling deceived, the withholding of information, the overprescribing of drugs that you don't need and the underprescribing of ones that you do (Ballard and O'Brien 1999). Lack of privacy, indignity, insensitivity, disrespect, stigmatization, disempowerment and disengagement are all very familiar features to service users and carers, particularly in long-term care (Ballard et al 2001; Innes and Surr 2001). The erosion of human and legal rights, and the overwhelming feeling that nothing personal is sacred, is still the day-to-day experience of people with dementia and their families.

Set within an inherently ageist and 'hypercognitive' society (Post 1995), the collusion of silence continues. Society places a high value on youth and intellectual capacity. Those who are elderly, particularly those with slowing mental powers, are at risk of prejudice. Services for people with dementia exist within society, and the individuals providing these services are subject to the same prejudice as the rest of society. The lack of human value attributed to those who are elderly, particularly those with failing mental powers, is evident in service provision, resource allocation, media coverage, policy priorities, professional training and status.

MY JOURNEY

I have, throughout my professional career, been interested in quality of care and how it affects people with dementia and older people generally. As a newly qualified clinical psychologist in the early 1980s working in the UK National Health Service (NHS), I was struck by the enormous impact that the social environment had upon patients' psychological state. This often outweighed the impact of the mental health problem that the individual had been referred for in the first place. The social environment on wards and in nursing homes heightened confusion, anxiety and depression rather than ameliorating them. As a psychologist seeing individual patients for therapy, I found myself listening to a whole range of stories that I found difficult to work with in a therapeutic frame. The behaviour of staff, as described by the patients, was neglectful of people's feelings and showed a huge lack of understanding for people's emotional needs and vulnerabilities. This was in contrast to what I knew of the staff groups on a personal level. By and large, I experienced the people I worked with as warm, gregarious, caring and terrifically hard-working – their behaviour and attitudes seemed at odds with patients' reports.

In the mid-1980s, I became involved in staff training and in observing patient levels of engagement. My early observational work had the impact of confirming what patients had told me and what research studies (Bond and Bond 1990; Bowie and Mountain 1993) were beginning to show. There was very little social interaction of any kind going on in these institutions. I wrote a paper, 'Looking at them, looking at me' (Brooker 1995), which reviewed the methods for observing the quality of care for people with dementia, for whom the only stimulating thing going on in the care environment was often the observer sitting in the corner of the day room with a clip board. Through staff training and various other changes in organizational and management practice, those we cared for generally became more interactive with the world outside themselves, and feedback from staff and service users improved to a more acceptable level (Brooker 1994). I still struggled however to articulate the underlying reasons for the poor quality of interpersonal care that I saw time and time again for people with dementia in institutional settings.

MALIGNANT SOCIAL PSYCHOLOGY

Kitwood's ideas (1990, 1993,1997) on malignant social psychology and the importance of the interpersonal process in dementia care (*see* Box 1.1 on page 10) completely tied in with my experience. Kitwood's premise was that these devaluing interpersonal interactions are commonplace in many care environments and undermine the personhood of those with dementia. Care staff and professionals do not usually do such things with malicious intent; instead, episodes of malignant social psychology have become an unchallenged and interwoven part of care culture. Malignant social psychology is society's response to people with dementia and, because of lack of training, it can also become the professional caring response (see Box 1.1).

Within formal care environments, there appears to be a link between the level of cognitive decline and the level of malignant social psychology. Developing earlier ideas of the Inverse Care Law, Bruce et al. (2002) observed that the most dependent people with dementia are the ones who spend least time in contact with staff. Staff tend to spend most time with those in their care who are least dependent (Brooker et al. 1998; Barnett 2000). This is also apparent in terms of the level of qualification of professional staff and their focus within dementia care: those with the greatest dependency needs are usually cared for by the least-qualified, lowest-status members of the various professional groups.

Figure 16.1 illustrates the direct relationship between general ageism and hypercognitivism in society and the expression of malignant social psychology in care environments. If ageism and hypercognitivism are left unchecked, malignant social psychology becomes manifest within care settings. At its worst, this leads to a radical depersonalization of people with dementia and reconfirms to wider society its belief that these people are less than human. An environment in which personhood is attacked at this level cannot be said to be providing good-quality care.

PROCESSES NECESSARY FOR THE MAINTENANCE OF PERSONHOOD AND QUALITY OF CARE

Given all this, it is surprising that are many care situations in which malignant social psychology has not taken root. A number of influences, detailed in Figure

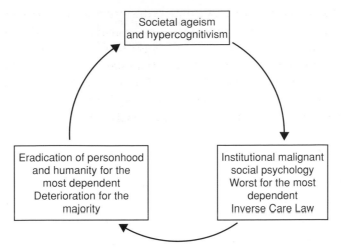

Figure 16.1 Malignant social psychology as a manifestation of ageism and hyper-cognitivism in care settings

16.2 and written about in earlier chapters, might work together to protect against this. Figure 16.2 shows a number of mediating factors that a partial evidence base suggests mediate against the worse ravages of malignant social psychology. It is not known which of these is the most important and whether it is possible to identify the absolute minimum standards in this arena, but all these processes have been postulated as being important in producing a better quality of life for people with dementia.

Experience suggests that these processes are quite fragile against the push of ageism and its manifestation in malignant social psychology. Care practice in dementia care is littered with the smoking shadows of 'hero-innovators' who took on the great dragon of institutionalization and were badly burnt (Georgiades and Phillimore 1975; Packer 2001).

PERSPECTIVES ON QUALITY IN DEMENTIA SERVICES

Coming up with a definition of quality of care for people with dementia is a challenge, not least because there are conflicting agendas on what should take priority. Policy-makers and politicians have to see the big picture. They have to categorize, generalize and make financial plans. People with dementia pose a problem for policy-makers because they comprise such a disparate and heterogeneous group in society. They are treated in policy terms as if they are a neat subsection of that even more heterogeneous group, 'the elderly'.

The service management perspective will often see working within a cash-restricted budget as the defining factor – much time will be devoted to calculating exactly which standards set out by policy-makers can be met within budget. Staff

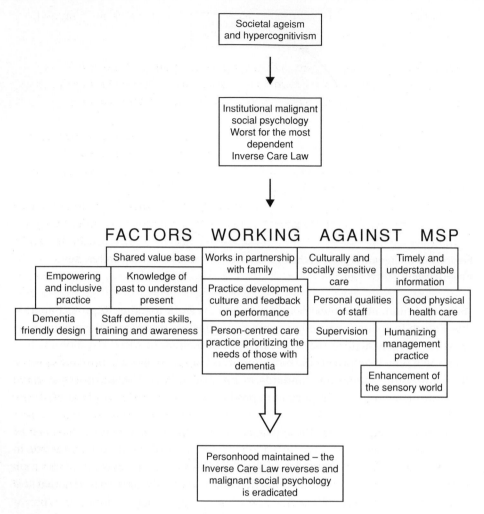

Figure 16.2 Protection from malignant social psychology

views on quality will relate to job satisfaction and supportive working environments, whereas families will often see safety and comfort as the key determinants of quality care. It is perhaps worth noting that many policy-makers will also have a dual role as family carer. They may also have had a previous role as a service manager or care practitioner. They will never have been a person with dementia.

So what about the perspective of people with dementia? What determines a good quality of life for a person with this condition? Kane (2001) proposes a move towards a more consumer-centred emphasis on quality of life. She argues that, in long-term care in the USA, and embedded in most rules and regulations governing care provision, is the assumption that:

> long-term care should aspire to the best possible quality of life *as it is consistent with health and safety*. But ordinary people may prefer the best health and safety outcomes possible *that are consistent with a meaningful quality of life*.

Most of us decide upon our lifestyle and pay attention to safety as part of that rather than defining our lifestyle by its safeness. If the focus were on quality of life rather than quality of care, on outcome rather than process, the lived experience of dementia might become less feared.

The most useful definition of quality may be that it is what the customer says it is. If the 'customers' in this context are those with dementia, what might they say is quality for them? Being able to get a direct answer from people with dementia, particularly those who live in long-term care, is difficult. Quality needs to be defined on a micro level for people with dementia before we can hope to have policies reflecting standards that make an impact on day-to-day lives. We first need to put ourselves in the shoes of someone with dementia. This is not easy as dementia affects people's sense of self in different ways, but there may, however, be some unifying factors.

A key aspect of helping staff and carers to become dementia-aware is to deepen their empathy with those who are being cared for. I have done this hundreds of times through a sensitive guided fantasy exercise to help staff to explore what care in 'their place' might feel like from the perspective of a person with dementia and what needs are paramount to their clients. At the end of this exercise, the specific things that people want vary according to their personal histories and personalities. The vast majority of people want gentle and kind human contact. Many wish to be held; a few do not. All wish that someone would take their fears seriously. All wish that someone would take the time to reach out to them as many feel disempowered to reach out to others. But none wants any of the things that appear in Box 1.1. People imagine they are in all kinds of places, but school, work and 'definitely not at home' are common responses. The behaviours that many describe are those used to escape or to search for something comforting and familiar. Others claim that they would become quite aggressive. The majority believe that they would sit quietly, tense and vigilant, hoping that no-one would hurt them.

This is where the definition of quality begins to equate with person-centred care and the outcome of the maintenance of personhood. The processes by which this might be achieved are detailed in Figure 16.2. The person-centred standards for care homes (Alzheimer's Society 2001) provide a comprehensive set of standards and key questions to help staff to reflect on their practice within such environments; many of these could also be very useful in day care and community settings. It is interesting that these were developed by working alongside staff and residents within a wide variety of care homes for many hours, and they can be seen to describe quality from this perspective. Kane (2001) defined 11 domains of quality of life for older people, generally in long-term care. These were a sense of safety, security and order, physical comfort, enjoyment, meaningful activity, relationships, functional competence, dignity, privacy, individuality, autonomy/choice and spiritual well-being. In a series of in-depth interviews undertaken in a long-term care setting (Bowers et al. 2001), 16 out of the 26 residents interviewed highlighted relationships, particularly friendships and reciprocity in care-givers, as being important.

Fundamental improvements in the quality of life for people with dementia living in long-term care will not occur until the policy agenda is aligned with the agenda for people with dementia. In the UK, the effects of the National Care Standards and the National Service Framework for Older People have yet to make their mark.

MEASURING AND IMPROVING THE QUALITY OF LIFE FOR PEOPLE WITH DEMENTIA

The question of how to measure and improve upon the outcome of care remains. A key element of any quality improvement programme is finding tools with which to monitor change in quality of life and quality of care. Selai and Trimble (1999) have usefully reviewed quality of life assessments in dementia and concluded that the area is, particularly from a research point of view, fraught with methodological issues. Quality of life measures take into account social as well as physical domains, alongside some of the wider aspects of social inclusion.

Because of the difficulties involved in engaging directly with people with dementia in terms of their quality of life, proxy methods, involving someone who knows the person with dementia well, have been used. A recent example of this is the ADRQL (Gonzalez-Salvador et al. 2000), a 47 item questionnaire administered as an interview with a direct care-giver, covering five domains of:

1. Relating to and being around others
2. Special identity and important relationships
3. Distress behaviour
4. Activities
5. Behaviour in the living environment.

The total score yields a measure of quality of life over the previous 2 weeks. It is not yet known whether the measure is sensitive to changes over time or how the relationship between care-giver and patient is rated, but it could prove a useful tool.

A number of writers (e.g. Selai and Trimble 1999) dismiss self-reporting for those with any significant degree of memory or language impairment. Some interesting work is being undertaken that involves interviewing people with dementia in nursing homes about their views (Allen 2000), but issues of reliability, generalizability, time and sensitivity to change need to be addressed. We also know from the vast literature on user feedback that people can apparently be very satisfied with appalling services, particularly where they are very dependent upon them.

Dementia care mapping (DCM) (Kitwood and Bredin 1992; Bradford Dementia Group 1997; Kuhn et al. 2000) is not a straightforward measure of quality of life or quality of care, instead purporting to measure the person-centredness of a care environment. It is the best known observational tool for this purpose in the UK (Audit Commision 2000) and, increasingly, internationally (Brooker 2002). Kitwood assumed that there was a direct relationship between quality of life and quality of care in dementia, DCM containing measures of both of these.

DCM began as an attempt to look at care from the perspective of those with dementia and was developed after many hundreds of hours of observation and work within various formal dementia care settings. Since that time, there have been a number of amendments and additions to the method and the process by which it is used. Through a process of preparation and feedback, staff are empowered to consider care from the point of view of the person with dementia. On the basis of these observations, changes are made to care plans and practice. DCM can be used to monitor change and provides positive reinforcement for the provision of person-centred care over time. The case study below used DCM as the main instrument for improving the quality of person-centred care so the process will be described in some detail here.

During a DCM evaluation, each mapper observes between five and ten participants continuously over a representative time period (e.g. 6 hours during the waking day in a residential setting). After each 5 minutes of observation, the mapper decides which of the main behavioural categories can be applied to each individual during the time frame. A number of guidelines help the mapper to determine the most appropriate behavioural category code. As well as quantifying activities using behavioural category codes, the mapper also makes a qualitative judgement on the relative state of ill-being or well-being experienced – the well/ill being value – during the 5 minute time frame. The method also provides an opportunity to record any personal detractors (episodes of malignant social psychology) as well as positive events that occur in the care process.

Through the process of DCM, many rich data are generated that can be analysed to monitor change over time at the level of both the individual resident and the organization. DCM has been used in a wide variety of formal care settings in the UK over the past 10 years, and in Germany and the USA for the past 4. The collective experience (Brooker and Rogers 2001), some of which has been published, but much of which has not, tells us that, when the setting conditions are favourable (Brooker 2002), the following objectives are achievable:

- A reduction in the level of ill-being and an increase in that of well-being
- The collection of quantitative and qualitative data demonstrating that this provides positive feedback on person-centred care that empowers staff
- A reduction in the number of, or an eradication of, examples of malignant social psychology
- Over progressive cycles of developmental evaluation, a shift in the focus of care to those who are most dependent
- A shared language and focus across professional disciplines, care staff and management teams
- Good face validity with front-line staff as well as those responsible for managing and commissioning care
- A positive influence on practice that results from the training itself
- Improved job satisfaction, which can in turn decrease staff turnover.

DCM is, however, not without its problems. It is labour intensive and needs updating. A revised version of DCM that will address a number of its shortfalls is expected in 2004 (Brooker 2002).

Case 1   IMPROVING AND MAINTAINING QUALITY

Background   The context for this case was a large busy urban NHS mental health care trust in the UK (Brooker et al. 1998). The trust had been formed by a merger between two smaller mental health care trusts, and standards of care were very variable. The large psychiatric hospital was in the process of closing, and units were being relocated to a number of different places. The trust had nine dementia care units on seven different geographical sites. These included four continuing care long-stay units that had been decanted from the big psychiatric hospital to smaller 'community units' within nursing homes. It addition to this, care for people with dementia was also provided at two day hospitals, two respite units and an assessment ward. There were three community teams, and the full range of services were also provided for those with functional mental health problems.

The decision to use DCM   During the mid 1990s, quality assurance systems emerged in UK health care with a focus on consumer and 'customer' care, and patients' charters. As an organization, we looked to DCM as a means of providing the consumer perspective on the care that this particular client group was receiving. With regards to the processes set out in Figure 16.2 above, the trust was attempting to establish all elements of good practice but was certainly not achieving a full commitment in any of them. Our other main feedback on consumer perspectives was a cycle of structured interviews with service users and carers (Brooker 1997; Brooker and Dinshaw 1998).

Training and preparation   DCM was used as part of our overall quality assurance and training strategy over a 4-year period. The first year was spent in preparation within the organization to ensure that, by the time the first mapping took place, people were keen for it to happen. Tom Kitwood provided the training in-house. Seventeen staff were funded to be trained, and an extra eight actually funded themselves (showing how keen they were to be involved). Clinical staff and direct operational management staff trained side by side, which ensured that both groups understood both the language and the process. At least one person from each clinical area, usually a member of the nursing staff, was trained. Because everyone trained at the same time, there was a culture shift that seemed to be important for bringing staff together. DCM provided a disparate group of staff with a focus – a common language and a pride in dementia care that many of them had never experienced before.

The process Formal Quality Assurance DCM evaluations were completed annually over a 3 year period on the nine units that catered for service users with dementia. Although DCM was used as part of the formal trust quality assurance programme, it was always emphasized that information from the individual maps was the property of the individual units. The mappers simply reported what they had observed; it was the responsibility of the unit staff to decide how they could use the information to improve care. The results of each map were confidential to the staff working on the unit, its direct operational manager, the quality assurance manager and, of course, the mappers. The results were provided only in aggregated or anonymous formats outside the unit feedback sessions.

All units had at least one DCM-trained member of staff (the quality co-ordinator). Each DCM evaluation was undertaken by a main mapper and an assistant mapper. In the first cycle, the main mapper role was taken on by an assistant psychologist who was employed specifically for this purpose. In the following cycles, however, this role became part of the work of two clinical nurse specialists. The assistant mapper was a qualified quality co-ordinator from a neighbouring unit. When more than 10 participants were mapped, a second assistant mapper was utilized. The following process was followed during each DCM evaluation:

1. Staff, service users and carers were prepared using meetings, posters and leaflets, this being carried out by the unit's quality co-ordinator.
2. Unit staff were responsible for selecting a sample of participants for DCM whom they considered to be representative of the service users on their unit. These generally spanned the range of cognitive abilities and diagnoses, and usually included those with physical or sensory disabilities. Between 9 and 18 participants were mapped in each evaluation.
3. The mappers undertook a pilot study to ensure that an interrater reliability (concordance coefficient, as described in the DCM manual) of at least 0.8 was achieved. This also enabled the mappers to become familiar with the participants.
4. The DCM evaluation was carried out over a period of 2 consecutive week days. There were at least 10 hours of observation time, which included a meal time, a couple of hours in the morning and a couple of hours in the afternoon or evening. In day hospital settings, participants were mapped throughout their attendance and while travelling on the hospital transport. The timing of the maps for individual units remained equivalent over the three cycles.
5. The results were analysed as quickly as possible after each map had been constructed and were fed back to as many unit staff as could be gathered together. The initial report and copies of the raw data were left with the staff.
6. Within the month after each evaluation, the unit team took part in an 'away-day' involving all the staff working on the unit, the mappers, the quality assurance manager and the operational manager responsible for that area. During this time, each participant's results were examined in detail and improvements were, if necessary, made to care plans. General care delivery was also analysed. The aim

of this day was to promote good care practice and give the whole team the opportunity to discuss any changes they felt would lead to an improved quality of life for service users.

7. During the away-day, each unit team developed an action plan of quality improvements for the following year. These were monitored closely by the clinical nurse specialists and formally reviewed on the following away-day.

The timing of the maps was planned 12 months in advance in full consultation with the units. From an organizational point of view, this involved the clinical nurse specialists and quality assurance manager in an away-day and a map approximately once a month, missing out peak annual leave times. The maps of individual units tended to occur at the same time each year.

An important aspect was to adhere to the principles of person-centred care for staff as much as for service users. Attempts were made to minimize the amount of threat felt by staff members. When a unit was mapped, the only people to know the results of the unit map were the unit staff team and their direct operational manager.

A system was set up whereby staff never mapped on their own unit. Instead, units were paired with each other, mappers from one unit mapping their sister unit and vice versa. When staff map their own unit, they are usually hypercritical, being much harder on their own care environment than they are on anybody else's. The approach adopted also meant that mappers were never in the position of giving feedback to their own unit.

In order to maintain confidentiality, the mappers had a confidential formal debriefing session after their mapping. Observing care practice for that length of time generates all sorts of emotion; it would have been appalling for mappers to talk about what they had mapped because that would have ruined everyone's trust in the system. The debrief was a means of guarding against this happening.

The results Data from DCM over the three annual cycles suggested that the quality of care improved significantly, with a general reduction in ill-being at all levels and in all settings. There was also a statistically significant reduction in the number of personal detractors that were recorded, five units achieving a score of zero. In addition, there was a significant weakening of the initial strong correlation that existed in the first cycle, which showed that very dependent service users usually achieved the lowest level of well-being. This suggests that care practice changed so that the most vulnerable received the more positive interactions, thus reversing the inverse care rule.

Changes in the frequency of occurrence of the main behavioural domains were also indicative of a more positive experience for service users over the cycles. There was a decrease in passive interest, sleeping and withdrawn behaviour and an increase in social interaction, eating and expressive activities.

A number of other audits of quality occurred regularly over the same time period, including audits of pressure area care, care plan audits and carer satisfaction interviews. There appeared to be a general clustering of performance on all these audits, and the performance on DCM of the different units followed a similar trend. In other words, those units which did well in terms of pressure care also had better care plans, more satisfied carers and better DCM scores.

THE REACTION OF STAFF, SERVICE USERS, FAMILY CARERS AND COMMISSIONERS

The obtrusive nature of observing care practice is probably the most daunting aspect of DCM. Although it is, in the strictest sense, individual service users who are being mapped, staff will recognize that it is their contribution to the experience of care which is under scrutiny. Questionnaires were used to assess how acceptable the process was for staff.

Within the present evaluation, the number of staff feeling 'a little anxious' or 'very anxious' decreased over successive evaluations. Staff did not, however, cease to be affected by the situation as an increasing number of staff classed themselves as 'a little bothered' by DCM evaluations over successive years, and a small percentage of staff continued to feel very anxious. Given that much information and many reassurances were provided about DCM in this context, one can imagine how high anxiety might have run had this not been the case. Any responsible user of DCM should be aware of the power of this tool. The impact of feeding back DCM results to staff is considered in the training of a basic user in DCM.

Staff were interested in the results from the first cycle, but all of them thought that the results would be useful in improving care by the third cycle, which is the real mark of success of the project. DCM was not seen as something tangential to care, like many quality tools, but as something that would directly improve patient care.

Service users appeared to tolerate the method well. Carers also seemed to appreciate the fact that quality was being monitored in this way. Commissioners commended the DCM project as an example of good practice. In the language of clinical effectiveness, DCM can be seen as measuring the outcome of the care process, which is a useful way to conceptualize it when the only other clinical outcomes in this area are depressingly negative. In the language of consumerism, DCM can be conceptualized as a form of user feedback on services for people with dementia. Both conceptualizations enable service purchasers to understand it in their terms.

WHAT HELPED IN DCM'S SUCCESS

This DCM project was set within a quality assurance strategy that had a strong commitment to a 'top-led, grass-roots-fed' approach. The decision to use DCM was taken in consultation with the quality co-ordinators (from each clinical area) after a series of presentations by the quality assurance manager. Quality co-ordinators, clinical nurse specialists and operational managers all learned the method together. The way in which the evaluations were carried out was negotiated fully with the various units. The maps always remained the 'confidential property' of the units themselves, and action plans based on their findings were the work of the entire unit team and their managers together.

Running any quality assurance programme in this way has costs attached to it. The initial costs were involved in training. Then, to get the project off the ground, an assistant psychologist was employed on an 18 month contract. DCM is, on the scale described here, time-consuming, and it would have been difficult for any existing member of staff to have taken on the additional duties at the start. Once the project had been running for a year, the initial systems had been well established and it was easier to see the nature and volume of the work involved. It became apparent that the clinical nurse specialists were the most appropriate personnel within the organizational structure to take on the role of main mappers. They spent approximately half of their time involved in work related to DCM, and the quality assurance manager spent approximately a quarter of her time on it. Although this may sound costly in terms of finance and staff time, it was a lot less than the trust devoted to information technology over the same time period, and the benefits of DCM were much more obvious to clinical staff.

The away-days incurred a financial cost in that staff had to be employed to cover inpatient units for the day. The meetings were held on trust premises, and staff provided their own lunch, so there was no cost in actually running the meetings. There were some suggestions over the years to cut these or to decrease them to half-day meetings, which was strongly resisted by individual unit staff. The away-days produced a wealth of quality improvements, many of which had no cost implications, with the additional benefit of their being owned by the staff providing the care. They also resulted in robust action plans that led to quality improvements in patient care. Without the opportunity for consultative feedback, it is difficult to see how else this could have been achieved in an organization of the size described here.

ORGANIZATIONAL REQUIREMENTS FOR OPTIMIZING THE QUALITY OF CARE FOR PEOPLE WITH DEMENTIA

Earlier in this chapter, reference was made to the improvements that can occur with DCM *if the setting conditions are favourable*. At the DCM think-tank meeting (Brooker and Rogers 2001) the following were seen as favourable setting conditions:

- A practice development framework should be in place within the organization. Reflective practice, a shared value base, supervision, training and staff development should be linked with the process of DCM.
- There needs to be a clear understanding, at all levels of the staffing hierarchy, of the philosophy underpinning DCM and the process involved in implementing an evaluation. This understanding should preferably extend beyond individual care unit boundaries.

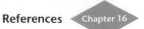

- DCM consists of a cycle of preparation, evaluation, feedback, reflection and action-planning. Resources need to be allocated to the whole of this process and not just the evaluation.
- A lead person or persons should be identified within the organization who have sufficient authority to allocate resources, organize the implementation, trouble-shoot and ensure that feedback is acted upon.
- It is surprisingly easy for trained mappers to be insensitive to the needs of staff who are present during a DCM evaluation. Sensitivity to the needs of both staff and those in receipt of care should have a high priority within any evaluation that seeks to improve person-centred care.
- Staff are particularly vulnerable within DCM evaluations if there has been no prior training in person-centred care. Observing care through mapping is an experience that can lead to some very powerful emotions, demanding debriefing for mappers.
- Giving feedback after a DCM evaluation takes considerable skill, and those undertaking this may require support and supervision at this time.

It is my opinion that these setting conditions apply not only to DCM, but also to any systematic review of quality monitoring and improvement. A practice development framework, a shared vision and value base, appropriate resources (including follow-through), a strong, credible leadership, appropriate training, supervision and support for staff are elements that are required in any organization that takes quality improvement seriously. The choice of measures and processes will depend upon the vision and value base to which the organization is committed. In long-term care, commitment needs to be made to the value base that the service user sees as most important. The challenge for service providers and commissioners is to align themselves to this value base.

REFERENCES

Allen, K. 2000: Drawing out views on services: a new staff-based approach. *Journal of Dementia Care* **8:** 16–19.

Alzheimer's Society. 2001: *Quality dementia care in care homes: person-centred standards.* London: Alzheimer's Society.

Audit Commission. 2000: *Forget me not. Mental health services for older people.* London: Audit Commission.

Ballard, C.G. and O'Brien, J. 1999: Pharmacological treatment of behavioural and psychological signs in Alzheimer's disease: how good is the evidence for current pharmacological treatments? *British Medical Journal* **319:** 138–9.

Ballard, C., Fossey, J., Chithramohan, R. et al. 2001: Quality of care in private sector and NHS facilities for people with dementia: cross sectional survey. *British Medical Journal* **323:** 426–7.

Barnett, E. 2000: *Including the person with dementia in designing and delivering care – 'I need to be me!'* London: Jessica Kingsley.

Bond, S. and Bond, J. 1990: Outcomes of care within a multiple-case study in the evaluation of the experimental National Health Service nursing homes. *Age and Ageing* **19:** 11–18.

Bowers, B.J., Fibich, B. and Jacobson, N. 2001: Care-as-service, care-as relating, care-as-comfort: understanding nursing home residents' definitions of quality. *Gerontologist* **4:** 539–45.

Bowie, P. and Mountain, G. 1993: Comment: Life on a long stay ward: extracts from the diary of an observing researcher. *International Journal of Geriatric Psychiatry* **8:** 1001–7.

Bradford Dementia Group. 1997: *Evaluating dementia care: the DCM method,* 7th edn. Bradford: University of Bradford.

Brooker, D.J.R. 1994: Quality assurance – lessons learnt about putting it into practice. *PSIGE Newsletter* **48:** 37–41.

Brooker, D.J.R. 1995: Looking at them, looking at me: a review of observational studies into the quality of institutional care for elderly people with dementia. *Journal of Mental Health* **4:** 145–56.

Brooker, D.J.R. 1997: Issues in user feedback on health services for elderly people. *British Journal of Nursing* **6:** 159–62.

Brooker, D. 2002: Dementia care mapping: a look at its past, present and future. *Journal of Dementia Care* **10:** 33–6.

Brooker, D.J.R. and Dinshaw, C.J. 1998: A comparison of staff and patient feedback on mental health services for older people. *Quality in Health Care* **7:** 70–6.

Brooker, D. and Rogers, L. eds. 2001: *DCM think tank transcripts 2001.* Bradford: University of Bradford.

Brooker, D.J.R., Foster, N., Banner, A., Payne, M. and Jackson, L. 1998: The efficacy of dementia care mapping as an audit tool: report of a three-year British NHS evaluation. *Ageing and Mental Health* **2:** 60–70.

Bruce, E., Surr, C. and Tibbs, M.A. 2002: *A special kind of care: improving well-being in people living with dementia.* Derby: Methodist Homes Association Care Group.

Cox, S. 2001: Developing quality in services. In: Cantley, C. ed. *A handbook of dementia care.* Buckingham: Open University Press, 258–77.

Georgiades, N. and Phillimore, L. 1975: The myth of the hero innovator and alternative strategies for organisational change. In: Kiernan, C. and Woodford, P. eds. *Behaviour modification for the severely retarded.* New York: Associated Scientific Publishers, 313–19.

Gonzalez-Salvador, T., Lyketsos, C., Baker, A. et al. 2000: Quality of life in dementia patients in long-term care. *International Journal of Geriatric Psychiatry* **15:** 181–9.

Innes, A. and Surr, C. 2001: Measuring the well-being of people with dementia living in formal care settings: the use of dementia care mapping. *Aging and Mental Health* **5:** 258–68.

Kane, R.A. 2001: Long-term care and a good quality of life: bringing the two closer together. *Gerontologist* **41:** 293–304.

Kitwood, T. 1990: The dialectics of dementia: with particular reference to Alzheimer's disease. *Ageing and Society* **10:** 177–96.

Kitwood, T. 1993: Towards a theory of dementia care: the interpersonal process. *Ageing and Society* **13:** 51–67.

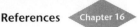

Kitwood, T. 1997: *Dementia reconsidered*. Buckingham: Open University Press.

Kitwood, T. and Bredin, K. 1992: A new approach to the evaluation of dementia care. *Journal of Advances in Health and Nursing Care* **1:** 41–60.

Kuhn, D., Ortigara, A. and Kasayka, R. 2000: Dementia care mapping: an innovative tool to measure person-centered care. *Alzheimer's Care Quarterly* **1:** 7–15.

MacDonald, A. and Dening, T. 2002: Dementia is being avoided in NHS and social care. *British Medical Journal* **324:** 548.

Marshall, M. 2001: The challenge of looking after people with dementia. *British Medical Journal* **323:** 410–11.

Packer, T. 2001: Obstacles to person-centred care delivery. 5: 'Everyone wants something': recognising your own needs. Journal of Dementia Care **9:** 26–7.

Post, S. 1995: *The moral challenge of Alzheimer's disease*. London: Johns Hopkins Press.

Selai, C. and Trimble, M.R. 1999: Assessing quality of life in dementia. *Aging and Mental Health* **3:** 101–11.

Index

abuse of elders *see* elder abuse
acetylcholinesterase inhibitors
    55, 56
ADRQL 246
ageism 51, 215–16, 226, 241,
    242–3
AIDS-related dementia 167
alcohol abuse 168
Alzheimer's disease
    anti-oxidants 56
    communication 74–83
    early stage 55, 56, 76, 171
    familial 173, 174
    family carers 188, 191,
        195–9
    function checklist 76–7
    group psychotherapy
        136–46
    herbal treatments 56
    medication 55, 171
    self-help 56
    support groups *see* self-help
        groups
    younger people 165, 166,
        171, 173, 174
analgesia 119–20, 129, 130
antibiotics 121
antifungal treatment 122
anti-oxidants 56–7
aphasia 73
Asian communities 204–5,
    206–7
associative learning 58

behaviour
    and communication 69–70,
        71, 80–81, 82–3
    in practice 159 60
    research evidence 155
    theory of 153–4
    dementia as problem of 7–8
    effects on carers 191–2,
        198–9
    explanations for 65–6
    food intake 105, 106–7, 130
bereavement 125–8, 130
bio-medical discourses 5–7, 9

body, discourses on 18
body temperature 110–111,
    120
bronchopneumonia 115, 120,
    121

cancer cachexia 123
capacity, mental 41, 236
care outcomes, identifying 26
care planning 128–31
care principles 42, 245
care services
    minority ethnic groups
        202–9
    palliative 114–15
    policy *see* policy
    politics of disability 17–19,
        42
    psychosocial approaches
        23–5
    quality 240–253
    young-onset dementia 165,
        174–6, 177
carers
    family *see* family care and
        carers
    formal
        communication 26
        dementia care mapping
            247–51, 253
        empathy 245
        interdependence 26
        supervision 213–23
'challenging' behaviour *see*
    behaviour
children 174
Chinese communities 205, 208
choices *see* decision-making
clinical supervision 213–23
cognitive-behavioural therapy
    195–9
cognitive rehabilitation 57–9
communication 148–9,
    160–161
    age-related change 71, 72, 73
    components 70–71
    during activities 156

early stage dementia 54,
    61–3, 64–5, 80–81
by failing to respond
    149–50
importance 25, 26
managing difficulties in
    69–71, 157–61
    assessments 157–8
    behaviour 69–70, 71,
        80–81, 82–3, 159–60
    communication theory
        153–4
    disease progression 74–7
    environment 72–3, 160
    hearing 71–2
    language disorders 73
    language therapy 81
    naming 71, 75, 77, 78–9,
        80
    pragmatics 70, 80–81
    relationships 158
    research evidence 155–6
    semantics 75–80
    skill contexts 74
    speech therapy 81
    symptom variation 74–5
    validation 82, 158–9
    vision 72, 79
mediating function 82
minority ethnic groups 206,
    207, 208
non-verbal 149, 156
person-centred care 62–3,
    155, 159, 161
with pictures 156
power 154
relational 158
reminiscence therapy 64–5,
    159
skill development 157, 160
theory of 151–4
through care environment
    150, 160
types of 149–51
validation therapy 61–2, 82,
    158–9
written 150–151

Index

community care
  bereavement services 128
  home care workers 216–17
  mental health legislation 41
  physical care needs 111–12
  post-war policy 39–40
  young-onset dementia 172,
    173, 175
consent issues 27, 28, 236
construction of dementia 3–5
  as behavioural problem 7–8
  bio-medical 5–7, 9
  disability 13–19
  subjective experience 8–11
  voice 12–13
conversational skills 64–5,
  80–81
coping skills training 198–9
coping strategies 25–6,
  99–100, 141, 194–5
coping styles 190
counselling 86–7
  after diagnosis 91–2, 95
  client-led 88
  clients' needs 92–100
  counsellor's role 87–88, 89,
    101
  desired outcomes 93, 94
  and family carers 88–9, 90,
    100–101
  general principles 87–9
  integrated model 89, 90
  pre-prescription 55
  process 89–91
  termination 89
  therapeutic engagement
    89–91
Creutzfeldt–Jacob disease 167
cultural groups 193, 202–9

day care 172, 175
death 115, 116–17, 125–6, 130
death rattle 124
decision-making
  counselling 99
  and elder abuse 236
  by people with dementia
    13, 22–32
  diagnosis-sharing 43, 54
  in early stages 54, 55
  legislation 40–42, 43
  medication 55
  policy contexts 23,
    40–43
  young-onset 169
decubitus ulcers 109–10, 121
dehydration 104, 105, 107–8,
  109, 122–4, 130
delirium 125
dementia
  causes of death in 116
  diseases causing 165–8

dementia care mapping
  (DCM) 24, 247–53
dementia counselling see
  counselling
depression, carers 188
diagnosis
  counselling after 91–2, 95
  differential effects on care
    191
  interventions after 53–7, 59
  reactions to 53–4, 59, 92, 95,
    187
  sharing of 43, 54, 59–60,
    62–3, 126–7
  young-onset dementia 166,
    170
disability discourse 13–19
disability movement 42–3
discomfort 118–20, 121, 124,
  129–30
discourses on dementia 3–19
double effect doctrine 125
Down's syndrome 168
drug treatment see medication
dying see palliative care
dysarthria 73
dysphagia 121
dysphasia (aphasia) 73

early stage dementia 51–3
  cognitive rehabilitation
    57–9
  coping strategies 25–6
  counselling see counselling
  future challenges 66–7
  information provision 54–5
  medication 53, 55–6, 171
  memory clinics 52, 90–91
  post-diagnostic interven-
    tions 53–7, 59, 171
  psychotherapeutic interven-
    tions 59–66, 171
  reactions to diagnosis 53–4,
    59
  self-help 56–7
  young-onset 170, 171
eating behaviour 105, 106–7
education 196–7, 209
  see also training
elder abuse 225–37
  causes 228, 232–3, 235
  and dementia 228–33,
    236–7
  forms of 227
  future research 237
  importance of naming
    226–7
  interventions 233–6, 237
  recognizing 235–6
  taboo nature of 226
employment 171–2, 189
empowerment 28, 29–31

end-stage dementia 105–6,
  107, 108, 109, 111, 122–4
  see also palliative care
environmental factors 72–3,
  111, 160, 241–2
errorless learning 58–9
ethnically sensitive practice
  202–9
ethnicity, definition 203
euthanasia 124–5
expanding rehearsal 57–8

faecal incontinence 109
familial diseases 166, 173–4
families
  bereavement 125–8, 130
  care by see family care and
    carers
  and diagnosis-sharing 126
  reactions to diagnosis 53–4,
    59, 187
  young-onset dementia 170,
    171–4, 176
family care and carers
  abuse 228, 229–31, 232–3,
    234, 235
  bereavement 127–8
  care principles 42
  cognitive-behavioural
    therapy 195–9
  cognitive rehabilitation
    57–8
  communication skills 157,
    160
  coping skills training 198–9
  and counselling 88–9, 90,
    100–101
  dementia care mapping 251
  early stage dementia 55–6,
    57–8, 59, 66–7
  education 196–7
  effects of caring 187–90
    abuse 228, 232–3, 235
    interventions 195–9
    mediating factors
      190–195
    minority ethnic groups
      193, 204–5, 206–7
  employment 171–2, 189
  financial security 172–3, 189
  gender differences 193
  information for 170, 173,
    196–7
  medication 55–6
  minority ethnic groups
    193, 204–5, 206–7
  physical care 106, 107,
    111–12
  post-war policy 38–40
  psychotherapeutic interven-
    tions 59
  satisfactions for 189
  stress management 197–8
  training 176, 198–9

young-onset dementia 170,
171–3, 176, 189
fever, palliative care 120–121
financial security 171–3, 189
fluid intake 104, 105, 107–8,
109, 122–4, 130
food intake 105–7, 123, 130
frontotemporal dementia 167,
173
fungal infections 122

genetic issues 166, 168, 173–4
Gingko biloba 56
group psychotherapy 136–46,
171
guilt 95–6, 127–8

haematoma-related dementia
167
health authorities 37–8
hearing 71–2
herbal treatments 56
HIV-related dementia 167
home care workers 216–17
hospice care 114, 123, 124–5
hospital-based care 37–9
deaths in 117
dementia care mapping
248–50
and eating behaviour 107
hydration 123
palliative 118, 123
housing 17–18, 40, 174–5
Huntington's disease 166, 167
hydration 104–5, 107–8, 109,
122–4, 130
hydrocephalus-related
dementia 167
hypercognitivism 241, 242
hypothermia 111
hypothyroidism 167–8

identity 4
incontinence 107–8, 109
independence 16
individualism 15–16
infections 115, 120–121, 122,
130, 167
information needs 54–5, 96–7,
169–70, 172–3, 196–7, 208,
209
informed consent 27, 28
institutions 37–8, 225–6, 227,
240–253
inverse care law 242, 250

labels, disability politics 17
language
age-related change 71, 72,
73
in construction of dementia
3–5, 16, 17, 18

managing difficulties in
69–83
minority ethnic groups 206,
207, 208
language therapy 81
legal security 173
legislation 40–42, 43
Lewy bodies, dementia with
165, 166–7
life, quality of 244–50
life expectancy 116
life histories 65, 95
life review 63, 159, 171
local authorities 37–8
location of dementia 17–18,
37–40
long-term care, quality
240 253
lung secretions 124

malignant social psychology
9, 10, 11, 62, 242–3
malnutrition 105–7, 121,
122–3, 130, 167–8
managerial supervision
214–15
medication
analgesia 119–20, 129, 130
at end of life 124–5
causing dysarthria 73
causing xerostomia 122
early stage dementia 53,
55–6, 97, 171
infections 121, 122, 130
lung secretions 124
sedation 124–5
young-onset dementia 171
memory aids 58
memory clinics 52, 90–91,
170–7
memory re-training 57–9
mental capacity 41, 236
mental health legislation
40–42, 43
mental health policy *see*
policy
mental hospitals 37–8
see also hospital-based care
minority ethnic groups 193,
202–9
mouth care 121–2, 130

naming ability 71, 75, 77,
78–9, 80, 153
nasogastric tube feeding 123
*National Service Framework for
Older People* 43–4, 51
neglect *see* elder abuse
nursing homes 38, 107,
116–17, 127–30
nutrition 56–7, 104–7, 121,
122–3, 130, 167–8

opioids 120, 125, 129
oral care 121–2, 130
outpacing 62–3

pain 118–20, 121, 122, 124,
129–30
palliative care 114–15
assessment 118
bereavement 125–8, 130
care planning 128–31
causes of death 115, 116,
117
death rattle 124
dehydration 122–4, 130
delirium 125
discomfort 118–20, 121, 124,
129–30
infections 120–121, 122, 130
lucidity before death 125
mouth care 121–2, 130
nutrition 122–3, 130
pain 118–20, 122, 124,
129–30
predicting imminent death
125–6
sedation 124–5
settings of death 116–17
Panax ginseng 56
Parkinson's disease 167
person-centred practice
communication 62–3, 155,
159, 161
dementia care mapping 247
early stage dementia 51–67
policy contexts 44
quality 245–6
personhood 9–11, 53, 62–3,
155, 242–3, 245
physical care needs 103–12
see also palliative care
Pick's disease 167
pictures, for communication
156
place of dementia 17–18,
37–40
policy 23, 35–7
chronology of 36
decision-making 23, 40–43
dementia care quality 243,
246
elder abuse 233–4, 235
future challenges 43–5
*National Service Framework
for Older People* 43–4
person-centred care 44
place of dementia 37–40
resource contexts 43, 44–5
young-onset dementia 176,
177
Polish communities 204, 205,
207–8
politics of disability 14–19, 42

power 13, 15–16, 23, 28, 29–32
  communication theory 154
  counselling 88–9, 99
pragmatics 70, 80–81
presenile dementia *see* young-
  onset dementia
pressure ulcers 109–10, 121
psychiatric hospitals 37–8
  see also hospital-based care
psychotherapeutic interven-
    tions
  early stage dementia 59–66
  family carers 195–9
  group work 136–46, 171
  life review 63, 159, 171
  reality orientation 60, 61,
    171
  reminiscence 63–7, 159, 171
  resolution therapy 62, 143–4
  validation therapy 60, 61–2,
    82, 136–7, 158–9
  young-onset dementia 171
  see also counselling; super-
    vision

quality in dementia care
    240–253

race, definition 203
racism 209
reality orientation 60, 61, 171
reflective listening 143–4
rehydration 123–4, 130
reminiscence therapy 63–7,
    159, 171
research, people with
    dementia as participants
    24–7, 28
residential care
  bereavement services 128,
    130
  deaths in 116–17, 127–8
  nutrition in 107
  person-centred standards
    245–6
  post-war policy 37–9
  young-onset dementia 174–5
resolution therapy 62, 143–4
resource contexts 43, 44–5
respiration, death rattle 124

sedation 124–5
self-esteem 92–5

self-help 56–7
self-help groups
  minority ethnic groups 208,
    209
  and post-war policy 39
  principles of care 42, 245
  problems facing 42–3
  written information 97
  young-onset dementia 170
semantics 70, 75–80
services *see* care services;
    policy
sexual relationships 174
signifiers 3–4, 5
skin care 108–10, 121
social construction of
    dementia *see* construction
    of dementia
social contexts 23–5
  dementia discourses 9–11
  minority ethnic groups
    206–10
  quality in dementia care
    241–3
  social contacts 97–8, 172
social model of disability 14
speech 73, 81, 149
starvation 122–3, 130
stereotypes 16–17
stigma 16–17
story-telling 63, 64, 144, 156
stress management 197–8
subjective experience 8–11
superstitious beliefs 66
supervision 213–23
support groups *see* self-help
    groups
swallowing 121, 122–3, 130
swearing 82–3
syphilis-related dementia 167

temperature, body 110–111,
    120
terminal illness *see* end-stage
    dementia; palliative care
thiamine deficiency 168
throat secretions 124
training
  dementia care mapping
    248–9
  family carers 176, 198–9
  for supervision 222
  see also education

tube feeding 108, 123
tumour-related dementia 167

urinary incontinence 107–8,
    109
user groups *see* self-help
    groups

validation therapy 60, 61–2,
    82, 136–7, 158–9
vanishing cues 57
vascular dementia 165, 166,
    191
violence *see* elder abuse
vision 72, 79
vitamin deficiencies 167–8
vitamin supplements 56–7
voice, people with dementia
    12–13, 25–32, 155, 169
  see also decision-making
voluntary sector 175
  see also self-help groups

wandering behaviour 191–2
weight loss 105–6, 107, 123
Wernicke–Korsakoff
    syndrome 168
World Health Organization
    (WHO) 14, 119–20

xerostomia 122

young-onset dementia 164–77
  assessment 170–171
  diagnosis 166, 170
  diseases causing 165–8
  employment 171–2
  epidemiology 168–9
  family life 173–4
  financial security 171–3, 189
  information needs 169–70,
    172–3
  legal security 172–3
  meaningful occupation 172
  medication 171
  psychotherapeutic interven-
    tions 171
  residential care 174–5
  service development 165,
    175–6, 177
  sexual relationships 174
  social needs 172
  specific needs 169–70